AF330058

1996
YEAR BOOK OF
INFERTILITY AND REPRODUCTIVE
ENDOCRINOLOGY

Statement of Purpose

The YEAR BOOK Service

The YEAR BOOK series was devised in 1901 by practicing health professionals who observed that the literature of medicine and related disciplines had become so voluminous that no one individual could read and place in perspective every potential advance in a major specialty. In the final decade of the 20th century, this recognition is more acutely true than it was in 1901.

More than merely a series of books, YEAR BOOK volumes are the tangible results of a unique service designed to accomplish the following:

- to *survey* a wide range of journals of proven value
- to *select* from those journals papers representing significant advances and statements of important clinical principles
- to provide *abstracts* of those articles that are readable, convenient summaries of their key points
- to provide *commentary* about those articles to place them in perspective

These publications grow out of a unique process that calls on the talents of outstanding authorities in clinical and fundamental disciplines, trained literature specialists, and professional writers, all supported by the resources of Mosby, the world's preeminent publisher for the health professions.

The Literature Base

Mosby and its editors survey more than 1,000 journals published worldwide, covering the full range of the health professions. On an annual basis, the publisher examines usage patterns and polls its expert authorities to add new journals to the literature base and to delete journals that are no longer useful as potential YEAR BOOK sources.

The Literature Survey

The publisher's team of literature specialists, all of whom are trained and experienced health professionals, examines every original, peer-reviewed article in each journal issue. More than 250,000 articles per year are scanned systematically, including title, text, illustrations, tables, and references. Each scan is compared, article by article, to the search strategies that the publisher has developed in consultation with the 270 outside experts who form the pool of YEAR BOOK editors. A given article may be reviewed by any number of editors, from one to a dozen or more, regardless of the discipline for which the paper was originally published. In turn, each editor who receives the article reviews it to determine whether or not the article should be included in the YEAR BOOK. This decision is based on the article's inherent quality, its probable usefulness to readers of that YEAR BOOK, and the editor's goal to represent a balanced picture of a given field in each volume of the YEAR BOOK. In addition, the editor indicates when to include figures and tables from the article to help the YEAR BOOK reader better understand the information.

Of the quarter million articles scanned each year, only 5% are selected for detailed analysis within the YEAR BOOK series, thereby assuring readers of the high value of every selection.

The Abstract

The publisher's abstracting staff is headed by a seasoned medical professional and includes individuals with training in the life sciences, medicine, and other areas, plus extensive experience in writing for the health professions and related industries. Each selected article is assigned to a specific writer on this abstracting staff. The abstracter, guided in many cases by notations supplied by the expert editor, writes a structured, condensed summary designed so that the reader can rapidly acquire the essential information contained in the article.

The Commentary

The YEAR BOOK editorial boards, sometimes assisted by guest commentators, write comments that place each article in perspective for the reader. This provides the reader with the equivalent of a personal consultation with a leading international authority—an opportunity to better understand the value of the article and to benefit from the authority's thought processes in assessing the article.

Additional Editorial Features

The editorial boards of each YEAR BOOK organize the abstracts and comments to provide a logical and satisfying sequence of information. To enhance the organization, editors also provide introductions to sections or individual chapters, comments linking a number of abstracts, citations to additional literature, and other features.

The published YEAR BOOK contains enhanced bibliographic citations for each selected article, including extended listings of multiple authors and identification of author affiliations. Each YEAR BOOK contains a Table of Contents specific to that year's volume. From year to year, the Table of Contents for a given YEAR BOOK will vary depending on developments within the field.

Every YEAR BOOK contains a list of the journals from which papers have been selected. This list represents a subset of the more than 1,000 journals surveyed by the publisher and occasionally reflects a particularly pertinent article from a journal that is not surveyed on a routine basis.

Finally, each volume contains a comprehensive subject index and an index to authors of each selected paper.

The 1996 Year Book Series

Year Book of Allergy, Asthma, and Clinical Immunology: Drs. Rosenwasser, Borish, Gelfand, Leung, Nelson, and Szefler

Year Book of Anesthesiology and Pain Management: Drs. Tinker, Abram, Chestnut, Roizen, Rothenberg, and Wood

Year Book of Cardiology®: Drs. Schlant, Collins, Engle, Gersh, Kaplan, and Waldo

Year Book of Chiropractic®: Dr. Lawrence

Year Book of Critical Care Medicine®: Drs. Parrillo, Balk, Calvin, Franklin, and Shapiro

Year Book of Dentistry®: Drs. Meskin, Berry, Kennedy, Leinfelder, Roser, Summitt, and Zakariasen

Year Book of Dermatologic Surgery®: Drs. Swanson, Glogau, and Salasche

Year Book of Dermatology®: Drs. Sober and Fitzpatrick

Year Book of Diagnostic Radiology®: Drs. Federle, Clark, Gross, Latchaw, Madewell, Maynard, and Young

Year Book of Digestive Diseases®: Drs. Greenberger and Moody

Year Book of Drug Therapy®: Drs. Lasagna and Weintraub

Year Book of Emergency Medicine®: Drs. Wagner, Dronen, Davidson, King, Niemann, and Roberts

Year Book of Endocrinology®: Drs. Bagdade, Braverman, Horton, Kannan, Landsberg, Molitch, Morley, Nathan, Odell, Poehlman, Rogol, and Ryan

Year Book of Family Practice®: Drs. Berg, Bowman, Davidson, Dexter, and Scherger

Year Book of Geriatrics and Gerontology®: Drs. Beck, Burton, Rabins, Reuben, Roth, Shapiro, and Whitehouse

Year Book of Hand Surgery®: Drs. Amadio and Hentz

Year Book of Hematology®: Drs. Spivak, Bell, Ness, Quesenberry, Wiernik, and Blume

Year Book of Infectious Diseases®: Drs. Keusch, Barza, Bennish, Klempner, Skolnik, and Snydman

Year Book of Infertility and Reproductive Endocrinology: Drs. Mishell, Lobo, and Sokol

Year Book of Medicine®: Drs. Bone, Cline, Epstein, Greenberger, Malawista, Mandell, O'Rourke, and Utiger

Year Book of Neonatal and Perinatal Medicine®: Drs. Fanaroff and Klaus

Year Book of Nephrology, Hypertension, and Mineral Metabolism: Drs. Coe, Curtis, Favus, Henderson, Kashgarian, Luke, and Myers

Year Book of Neurology and Neurosurgery®: Drs. Bradley and Wilkins

Year Book of Neuroradiology: Drs. Osborn, Eskridge, Grossman, Hudgins, and Ross

Year Book of Nuclear Medicine®: Drs. Gottschalk, Blaufox, McAfee, Wackers, and Zubal

Year Book of Obstetrics and Gynecology®: Drs. Mishell, Herbst, and Kirschbaum

Year Book of Occupational and Environmental Medicine®: Drs. Emmett, Frank, Gochfeld, and Hessl

Year Book of Oncology®: Drs. Simone, Bosl, Cohen, Glatstein, Ozols, and Tallman

Year Book of Ophthalmology®: Drs. Cohen, Augsburger, Eagle, Flanagan, Grossman, Laibson, Maguire, Nelson, Rapuano, Sergott, Tasman, Tipperman, and Wilson

Year Book of Orthopedics®: Drs. Sledge, Cofield, Dobyns, Griffin, Poss, Springfield, Swiontkowski, Wiesel, and Wilson

Year Book of Otolaryngology–Head and Neck Surgery®: Drs. Paparella, and Holt

Year Book of Pain: Drs. Gebhart, Haddox, Jacox, Janjan, Marcus, Rudy, and Shapiro

Year Book of Pathology and Laboratory Medicine: Drs. Mills, Bruns, Gaffey, and Stoler

Year Book of Pediatrics®: Dr. Stockman

Year Book of Plastic, Reconstructive, and Aesthetic Surgery®: Drs. Miller, Cohen, McKinney, Robson, Ruberg, and Whitaker

Year Book of Podiatric Medicine and Surgery®: Dr. Kominsky

Year Book of Psychiatry and Applied Mental Health®: Drs. Talbott, Ballenger, Breier, Frances, Meltzer, Schowalter, and Tasman

Year Book of Pulmonary Disease®: Drs. Bone and Petty

Year Book of Rheumatology®: Drs. Sergent, LeRoy, Meenan, Panush, and Reichlin

Year Book of Sports Medicine®: Drs. Shephard, Drinkwater, Eichner, Torg, Col. Anderson, and Mr. George

Year Book of Surgery®: Drs. Copeland, Bland, Deitch, Eberlein, Howard, Luce, Seeger, Souba, and Sugarbaker

Year Book of Thoracic and Cardiovascular Surgery®: Drs. Ginsberg, Wechsler, and Williams

Year Book of Ultrasound®: Drs. Merritt, Carroll, and Fleischer

Year Book of Urology®: Drs. DeKernion and Howards

Year Book of Vascular Surgery®: Dr. Porter

1996

The Year Book of INFERTILITY AND REPRODUCTIVE ENDOCRINOLOGY

Editors

Daniel R. Mishell, Jr., M.D.

The Lyle G. McNeile Professor and Chairman, Department of Obstetrics and Gynecology, University of Southern California School of Medicine; Chief of Professional Services, LAC & USC Medical Center Women and Children's Hospital, Los Angeles

Rogerio A. Lobo, M.D.

Willard C. Rappleye Professor of Obstetrics and Gynecology, Columbia University College of Physicians and Surgery; Chairman of the Department of Obstetrics and Gynecology; The Presbyterian Hospital Director, Sloane Hospital for Women, New York, New York

Rebecca Z. Sokol, M.D., F.A.C.P.

Professor of Medicine and Obstetrics and Gynecology, and Director of Andrology, University of Southern California School of Medicine, Los Angeles

Editorial Coordinator

Shirley J. Davenport

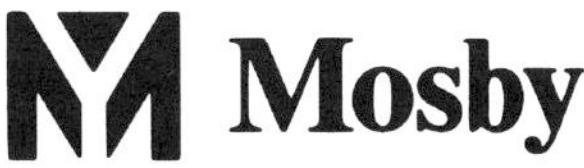

St. Louis Baltimore Boston Carlsbad Chicago Naples New York Philadelphia Portland
London Madrid Mexico City Singapore Sydney Tokyo Toronto Wiesbaden

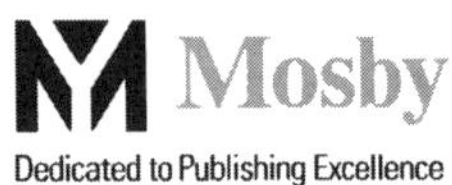

Mosby

Dedicated to Publishing Excellence

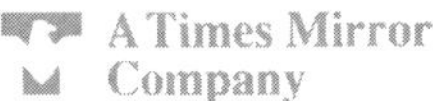

A Times Mirror
Company

Vice President and Publisher, Continuity Publishing: Kenneth H. Killion
Director, Editorial Development: Gretchen C. Murphy
Developmental Editor, Continuity: Donna Steinhagen
Acquisitions Editor: Linda Sheehan
Illustrations and Permissions Coordinator: Nancy Dunne
Manager, Continuity—EDP: Maria Nevinger
Project Supervisor, Editing: Rebecca Nordbrock
Assistant Project Supervisor: Sandra Rogers
Freelance Staff Supervisor: Barbara M. Kelly
Director, Editorial Services: Edith M. Podrazik, B.S.N., R.N.
Information Specialist: Kathleen Moss, R.N.
Circulation Manager: Lynn D. Stevenson

1996 EDITION
Copyright © October 1996 by Mosby–Year Book, Inc.

Printed in the United States of America
Composition by Reed Technology and Information Services, Inc.
Printing/binding by Maple-Vail

Mosby–Year Book, Inc.
11830 Westline Industrial Drive
St. Louis, MO 63146

Editorial Office:
Mosby–Year Book, Inc.
161 North Clark Street
Chicago, IL 60601

International Standard Serial Number: 0896-4475
International Standard Book Number: 0-8151-6007-0

Table of Contents

Journals Represented

Mosby and its editors survey more than 1,000 journals for its abstract and commentary publications. From these journals, the Editors select the articles to be abstracted. Journals represented in this YEAR BOOK are listed below.

Acta Obstetricia et Gynecologica Scandinavica
American Journal of Human Genetics
American Journal of Obstetrics and Gynecology
Andrologia
Archives of Andrology
Archives of Ophthalmology
British Journal of Obstetrics and Gynaecology
British Journal of Urology
Clinical Endocrinology (Oxford)
Endocrinology
European Journal of Obstetrics, Gynecology and Reproductive Biology
Fertility and Sterility
Gynecologic and Obstetric Investigation
Gynecological Endocrinology
Human Reproduction
Human Reproduction Uptake
International Journal of Gynaecology and Obstetrics
International Journal of Sports Medicine
Journal of Andrology
Journal of Assisted Reproduction and Genetics
Journal of Clinical Endocrinology and Metabolism
Journal of Reproductive Medicine
Journal of Urology
Journal of the American Medical Association
Lancet
Maturitas
Nature Medicine
New England Journal of Medicine
Obstetrics and Gynecology

STANDARD ABBREVIATIONS

The following terms are abbreviated in this edition: acquired immunodeficiency syndrome (AIDS), cardiopulmonary resuscitation (CPR), central nervous system (CNS), cerebrospinal fluid (CSF), computed tomography (CT), deoxyribonucleic acid (DNA), electrocardiography (ECG), health maintenance organization (HMO), human immunodeficiency virus (HIV), intensive care unit (ICU), intramuscular (IM), intravenous (IV), magnetic resonance (MR) imaging (MRI), and ribonucleic acid (RNA).

NOTE

The YEAR BOOK OF INFERTILITY AND REPRODUCTIVE ENDOCRINOLOGY is a literature survey service providing abstracts of articles published in the professional literature. Every effort is made to assure the accuracy of the information presented in these pages. Neither the editors nor the publisher of the YEAR BOOK OF INFERTILITY AND REPRODUCTIVE ENDOCRINOLOGY can be responsible for errors in the original materials. The editors' comments are their own opinions. Mention of specific products within this publication does not constitute endorsement.

To facilitate the use of the YEAR BOOK OF INFERTILITY AND REPRODUCTIVE ENDOCRINOLOGY as a reference tool, all illustrations and tables included in this publication are now identified as they appear in the original article. This change is meant to help the reader recognize that any illustration or table appearing in the YEAR BOOK OF INFERTILITY AND REPRODUCTIVE ENDOCRINOLOGY may be only one of many in the original article. For this reason, figure and table numbers will often appear to be out of sequence within the YEAR BOOK OF INFERTILITY AND REPRODUCTIVE ENDOCRINOLOGY.

Publisher's Preface

The 1996 YEAR BOOK OF INFERTILITY AND REPRODUCTIVE ENDOCRI-NOLOGY marks the conclusion of an outstanding publication and tenure of editorship by Daniel R. Mishell, Jr., M.D., and his associate editors, Rogerio A. Lobo, M.D., and Rebecca Z. Sokol, M.D. Although it is no longer viable for Mosby–Year Book, Inc. to publish this series, we want to extend our sincere thanks to the entire editorial board for all of their hard work and enthusiasm. We are fortunate to continue our association with Dr. Mishell, who remains editor of the YEAR BOOK OF OBSTETRICS AND GYNECOLOGY.

During the eight years of this series, YEAR BOOK readers were provided with informative literature selections and insightful editorial commentary of the highest caliber. Moreover, we at Mosby–Year Book, Inc. have been treated to a most enjoyable and rewarding editorial association. A special thanks goes out to Shirley Davenport, editorial coordinator for Dr. Mishell, who helped us guide all of the editors through the YEAR BOOK'S development process.

Although we will miss publishing the YEAR BOOK OF INFERTILITY AND REPRODUCTIVE ENDOCRINOLOGY and working with the members of this fine team, we wish them the very best in all their future endeavors and extend out heartfelt thanks and appreciation for their excellent service.

Introduction

It has been estimated that the incidence of infertility has nearly doubled in the United States in the past 2 decades as more women postpone their initial attempts to conceive until they are older than age 30 years. Several studies have shown that the percentage of infertile couples starts to significantly increase when the female partner reaches 31 years of age and steadily increases thereafter. It has been estimated that in the United States 30% of these couples seek assistance from clinicians to aid their chances of conceiving. Numerous scientific articles are written each year that report the result of studies using various techniques to diagnose and treat the multiple causes of infertility. Busy practitioners can read only a small percentage of these articles. To assist these clinicians, the annual volumes of the YEAR BOOK OF INFERTILITY AND REPRODUCTIVE ENDOCRINOLOGY are integrated to provide them with an opportunity to rapidly survey the world's most relevant literature dealing with infertility. A critical analysis of the articles by one of the three editors is also provided to interpret the relevance of the articles in order to assist clinicians to better diagnose and treat the infertile couple.

Each editor has reviewed the entire scientific literature published in his or her area, has selected the most important relevant articles for abstracting, and has then written a descriptive comment. Dr. Rebecca Sokol, an expert in the area of male infertility, has selected the articles dealing with this subject and offers critical comments. Dr. Rogerio Lobo has selected the articles relating to reproductive endocrinology, and I have selected the articles concerned with female infertility. In this volume, we also are fortunate to have an excellent summary of the current knowledge of the etiology and treatment of infertility. This information was assembled by a group of international experts in the field of infertility and represents a synthesis of results of evidence-based research in this area.

The editors believe that the information contained in this volume will be of great aid to practitioners when couples who have problems conceiving children seek their assistance.

Daniel R. Mishell, Jr., M.D.

Infertility Revisited: The State of the Art Today and Tomorrow*†

THE ESHRE CAPRI WORKSHOP GROUP

The ESHRE Capri Workshop group first arrived at the working definitions, then discussed the diagnoses prevalence, untreated prognosis and the advantages and disadvantages of the available treatments for the various categories of infertility, namely anovulatory, tuboperitoneal, male, and unexplained infertility.

Infertility

DEFINITIONS

Fertility—Based on the distribution of fecundity observed in a "normal" population, normal fertility was defined by the group as achieving a pregnancy within 2 years by regular coital exposure.

Sterility, subfertility, infertility—Those couples who do not achieve a pregnancy within 2 years include the sterile members of the population, for whom there is no possibility of natural pregnancy, and the remainder, who are subfertile. Together, these comprise the infertile population. The term "sterile" may refer to either the male or the female, whereas the term "subfertile" refers to the couple.

Fecundability, fecundity—Fecundability is the probability of achieving a pregnancy within 1 menstrual cycle. Fecundity is the ability to achieve a live birth from 1 cycle's exposure to the risk of pregnancy.

PREVALENCE AND EPIDEMIOLOGY OF INFERTILITY

Infertility is a condition that affects the couple. Male or female infertility cannot be considered in isolation. Because most demographic measures of fertility are based on the woman, estimates of the prevalence of infertility are usually based on the female. In a strictly monogamous society, these measures will reflect couple infertility, whereas in a society in which men have many partners, such measures can only refer to female infertility. One limitation of such demographic measures is that voluntary and involuntary childlessness cannot easily be distinguished.

Table 1 gives regional and country estimates of primary infertility rates, but there is considerable variation in rates between different age cohorts, both within and between countries. Estimates of secondary infertility must include an assessment of the woman's exposure to the risk of pregnancy (i.e., whether she is using any contraceptive method or lactating, etc.) and are much more difficult to interpret.

Consideration of the patterns of diagnoses for both partners of the infertile couple shows that minor degrees of fertility impairment are seen in both partners more frequently than expected. Such fertility impairments are not necessarily associated with infertility when present in only one

---

*Based on recommendations of the ESHRE Workshops, held in Anacapri, August 1992, 1993, 1994, and 1995.
†Adapted from *Human Reproduction* 11(8):1779–1807, 1996. Reprinted with permission.

partner but may become important when present in both partners.[1] These observations led the group to highlight the distinction between sterility and subfertility. Whereas subfertility can only be identified in a couple, it is possible to define male or female sterility. In men, conditions associated with sterility include azoospermia and lack of ejaculation; in women, ovarian failure, complete occlusion of the oviducts, and the absence of the uterus are associated with sterility. In these situations there is no possibility

TABLE 1.—Estimates of the Prevalence of Primary Infertility (Percent) by Region and Country

Africa	10.1		**Latin America**	3.1
Angola	12		Colombia	4
Burkino Faso	6		Costa Rica	2
Burundi	3		Guyana	9
Cameroon	15		Mexico	3
C. African Rep.	17		Panama	3
Chad	11		Paráguay	3
Congo	21		Peru	3
Gabon	32		Venezuela	2
Ghana	3			
Guinea	6		**Middle East**	3.0
Ivory Coast	10		Jordan	3
Kenya	7		Egypt	4
Lesotho	4		Turkey	2
Mali	8		Syria	3
Mozambique	14			
Niger	9		**Europe**	5.4
Nigeria	8		Belgium	7
Senegal	4		Bulgaria	6
Sudan	9		Czechoslovakia	4
Tanzania	10		Denmark	6
Zaire	21		Finland	5
Zambia	14		France	6
			Great Britain	6
Caribbean	6.5		Italy	6
Dominican Rep.	6		Norway	5
Haiti	7		Poland	3
Jamaica	7		Romania	6
Trinidad & Tob.	5		Spain	4
			Sweden	11
Asia & Oceania	4.8		Yugoslavia	5
Bangladesh	4			
Fiji	4		**North America**	6
Indonesia	7		USA	6
Korea	2			
Malaysia	4			
Nepal	6			
Pakistan	5			
Philippines	2			
Sri Lanka	4			
Thailand	2			

Definitions: Africa—percent childless women aged 45–49 years; *Europe and USA*—percent currently married women aged 40–44 years who are childless, except *Sweden*—percent women aged 40–45 years who are childless; *Other regions*—percent women aged 40–44 years married for at least 5 years who are childless, except *Egypt*—percent currently married women aged 45–49 years who are childless.

Note: Regional figures are weighted average of country-specific rates (1985 population).

(Adapted from Farley TMM, Belsey EM: The prevalence and aetiology of infertility, in *Biological Components of Fertility. The Proceedings of the African Population Conference.* Dakar, Senegal, November 1988. International Union for the Scientific Study of Population, Liege, Belgium, 1988, Vol. 1, pp 2.1.15–2.1.30.)

of natural conception. Using the concepts of subfertility and sterility, the distribution of couple diagnoses observed in the World Health Organization (WHO) Standardized Investigation of the Infertile Couple is shown in Table 2. That the number of couples in whom there are fertility impairments in both partners is higher than would be expected suggests that the factors that make a couple infertile and consult for infertility are different for the different types of couples in the population. It is probable that there are large numbers of couples in the general population in which only one partner has impaired fertility and who never seek medical help because fertility is not delayed enough to be a problem; however, if both partners have impaired conditions, then delays are unacceptably long and the couple usually seeks help.

A practical example of this interaction is the following: when a clinician sees an infertile couple in which the man has a low sperm count and a varicocele, there is a greater than normal probability that the female partner will be found to have an ovulation problem as well. There is thus a strong case for investigating both partners except when there is a condition associated with sterility.

DIAGNOSIS

Diagnosis of sterility is, in general, easy, whereas diagnosis of subfertility can be very difficult. The difficulty is compounded by a lack of agreement on the diagnostic tests to be performed. Such agreement is not readily obtained because of different views about the value of certain diagnostic tests and the variety of clinical experience. Although some believe that any abnormal diagnostic test result defines a cause of infertility, it is more probable that abnormal test results define a cause of infertility only if treatment of this cause enhances fecundability as compared with no treatment. Based on the latter view, diagnostic tests for infertility can be sorted into 3 categories:

1. Abnormal test results that have an established correlation with impaired fecundability: semen analysis, tubal patency by hysterosalpingogram or laparoscopy, laboratory assessment of ovulation. In each case, when the test result is unequivocally abnormal (azoospermia, bilateral tubal occlusion, or anovulation), fertility is unarguably impaired without therapy.

2. Abnormal test results that are not consistently correlated with impaired fecundability: postcoital test,[2] laparoscopic finding of mild endometriosis,[3] cervical mucus penetration test,[4] hysteroscopy,[5] antisperm antibody assays,[6] and the zona-free hamster egg penetration test.[7] For these diagnostic tests, abnormal results frequently are associated with subsequent fertility without therapy.

3. Abnormal test results that do not appear to be correlated with impaired fecundability: endometrial dating,[8] varicocele assessment,[9] falloposcopy.[10] For these diagnostic tests, either there are data that confirm the lack of a correlation with pregnancy or such follow-up studies do not exist.

TABLE 2.—Interaction Between the Partners of the Infertile Couple. Percentage Distribution of Couple Diagnoses

Female Partner	Male Partner			
	Fertile	Subfertile		Sterile
		No demonstrable cause	Minor factors	
Fertile	—	—	—	3.2
Subfertile				
No demonstrable cause	—	14.1	20.3	
		78.6		
Minor factors		25.2	19.0	2.4
Sterile	10.1		5.5	0.3
Definitions	Male partner	Female partner		
No demonstrable cause	Normal semen quality	Regular ovulation and menses		
	Normal sexual function	Normal endocrine profile		
		Tubal patency		
Sterile	Aspermia	Bilateral tubal occlusion		
	Azoospermia	Amenorrhea with elevated FSH		
Minor factors	All other diagnoses	All other diagnoses		

Note: Includes data from 5,713 infertile couples from the WHO standardized investigation.
Abbreviation: FSH, follicle-stimulating hormone.
(Courtesy of Farley TMM: The WHO standardized investigation of the infertile couple in Ratnam SS, Reoh E-S, Anandakumar C (eds): *Infertility Male and Female*, Vol. 4. The Proceedings of the 12th World Congress on Fertility and Sterility, Singapore, October 1986, The Parthenon Publishing Group, Carnforth, Lancs., UK, 1987, pp 123–135.)

Standard investigations aimed to evaluate infertility in a couple include laboratory assessment of ovulation, evaluation of tubal patency, and semen analysis. At present, other additional investigations contribute relatively little to effective diagnosis of unexplained infertility and are not recommended by the group.

No assessment of ovulation available today confirms the completion of a normal ovulatory process. In the absence of an ideal method, the measurement of midluteal progesterone levels in plasma is the most cost-effective compromise. More than one assay may need to be done to confirm that the concentrations are around the peak. The values most often suggested as indicative of ovulation are levels exceeding 16 nmol/L, equivalent to 5 ng/mL, for a minimum of 5 days or a single value exceeding 32 nmol/L, corresponding to 10 ng/mL.[11, 12] Tubal patency can be evaluated by hysterosalpingography and/or laparoscopy. Because tubal patency may not be the only cause, laparoscopy also may help detect other factors (e.g., endometriosis, adhesions).

Semen analysis consists at present of applying the recommendations of the WHO Laboratory Manual for the Examination of Human Semen and Sperm-Cervical Mucus Interaction.[13]

TREATMENT

When the clinician has completed the diagnostic assessment of infertility, the next step is to estimate the baseline prognosis without therapy, and then determine whether treatment can increase the likelihood of pregnancy. The decision about treatment may involve choosing from several options, and for each option, the couple should be given information about the benefits, side effects, and costs. Infertility causes varying degrees of urgency and concern in different couples, and individuals may have different approaches to risk taking. Thus, continuing without treatment is a valid choice in many cases. If treatment is preferred, the final choice of treatment should be made by the couple.

Knowledge of the untreated prognosis is helpful in advising couples, because surveys indicate that a large proportion of infertile couples do not seek therapy. In data from the United States, fewer than 50% of couples seek medical advice, and only half of those consulting physicians decide to undergo treatment.[14] Ongoing surveys seem likely to confirm that these figures also apply to European populations. The untreated prognosis in some cases is very reassuring, but infertility can be difficult to treat, and fewer than 50% of treated infertile women are successful in achieving a live birth. Thus, it is desirable to consider the particular prognostic factors in each case. Of course, if there is azoospermia, bilateral tubal obstruction, or prolonged amenorrhea, the likelihood of conception is close to zero, but these cases form only a minority of infertile couples. For more typical cases, the untreated prognosis depends on both diagnostic and clinical factors.

Observations of couples with unexplained infertility under follow-up in specialized clinics indicate that without treatment, 14% to 20% will have successful conceptions within 1 year and 25% to 30% within 2 years.[15, 16] Successful in this instance means that only conceptions leading to live births are included in the figures. If the duration of infertility is less than 3 years, the couple has secondary infertility, or the female partner is younger than 30 years of age, the prognosis is better than average. If the diagnosis is male factor, tubal defect, or endometriosis, however, the untreated prognosis is much worse.[15, 16]

Although effectiveness, side effects, costs, and personal choice all are considered in making infertility treatment decisions, the effectiveness of a given treatment compared with other options often will be the critical issue. Thus, estimates of effectiveness dominate the literature on treatments for infertility. Treatment effectiveness can be judged fairly only in randomized clinical trials because conception without therapy can occur in most subfertile couples over time. Randomization isolates the effects of treatment from the effects of other variables that might affect patient outcomes. Other study designs provide inferior evidence for several reasons. With nonrandom allocation methods, the baseline characteristics of the historical or contemporary control groups may account for the increased pregnancy rates that are thought to be caused by a treatment effect. Prognostic variables are maldistributed more often in nonrandomized studies than in randomized studies.[17] Also, the existence of the infertile state cannot remove the need for controlled studies, because even when the infertile state is of long duration, conceptions may sometimes occur without treatment.[15, 16] Therefore, case series without control groups have little value in establishing the true effect of a given treatment.

MANAGEMENT

Finally, the group agreed that in management of infertility, the effectiveness of treatment is only one component of the treatment decision. Also important are the cost of an individual therapy, the time required to participate in a therapy program, and the severity of any side effects. Furthermore, characteristics of the couple may influence the treatment decision; the desire to have a child varies from couple to couple, as does the willingness to take any given risk. Finally, even in the absence of a perceived benefit, some couples may prefer action to continued inaction. Therefore, each couple should enter into the development of a treatment plan that will optimally meet its own needs. The physician's role is to provide clinical information (counseling on optimal time of intercourse) and a choice of treatment programs.

RESULTS

In each of the following chapters on individual diagnostic categories, treatment effectiveness is judged on the basis of the highest quality of evidence that was available at the time this material was prepared. Randomized clinical trials (RCTs), represent the best evidence from individual studies, followed at some distance by cohort studies. Case series are much lower in the hierarchy.[18] Meta-analysis of randomized clinical trials can further improve the value of the evidence from single studies.[19] With the use of meta-analysis, the results of several small studies that lack sufficient power may be combined to yield or rule out a significant effect of treatment. Also, meta-analytic techniques include an assessment of the variability in the published study results. If treatment effects vary significantly from study to study, one would place less confidence in both the combined and individual results.

Therefore, the following guidelines governed the collection of evidence for the effectiveness of treatment.[17] The publications selected were those which represented the highest level of clinical evidence: meta-analysis of RCTs, individual RCTs, and cohort studies.[15] If a treatment has been evaluated only in case series, an attempt has been made to select the largest of these and present aggregate results. Readers should take note, however, that pregnancy rates in case series may be inflated by numerous selection factors and these rates are not strictly comparable to the results from more rigorous study designs.[19] Studies were selected in which treatment was evaluated with respect to the most relevant outcome. Although live birth rates would be preferable, in most cases the measure of effectiveness was pregnancy rate.[16] Where possible, the data chosen have been drawn from accessible peer-reviewed journals so that interested readers may consult the original sources.

Anovulatory Infertility

Anovulatory infertility is a condition in which there is no rupture of the follicle with subsequent release of an ovum. Unfortunately, there is no established method to ascertain the completion of a normal ovulatory process, and the only absolute proof of normal ovulation is a subsequent pregnancy. In the absence of an ideal method, the measurement of mid-luteal progesterone levels in plasma is the most cost-effective compromise. More than one assay may need to be done to confirm the determination around the peak. The values suggested as indicative are levels greater than 16 nmol/L, equivalent to 5 ng/mL, for a minimum of 5 days.[11] Several factors are involved in the process leading to the release of an ovum. A blockade during one of these stages could interfere with ovulation or the capacity of a mature oocyte to develop into an embryo.

DIAGNOSIS

Various causes of anovulation have been identified in women. These are indicated in Table 3. Each of the causes listed in Table 3 should be considered in clinical practice. In addition, the following information should also be obtained: a medical history; the duration of infertility; physical and laboratory examinations to rule out other health problems (e.g., diabetes, thyroid dysfunction); further diagnostic studies of the couple, because failure to achieve a pregnancy may be related to some male factors (a spermiogram should be obtained); or tubal problems (test for tubal patency). Other useful general information includes the age of the

---

TABLE 3.—Causes of Anovulation

Intrinsic ovarian failure
- —Genetic
- —Autoimmune disease
- —Others (e.g., cytotoxic chemotherapy)

Secondary ovarian dysfunction
- —Disorders of gonadotropin regulation
  - *a) Specific*
    - hyperprolactinemia
    - Kallmann's syndrome
  - *b) Functional*
    - weight loss
    - exercise
    - idiopathic
    - drugs

Gonadotropin deficiency
- —Pituitary tumor
- —Pituitary necrosis or thrombosis

Disorders of gonadotropin action
- —Polycystic ovary syndrome

(Courtesy of Franks S: Diagnosis and treatment of anovulation, in Hillier SG (ed): *Ovarian Endocrinology*. Blackwell Scientific Publications, Oxford, pp 227–238, 1991.)

---

patient, body mass index (both overweight[20] and underweight[21] can affect ovulation), and evidence of acne and/or hirsutism.

Four conditions are found with relatively high frequency in women with suspected ovulatory failure attending infertility clinics. These include: hyperprolactinemic anovulation, hypogonadotropic anovulation, hypergonadotropic anovulation, "normogonadotropic" anovulation.

Hyperprolactinemia

The upper limit of normal prolactin (PRL) levels in plasma for a hypoestrogenic, amenorrheic, gestagen-negative woman is 400–500 mIU/mL (20–25 ng/mL). When estrogen levels are normal, the maximal normal PRL level is 600–800 mIU/mL (30–40 ng/mL).[22] If elevated, the measurement should be repeated under basal conditions. If the patient is hyperprolactinemic, thyroid-stimulating hormone (TSH) should be measured to exclude hypothyroidism.[23] If PRL levels are confirmed to be elevated, some type of pituitary imaging should be carried out (radiography, CT, nuclear MR) to diagnose an empty sella, a microadenoma, and to rule out a macroadenoma, which usually but not always produce very high levels of PRL.[24]

Hypogonadotropic Hypogonadism

The best indirect evidence is the estrogen status. Serum estradiol levels are lower than 40 pg/mL (110 pmol/L),[25] and there should be no withdrawal bleeding after a gestagen challenge.[26]

Hypergonadotropic Hypogonadism

Plasma levels of follicle-stimulating hormone (FSH) should be higher than 20 mIU/mL in repeated measurements.[27] The patient is usually hypoestrogenic and does not respond to the gestagen challenge. If she is younger than 40 years of age, this finding indicates premature ovarian failure. An ovarian biopsy is not necessary. In women younger than age 25, a karyotype should be performed. If karyotyping reveals the presence of a Y chromosome, surgical removal of the gonad is recommended because there is a risk of malignant transformation.[28]

"Normogonadotropic" Anovulation

In these women, concentrations of FSH and luteinizing hormone (LH) in a random blood sample are usually within the normal range. However, there is usually some disturbance in the pattern of pulsatile gonadotropin-releasing hormone (GnRH) secretion.[29] Defining that condition requires frequent collection of multiple blood samples, which is impractical and expensive in routine clinical practice. Because these women have some ovarian activity, they are not hypoestrogenic and will bleed in response to a gestagen challenge. The majority of these patients are likely to have polycystic ovaries (PCOs), and these can usually be detected by ultrasound examination. When these women are hirsute, their blood androgen levels may be high. High androgen levels may be useful to differentiate PCOs from multifollicular ovaries (MFOs),[30] which have upper normal or enlarged ovaries with numerous follicles and normal androgen levels.

TREATMENT

There is a spectrum of conditions between total anovulation and normal ovulation. In vitro fertilization data indicate that the best results for fecundity can be obtained by the "timely release of a mature ovum." If the fallopian tubes are compromised or if the semen analysis indicates poor semen quality, the couple should be offered assisted reproduction techniques. Any suspicious ovarian mass should be investigated before initiation of stimulation. General measures to start or reestablish ovulation include changes in lifestyle when necessary (obesity, malnutrition, overexercise, alcoholism, etc.), whereas specific treatments apply to the following 4 types of anovulation.

Hyperprolactinemia

These patients should be treated with a drug that lowers plasma PRL levels. The most widely used of these is bromocriptine. The average dose given is 2.5 mg twice a day. Treatment should be continued until plasma PRL levels are normal and be monitored by PRL and progesterone assays. If ovulation does not occur, the dose of bromocriptine can be increased to as much as 25 mg/day, divided into 2–3 doses per day, on the basis of individual responses.[31] Bromocriptine can also be administered intravaginally. Because absorption is slower, the effective blood levels persist longer and the drug can therefore be administered less frequently and at a lower dose.[32] Also, side effects are less frequent with vaginal than with oral administration. Other possible drugs are lisuride, pergolide, other ergot derivatives, CV 205-502[33] and, more recently, the long-acting drug cabergoline.[34] These drugs can be combined, as suggested by Diamant et al.,[35] with antiestrogens if ovulation does not occur despite normalized PRL levels. If ovulation still does not occur, attempts can be made to induce it with gonadotropins or with pulsatile GnRH administration.

A major advantage of the PRL-lowering drugs is that, in contradistinction to gonadotropin therapy, they do not increase the incidence of multiple pregnancies or early pregnancy loss.[36] If pregnancy does not occur after 6–8 months of ovulatory cycles, the couple must be reinvestigated.

Hypogonadotropic Hypogonadism (WHO Group 1)

The most common type of hypogonadotropic hypogonadism is idiopathic. Known causes include being underweight, malnutrition, and excessive exercise. If one of these latter conditions is present, the patient should be counseled. If, instead, the cause is primary pituitary failure, ovulation may be induced with gonadotropins.

If the pituitary failure is secondary to hypothalamic dysfunction, the best treatment is pulsatile GnRH (5 µg, intravenously, 60–90 minutes or 10 µg, subcutaneously, every 90 minutes). The patient should be referred to a specialist for these treatments. Pulsatile GnRH treatment can be monitored by ovarian ultrasound. Otherwise, it can be monitored by basal body temperature and/or plasma progesterone levels (1–3 measurements in the luteal phase of the cycle). After ovulation has occurred, one can give 1,000–2,000 IU of human chorionic gonadotropin (hCG) every third day for 3 times to support the corpus luteum (after the pump has been removed).[37] The advantages of pulsatile GnRH over human menopausal gonadotropin (hMG) are that there is little risk of hyperstimulation and the need for monitoring is minimal. The disadvantages are that treatment is more complex and not all patients like to wear the pump necessary for intermittent administration.

An alternative treatment is administration of hMG followed by hCG. The normal starting dose of hMG is 150 IU/day, which usually is increased until there is a response. The patient should be monitored every 1–2 days by ultrasound and/or plasma estradiol levels, starting on the fourth or fifth day of treatment. Ovarian hyperstimulation is a recognized complication and can have serious consequences (see below). Even with the closest monitoring, it is difficult to reduce the incidence of multiple pregnancies, which is at least 20%. Their incidence and the incidence of ovarian hyperstimulation can be lowered by withholding hCG if there are more than 3 follicles greater than 16 mm in diameter.[38]

Pure FSH is not indicated for this group of patients because some LH is required for ovulation.[39] Antiestrogens are not effective.

Hypergonadotropic Hypogonadism

Although FSH levels in these women may fluctuate for months, and there have even been cases of women who became pregnant after the diagnosis was confirmed by biopsy,[40] for all practical purposes they cannot be treated. Therefore, ovulation induction is not indicated. Hypergonadotropic women have either the so-called resistant ovary syndrome (a rare condition in which ovaries contain thousands of primordial follicles)[41] or incipient ovarian failure.

When high FSH is persistent, there is no need for a biopsy to confirm the diagnosis, nor is it useful to apply any of the ovulation-inducing regimens recommended for the other groups discussed in this report. However, the long-term hypoestrogenic condition should be treated with estrogen to prevent osteoporosis and an increased risk of cardiovascular disease, etc. These patients can achieve pregnancy through a program of egg donation.

"Normogonadotropic" Anovulation (WHO Group 2)

These patients have normal FSH, but LH may be elevated. The majority of these women have PCOs,[42] and a smaller subgroup have MFOs.[30] They have in common a less favorable response to all forms of ovulation induction than patients already mentioned in groups 1 and 2. They also have a greater risk of ovarian hyperstimulation when they do respond.

After weight reduction of overweight patients (body mass index greater than 25), the treatment of choice is an antiestrogen such as clomiphene citrate or tamoxifen. The usual starting dose of clomiphene citrate is 50 mg/day for 5 days, beginning on the second to sixth day after induced or spontaneous bleeding. If, according to plasma progesterone monitoring, there is no ovulation, this dose should be increased by 50 mg each cycle up to 250 mg/day for 5 days in each treatment schedule. If ovulation is accomplished, the same dose should be continued for at least 10 cycles or until pregnancy occurs.[43] The patient should be monitored monthly by ultrasound and, if there is persistent ovarian follicular enlargement, treatment should be postponed until it regresses. If ovulation and/or pregnancy does not occur with clomiphene citrate, tamoxifen may be used if the adrenal androgen levels are not elevated. The suggested tamoxifen dosage is 20–40 mg/day, beginning on cycle day 3, for 5 days.[44] If ovulation does not occur and the adrenal androgens are high, dehydroepiandrosterone sulfate greater than 30 pg/mL, addition of daily dexamethasone to cyclic clomiphene may be helpful.[45] Cyclofenil, another weak antiestrogen, has not been shown to be effective.[46]

There are several advantages of clomiphene treatment over conventional hMG stimulation. With clomiphene, there is practically no risk of hyperstimulation and only a small increase in the incidence of twin pregnancies (about 5%),[47] whereas the risks of spontaneous abortion or tubal pregnancy do not seem to be increased, nor are there more fetal malformations (although a possible increased risk of neural tube defect is still arguable). There is no documented advantage for sequentially combining clomiphene with hCG or estrogen.[48] The effects of these additional therapies have not been well investigated and hCG might only worsen the risk of multiple pregnancy because of its very long half-life. Clomiphene is probably the most cost-effective and easiest treatment available.

The side effects of clomiphene citrate, in addition to persistent ovarian enlargement, may include vasomotor disturbances, visual disturbances, urticaria, and alopecia. These require interruption or discontinuation of treatment for only a small percentage of patients. If a patient does not ovulate after clomiphene treatment, other, more complicated, modalities include the use of pulsatile GnRH or human gonadotropins. The latter provide a good cumulative pregnancy rate but a higher risk of multiple pregnancies and ovarian hyperstimulation. Low-dose hMG or FSH regimens[49, 50] and the stepdown regimens[51] produce fewer multiple pregnancies, but the overall pregnancy rate is low and they are very labor intensive. The low-dose FSH regimen is presently the most widely used hMG treatment worldwide.

Another alternative treatment suggested for patients with PCOs who are resistant to clomiphene is laparoscopic ovarian electrocautery. The spontaneous cumulative pregnancy rate over many cycles has been reported to be around 50%. The risk of multiple pregnancy is not increased, and the abortion rate is low.[52] The mechanism of action of this therapy is still obscure, but it seems to be linked to an immediate decrease in ovarian androgen. The efficacy of this treatment has yet to be evaluated in a formal prospective comparative study.[53] Applying this technique, with the ensuing risks of postoperative adhesions,[54] is a choice for the individual physician, who should decide whether clomiphene-unresponsive patients with PCOs who are undergoing laparoscopic examination for any reason should be cauterized at that time. It should be remembered that abortion rates in patients with PCOs are relatively high regardless of which induction procedure is used.

RESULTS

Bromocriptine

Selection of data: The largest case series were selected.

Description of Data

Level of evidence	case series
Publication dates	1983–1989
Number of studies	2[55, 56]
Number of patients	131
Outcome evaluated	pregnancy
Treatment effect	pregnancy rate

Among infertile women with hyperprolactinemia, menses generally return within 6 months. Pregnancy rates in large-scale outcome studies range from 34% to 70%.[55, 56] Long-acting injectable (monthly) and oral (daily) preparations of bromocriptine may facilitate long-term treatment. Chemically related dopamine agonists such as pergolide and cabergoline may be tolerated better. When taken only twice weekly, cabergoline is at least as effective as bromocriptine.[34]

Clomiphene Treatment

Selection of Data: Four randomized clinical trials evaluated ovulation rates among anovulatory women using clomiphene or placebo tablets.

Description of data

Level of evidence	randomized clinical trials
Publication dates	1966–1985
Number of studies	4[57–60]
Number of patients	279
Outcome evaluated	ovulation, pregnancy
Treatment effect	odds ratio

In randomized clinical trials, the likelihood of ovulation was 5.5 times higher (95% confidence interval [CI], 3.1–9.5) after clomiphene use than in placebo-treated patients (Table 4).[57–60] The likelihood of conception was similarly increased in the trial that evaluated pregnancy rates (typical odds ratio, 4.0, 95% CI, 1.0–16.1).[59] The pregnancy rates were 9% in 5 cycles of placebo treatment and 33% in 5 cycles of clomiphene treatment.

Gonadotropin

Selection of data: Four studies reported on the effectiveness of the induction of ovulation with hMG in women with infertility caused by ovulatory defects. These studies included more than 50 subjects and reported outcome data by WHO group 1 and 2. All 4 studies were case series rather than randomized, controlled trials.

Description of Data

Level of evidence	case series
Publication dates	1974–1994
Number of studies	4[61–64]
Number of cycles	2,613
Outcome evaluated	ovulation, pregnancy
Treatment effect	pregnancy rate

The pregnancy rates in these 4 studies spanning 20 years of experience are remarkably similar (Table 5).[61–64] The aggregate pregnancy rate among patients in WHO group 1 was 25% per cycle, compared with 8% per cycle among women with WHO group 2 ovulatory problems. The high proportion of women with hyperandrogenicity contributes to the lower success rates in the patients with group 2 ovulatory problems.[64]

TABLE 4.—Clomiphene Treatment for Anovulatory Infertility: Effects on Ovulation

Authors	Odds ratio (95% CI)	Number of patients
Connaughton et al., 1974	1.3 (0.4–4.0)	62
Cudmore and Tupper, 1966	7.5 (1.6–39)	41
Garcia et al., 1985	8.8 (1.9–45)	46
Johnson et al., 1966	13 (4.8–38)	130
Odds ratio	5.5 (3.1–9.5)	279

Abbreviation: CI, confidence interval.

TABLE 5.—Pregnancy Rate Per Cycle of Human
Menopausal Gonadotropin Treatment in
Women With Anovulatory Infertility

Authors	Number of pregnancies per cycle (%)	
	WHO Group I	WHO Group II
Caspi et al., 1974	18/77 (23%)	10/34 (29%)
Ellis & Williamson, 1975	24/147 (16%)	19/175 (11%)
Lunenfeld et al., 1981	220/826 (27%)	137/2,064 (7%)
Fluker et al., 1994	18/72 (25%)	34/318 (11%)
Aggregate results	280/1,122 (25%)	200/2,591 (8%)

Gonadotropin-Releasing Hormone (GnRH)

Selection of data: A cohort comparative study[65] and previous case series that were aggregated in an overview.[37]

Description of Data

Level of evidence	case series, cohort comparison
Publication dates	1991–1994
Number of studies	2[37, 65]
Number of patients	344
Outcome evaluated	Ovulation, pregnancy
Treatment effect	pregnancy rate

In the literature to 1991, 80% of the GnRH-treated cycles were ovulatory and the conception rate was 27% per cycle (Table 6).[37] In a recent nonrandomized comparison of exogenous gonadotropins and pulsatile GnRH for the induction of ovulation in women with amenorrhea, ovulation and conception rates were similar (see Table 6).[65] The cumulative chance of conceiving after 6 treatment cycles, however, was 72% for hMG and 96% for pulsatile GnRH. Gonadotropin-releasing hormone induction of ovulation in patients with polycystic ovarian syndrome is less successful. Among 131 patients summarized by Filicori et al., ovulation occurred in 240 (41.7%) of 414 cycles, and pregnancy occurred in only 54 (13.0%).[37]

TABLE 6.—Pulsatile GnRH Use for the Induction of Ovulation

Agent	Authors	Patients	Cycles initiated	Ovulation rate (% per cycle)	Pregnancy rate (% per cycle)
GnRH	Filicori et al., 1991	273	683	544 (80%)	183 (27%)
GnRH	Martin et al., 1993	41	118	110 (93%)	34 (29%)
hMG	Martin et al., 1993	30	111	108 (97%)	28 (25%)

Note: Aggregate published results and a comparative study.
Abbreviations: GnRH, gonadotropin-releasing hormone; *hMG*, human menopausal gonadotropin.

RISKS OF OVARIAN STIMULATION

Risks of Ovarian Stimulation

Ovarian Hyperstimulation Syndrome

The ovarian hyperstimulation syndrome is an iatrogenic condition of increased vascular permeability causing an exudate of fluid from the intravascular to the extravascular compartment leading to ascites, decreased intravascular volume and hemoconcentration. This condition was originally described in the 1960s following use of ovulation induction techniques in anovulatory women. This syndrome also occurs after controlled ovarian hyperstimulation for artificial reproductive techniques. Although mild to moderate ovarian hyperstimulation is relatively common, the incidence of the severe syndrome in controlled ovarian hyperstimulation is about 0.5%. In contrast to ovulation induction in anovulatory women, with controlled ovarian hyperstimulation, hyperstimulation is deliberate, multiple follicles are enlarged, the follicular wall is punctured with aspiration of granulosa cells, and the time of embryo transfer can be regulated or avoided entirely. There have been numerous classification systems of the degrees of ovarian hyperstimulation syndrome, most relating to ovulation induction. Navot et al.[66] suggest that when the syndrome occurs with controlled ovarian hyperstimulation, the symptom complex should be divided into severe and critical, as both of these categories require hospitalization and intensive care. The ovarian hyperstimulation syndrome is severe when there is massive ascites with or without hydrothorax, a hematocrit greater than 45% or a 30% increase over baseline, white blood cell count greater than 15 mg/100 mL, oliguria, creatinine levels between 1 and 1.5, and a creatinine clearance of greater than 50 mL per minute together with liver dysfunction and anasarca. The level of ovarian hyperstimulation is critical when the ascites becomes tense, the hematocrit rises above 55, the white blood cell count is above 25,000, creatinine levels are greater than 1.6, creatinine clearance is less than 50 mL per minute, and either renal failure, trombophlebitis, or the acute respiratory distress syndrome is present.

Major risk factors for the development of ovarian hyperstimulation syndrome are administration of exogenous hCG, especially in the luteal phase, and endogenous hCG occurring with pregnancy. It has been suggested that there are two types of the syndrome: early and late. Early development of the syndrome occurs 3–7 days after the ovulatory hCG injection and the likelihood of occurrence is related to the serum estradiol level as well as to the number of oocytes retrieved. Late onset of this syndrome usually occurs 12–17 days after the hCG injection and its incidence and severity are related to the number of gestational sacs present. Individuals at high risk for developing the syndrome with controlled ovarian hyperstimulation have estradiol levels above 12.8 pmol/L (4,000 pg/L) at the time of induced ovulation, multiple follicles (more than 35), ultrasound evidence of multiple early antral follicles, pregnancy, luteal hCG administration, and the use of GnRH agonists before ovulation. Individuals are at low risk if estradiol levels are under 4,000 ng/L, there are few dominant follicles (fewer than 20), no pregnancy, poor or no luteal support, and only clomiphene citrate or hMG used for ovarian stimulation. Various techniques are advocated for prevention of this syndrome. These include prolonged use of GnRH agonists or withholding hCG until the estradiol levels fall (drift), use of a lower dose of hMG and a shorter stimulation interval, decreasing the ovulatory hCG dose or withholding it entirely, withholding luteal phase hCG, and avoiding endogenous hCG by cryopreservation of the embryos. If the syndrome does occur, the treatment for moderate hyperstimulation, with hematocrit under 44% and only moderate ascites, is bed rest and increased oral intake of liquids containing sodium chloride and other electrolytes. When the syndrome becomes severe, with hematocrit greater than 45% or a 30% increase, patients should be hospitalized, with frequent monitoring of electrolytes, blood urea nitrogen, and creatinine as well as liver enzymes and the coagulation profile. Fluid balance should be maintained and one should monitor the daily intake and output, body weight, hematocrit and abdominal girth. Infusion of fluids, including sodium chloride and glucose, from 1.5 to more than 3 L per day as well as infusion of low salt human abumin, 50–100 g every 2–12 hours, has been advocated. If the ascites becomes tense, infusion of Lasix and paracentesis are beneficial. When the condition becomes critical, with impending renal failure, dopamine should be given. If thrombosis is present, heparin should be administered and, if impending renal failure or acute respiratory stress syndrome occur and the patient is pregnant, termination of the pregnancy may be indicated.

The cause of ovarian hyperstimulation syndrome has not been completely elucidated. Elevated levels of estrogen, progesterone, PRL, renin, and prostaglandins have all been considered to be the agents that increase capillary permeability and lead to exudation of fluid from the intravascular to extravascular compartments. The main etiologic factor is now believed to be angiotensin II, which increases vascular permeability as well as causing vasoconstriction and neovascular proliferation. Navot et al.[66] reported that levels of plasma renin activity were increased and directly related to the severity of the syndrome. It is possible that angiotensin-converting enzyme inhibitors may be useful in the prevention of this problem.

In conclusion, ovarian hyperstimulation syndrome is a rare but dangerous consequence of gonadotropin therapy. Its incidence can be reduced but not eliminated by various modifications of ovarian stimulation.

Ovarian Cancer

There is speculation that increased incidence of ovulation with controlled ovarian hyperstimulation may lead to an increased risk of ovarian epithelial cancer later in life. The basis for this speculation is the fact that the risk of ovarian epithelial cancer is inversely related to parity, and use of oral contraceptives while young protects against the development of ovarian cancer after their use is discontinued, up to age 55 years. Furthermore, the magnitude of the reduction in the risk of ovarian cancer related to oral contraceptive use is directly related to the duration of use of these agents. There have been several single case reports of development of ovarian cancer after the use of fertility drugs. In 1992, Whittemore et al.[67] combined the results of 12 case control studies conducted between 1956 and 1986 and reported that there was an increased risk of ovarian cancer among infertile women using profertility drugs. The overall relative risk was increased 2.8 times, which was statistically significant. The problem with this study was the fact that the women developed cancer in their perimenopausal or postmenopausal years and thus had had to use fertility drugs many years previously, so recall bias was likely. In addition, clomiphene citrate was only approved for marketing in the United States in 1966, and the cancers that developed perimenopausally or postmenopausally in the 1960s and the 1970s make it unlikely that clomiphene was the fertility drug used. There was no information in the article regarding the type of fertilty drugs used. Another case control study was published by Rossing et al.[68] in 1994. This study consisted of a group of 3,837 women evaluated for infertility. Among this group there were 11 ovarian invasive or borderline tumors, and 9 of these women had used clomiphene citrate. The relative risk of ovarian cancers with use of this drug was 2.3 times that for infertile women not using the drug. When clomiphene was used for 1–11 cycles, there was a slightly decreased nonsignificant relative risk (0.7) of ovarian tumors developing, whereas when clomiphene citrate was used for more than 12 cycles, there was a sevenfold increase, which was statistically significant. The types of tumors found in this study were 4 epithelial carcinomas, 5 with low malignant potential and 2 granulosa cell tumors. In the discussion of this paper, the authors stated that the study had a number of limitations. They further concluded that although the findings raise the possibility that prolonged use of clomiphene citrate increases the risk of ovarian tumors, additional larger studies are needed to test this hypothesis. In an editorial, Whittemore stated that the distinction between an association and a causal effect is critical, as an association can occur by chance and does not necessarily indicate a causal link. To prove a causal association, large collaborative multicenter studies are needed. Until such studies are carried out, the results of these two studies cannot be used to demonstrate that there is a true causal relationship between the use of ovulation-inducing agents and an increased risk of ovarian cancer.

Tuboperitoneal Infertility

PREVENTION OF SEXUALLY TRANSMITTED DISEASE (STD)-RELATED INFERTILITY

Sequelae to genital infections are one cause of impaired fertility. In contrast to many other causes, postinfection infertility in general and STD-related infertility in particular are acquired and, hence, preventable. Although many STDs might be indirectly associated with infertility or be present in couples consulting for infertility, only 2 organisms have proven direct effects on postinfection fertility and are of importance to discuss in this context: *Neisseria gonorrhoeae* and *Chlamydia trachomatis*.

TABLE 7.—Salpingitis Related to STD Agents

	Percent of all %	STD-associated %	Other etiology %
Acute salpingitis			
Age ≤ 25	75	60	40
Age > 25	25	15	85

Abbreviation: STD, sexually transmitted disease.

(Data from Mårdh P-A: An overview of infectious agents in acute salpingitis, their biology, and recent advances in methods of detection. *Am J Obstet Gynecol* 138:933–951, 1980; and Weström L, Wolner-Hanssen P: Pathogenesis of pelvic inflammatory disease (review). *Genitourin Med* 69:9–17, 1993.)

Infections caused by these agents are common and endemic worldwide. In industrialized countries, genital chlamydial infections are 4–6 times more common than gonorrhea.[69] Indeed, genital chlamydial infection is currently the most common bacterial STD. Both of these infections may have an impact on fertility by postinfection damage to the fallopian tubes in the female. Many studies have documented that gonococci and chlamydiae account for the majority of these infections among women of fertile age (Table 7).[70, 71] During the past century, it has been documented that tubal factor infertility (TFI) in women is a sequela to pelvic infections.[72, 73] During the epidemics of gonorrhea and genital chlamydial infection in the past decades, these STDs have accounted for up to 60% of cases of acute salpingitis in young women.[70, 71] The extent to which acute salpingitis leads to TFI has been evaluated in a large prospective cohort study from the University of Lund in Sweden. The study comprised more than 2,500 women subjected to routine diagnostic laparoscopy because of clinical suspicion of acute salpingitis during the 25-year period from 1960 through 1984. After the index laparoscopy, 1,309 patients and 451 control women exposed themselves to a chance of pregnancy at some time during the follow-up period and either conceived or were examined for infertility.[73–75] An analysis of the material gives numerical values for the risk of infertility and ectopic pregnancy after acute salpingitis (Table 8). In the results presented below, there were no differences between STD-associated and non–STD-associated salpingitis.[76] Overall, 2% of the control women and 14% of the patients were involuntarily infertile after the index laparoscopy. Postinfection TFI was diagnosed in 0.8% of the control women and 12% of the patients. One of 11 patients and 1 of 73 control women experienced first pregnancies after the infection that were ectopic (see Table 8).[73] The material permits identification of variables of importance for the fertility prognosis and that can be modified to lower the rates of postinfection infertility.[73–75]

Number of infections: Both tubal factor infertility and ectopic pregnancy increased significantly with each new episode (see Table 8). In a recent study, examinations of sex partners of women with salpingitis revealed an STD and/or objective signs of urethritis in over half of those

TABLE 8.—Infertility and First Pregnancy in 1,730 Women Followed After Laparoscopy for Suspected Salpingitis

| | Numbers of salpingitis episodes | | | | |
	None (controls)	One	Two	Three or more	All salpingitis
Pregnant					
Intrauterine	433	852	124	24	1,000
Ectopic	6	61	24	15	100
Not pregnant					
TFI	4	79	46	30	155
Non-TFI	5	23	4	0	27
Total	448	1,015	198	69	1,282

Abbbreviation: TFI, tubal factor infertility.
(Courtesy of Weström L: Sexually transmitted diseases and infertility. *Sex Transm Dis* 21:532–537, 1994.)

men, regardless of the cause of the salpingitis in his partner.[77] This observation suggests that salpingitis in a woman often indicates a genital infection in the couple.

In the Lund study, surveillance and control of gonorrhea and genital chlamydial infections as well as examination and treatment of sex partners of women with salpingitis reduced the rate of repeated episodes of salpingitis from 27.5% in the 1960s to 9% in the 1980s.[73] The corresponding decrease in postinfection TFI was from 14.6% to 8.9%.[78]

Severity of the infection: The impact of this factor could be evaluated only in the 1,015 women with only one salpingitis episode. After a laparoscopically mild tubal infection, 1.8% of the women had either TFI or an ectopic first pregnancy (relative risk [RR], 1). After a moderately severe or severe infection, the RR for TFI was 1.8 and for ectopic first pregnancy was 5.6.[73]

Factors influencing the severity of the infection: For salpingitis as for other infections, the progress from mild to severe disease is a function of time. In 443 women with STD-associated salpingitis, it was found that women who initially sought treatment after 3 days of symptoms had an almost 3 times greater risk (RR, 2.8) of impaired fertility after the infection than those who sought treatment promptly.[79]

Earlier studies have documented that women who used oral contraceptives to a certain extent were protected from ascending infection,[71] and, if salpingitis was indeed present, had a laparoscopically mild salpingitis more often than non–contraceptive users or users of other methods.[80] The eventual impact on postinfection TFI of the contraceptive method used at the time of the disease episode was therefore evaluated. With non–contraceptive users as a reference group (RR, 1), the RR for TFI after salpingitis for pill users was 0.3 ($P < 0.01$), for users of an intrauterine device (IUD) 0.5 ($P < 0.05$), and for users of barrier or other contraception 0.9 and 0.8.[73, 75] Explanations for the lower risk in IUD users might be that, in contrast to the other groups, the majority of IUD users had proven fertility before the salpingitis episode, or that the etiology and pathogenesis of IUD-associated salpingitis is often different from that of STD-associated infection. The results presented should be interpreted with caution because there is no information about use of contraception after the disease episode. Furthermore, the oral contraceptives used by these women were all first- and second-generation combined pills, with higher contents of steroids than the pills used today. From available data, we can calculate that if we could halve the proportion of women with moderately severe and severe salpingitis, postsalpingitis infertility would be reduced.[73, 78]

Parallel with the epidemic of overt salpingitis, there is an epidemic of atypical (chlamydia-associated) tubal infection[81] that may lead to infertility.[82] The magnitude of such a series of events is not known. From what is stated above, it is obvious that *N. gonorrhoeae* and *C. trachomatis* cause impaired infertility in women via irreversible damage to the fallopian tubes by salpingitis. It is also obvious that prevention of STD-related infertility should operate along 2 lines, the first of which is surveillance and control of the epidemics of salpingitis-producing STDs.

Encourage use of condoms (to prevent transmission) and combined contraceptive pills (to prevent ascent of STD agents to the fallopian tubes) in women younger than 25 years of age, because the majority of TFIs are consequences of infections during this period of life. The second line of prevention is prompt evaluation and treatment of suspected cases of salpingitis. Examination and treatment of the couple, not just the woman with salpingitis, is essential in order to prevent reinfection.

DIAGNOSIS

Hysterosalpingography (HSG)

Hysterosalpingography is the simplest preliminary test to investigate uterine and tubal disease. It is performed at the beginning of the cycle (days 7–10) by transcervical injection into the uterine cavity of radiopaque dye (oil- or water-soluble) under fluoroscopic visualization.[83] Hysterosalpingography causes very few complications (infection, bleeding, etc.) and is useful for locating tubal occlusion, measuring tubal diameter and the length of the proximal segment, and determining the presence of rugae. In a recent meta-analysis of 20 studies comparing HSG and laparoscopy, it was found that for tubal patency the sensitivity of HSG was 0.65 and the specificity 0.83, whereas for peritubal adhesions, HSG was not reliable.[84] In fact, because the findings of the 2 methods can be significantly different,[85] HSG cannot be used as the sole diagnostic test for tubal normality. In addition to its diagnostic value, HSG may have a therapeutic effect as well, because some studies have reported the achievement of pregnancy immediately after the procedure, especially when oil-soluble dyes were used.[86]

Endoscopy

Laparoscopy is performed under general anesthesia and provides direct visualization of the pelvis. Hence, it is possible to assess tubal patency and the extraluminal and peritubal condition, as well as the existence of other associated pathologies, e.g., endometriosis.

Based on the laparoscopic findings, several efforts have been made to create a scoring system that could predict the reproductive potential of tubal infertility patients and would help the surgeon to decide between surgical correction and in vitro fertilization (IVF).[87, 88] One of the main limitations of laparoscopy is that it does not provide information about the lumen and the mucosa of the tubes, which might be useful prognostic factors.[89] In view of the discrepancies between HSG and laparoscopy, efforts have been made to achieve direct visualization of the tubal lumen by salpingoscopy. Tubal catheterization can be performed via laparoscopy,[90] hysteroscopy,[91] or, more recently, transcervically as an outpatient procedure.[92] This latter procedure is called falloposcopy.

TREATMENT

Treatment of Tubal Diseases

Microsurgery (distal + proximal disease)—The introduction of microsurgical techniques, e.g., adhesiolysis, fimbrioplasty, neosalpingostomy, and anastomosis, for the treatment of tuboperitoneal infertility has significantly improved pregnancy rates compared with those after conventional macrosurgical techniques. However, the postoperative results, even with microsurgery, depend to a great extent on the degree of preexisting tubal damage and the severity of mucosal distortion, as well as on the cause of the lesions.[93] Another factor that significantly influences the prognosis of these patients is the woman's age.[94]

Laparoscopic surgery (distal + proximal disease)—From the published results, the reproductive outcome after laparoscopic surgery is similar to that after microsurgery, although a prospective, randomized comparison of the 2 procedures has not yet been performed.[95, 96]

Transcervical tubal recanalization (proximal disease)—To minimize surgical intervention, efforts were made to achieve tubal recanalization in women with proximal occlusion by transcervical tubal catheterization. This can be performed hysteroscopically or under fluoroscopic control, using balloons, wires, or simple catheters. The procedure is a technically simple, safe, cost-effective and minimally invasive procedure that is associated with satisfactory patency and pregnancy rates and should be used as the first treatment option for women with proximal tubal occlusion.[97]

Treatment of Endometriosis Lesions

Endometriosis can be treated medically with ovulation-suppressing drugs or by surgical ablation of the pelvic implants. If diseased tubes or severe pelvic endometriosis cannot be corrected, mechanical causes of infertility may be circumvented by IVF (as described later).

RESULTS

Controlled studies of treatment for tubal infertility are scarce. It is not possible from the data to determine whether the variability of the study results arises from differences in the baseline characteristics of the patients, from the efficacy of the methods, or from different approaches.

Tuboplasty Surgery

Selection of data: A 1988 review assembled the results of surgical procedures for distal tubal occlusion. Few studies since 1988 have addressed this issue.

Description of Data

Level of evidence	case series
Publication dates	1975–1986
Number of studies	14[98]
Number of patients	1,275
Outcome evaluated	pregnancy
Treatment effect	pregnancy rate

Of 1,275 patients who underwent surgery, 422 (33%) conceived, and the conceptions yielded 326 (26%) intrauterine pregnancies and 96 (8%) ectopic pregnancies. In the studies reporting on the outcome of the intrauterine pregnancies, there were 239 of 1,158 (21%) term pregnancies and 55 of 1,128 (5%) spontaneous abortions.[98] The pregnancy rate in a given case depends on diameter, extent of adhesions, and presence of fimbria.

Although tuboplasty and IVF have not been compared in a formal meta-analysis, IVF appears to be superior to surgical treatment for women with tubal disease.[99, 100] In a Dutch study, although IVF success rates were only 10% per initiated cycle, the cost-effectiveness of IVF treatment was equivalent to that of tubal surgery and in some subgroups of patients IVF was superior.[100] In a Norwegian study, the availability of IVF treatment reduced tubal operations by 50% and the calculated cost per live birth was $17,000 for tubal surgery, compared with $12,000 after IVF treatment.[99]

Selective Salpingography

Selection of data: Transvaginal tubal catheterization has become the standard treatment for proximal tubal occlusion. The methods fall under two general headings: selective salpingography and transcervical balloon tuboplasty (TBT). The selected data for the former come from an aggregation of 11 published selective salpingography results.[101]

Description of Data

Level of evidence	case series
Publication dates	1990–1994
Number of studies	11[101]
Number of patients	479
Outcome evaluated	pregnancy
Treatment effect	pregnancy rate

Fallopian tubes were visualized to the fimbria in 661 of 809 instances (82%). Variability among the studies in tubal visualization may be the result of different proportions of true proximal tubal obstruction or at technical failure to opacify one or both tubes. In the 11 reports, 117 of 479 patients (24%) conceived. The pregnancy rates ranged from 9% to 37%.[101]

Transvaginal Balloon Tuboplasty

Selection of data: Selective salpingography is considered by some authors to be a preliminary procedure, to be followed if unsuccessful by TBT. The selected data come from a multicenter international trial of TBT.

Description of Data

Level of evidence	case series
Publication date	1993
Number of studies	1[102]
Number of patients	106
Outcome evaluated	pregnancy
Treatment effect	pregnancy rate

In the 134 patients with reconfirmed bilateral (or unilateral with a single tube) proximal tubal obstruction, preliminary HSG with special techniques or selective salpingography were successful in showing tubal patency in 28 patients. In the remaining 106 patients, both tubes were recanalized by TBT in 72 (68%) and one tube in 23 (22%). Pregnancy occurred in 8 (29%) of the 28 patients who did not require TBT and in 37 (35%) of the 106 patients who had TBT performed. In the latter group, there were only 2 (11%) pregnancies in the 18 patients who also had distal tubal disease.

In Vitro Fertilization Treatments

Selection of data: The highest quality of evidence would be preferred, but many IVF randomized controlled trials report high pregnancy rates. In part because the trials tested protocol modifications and excluded incomplete cycles and protocol deviations, collected national data may be more representative of the success rate than would be expected among typical couples. It is worth noting that IVF treatment was originally developed for the management of untreatable tubal infertility. The selected data come from the international registry and from recent American Society of Reproductive Medicine, Society for Assisted Reproductive Technology (ASRM-SART) data.[103, 104]

Description of Data

Level of evidence	Registry results
Publication date	1994
Number of studies	2[103, 104]
Number of cycles	161,677
Outcome evaluated	term delivery
Treatment effect	term delivery per cycle initiated

If the other clinical characteristics are reasonable, IVF is a successful therapy (Table 9).

TABLE 9.—In Vitro Fertilization Cycles Initiated and Delivery Per Cycle, by Female Age and Presence of Male Factor (MF)

Patient category	Cycles initiated	Cancellation rate	Transfer rate per retrieval	Deliveries/cycle (%)	
<40 y no MF	18,694	14.0	91.4	3,198	(17.1)
≥40 y no MF	3,687	25.2	86.6	199	(5.4)
<40 y MF	5,444	10.1	78.7	747	(13.7)
≥40 y MF	1,159	21.8	74.6	44	(3.8)
Unstimulated	420	33.6	65.2	14	(3.3)
All cycles*	29,404	14.7	87.7	4,188	(14.2)
All cycles**	132,273	12.8	83.9	17,021	(12.9)

* The American Fertility Society, Society for Assisted Reproductive Technology, 1994.
** International Working Group for Registers on Assisted Reproduction, 1995.

ENDOMETRIOSIS

Endometriosis-associated infertility has been the subject of many trials of ovulation suppression therapy and cohort studies of laparoscopic ablation of endometriosis implants.[3] At this time a large randomized clinical trial of laparoscopic ablation is nearing completion. The results of the cohort studies are shown in this review, but it seems prudent to await the publication of the results of the current trial before commenting on the usefulness of laparoscopic ablation.

Ovulation Suppression

Selection of data: Three randomized clinical trials have compared ovulation suppression with placebo therapy. The trials evaluated the use of danazol, medroxyprogesterone acetate (MPA), and gestrinone. Five additional trials have compared gestrinone and GnRH agonist (GnRHa) ovulation suppression with danazol therapy. One further trial has compared oral contraceptive ovulation suppression with danazol. All of these trials were limited to patients with minimal to mild endometriosis, a group who comprise the majority of endometriosis-associated infertility.[105]

TABLE 10.—Treatment of Endometriosis-Associated Infertility by Means of Ovulation Suppression in Placebo-Controlled Randomized Clinical Trials

Authors	Exper.		Control		Odds Ratio	95% CI
	Preg.	Total	Preg.	Total		
Thomas & Cooke, 1987	5	20	4	17	1.08	0.24–4.78
Bayer et al., 1988	13	37	17	36	0.61	0.24–1.54
Telimaa et al., 1988	6	18	6	14	0.67	0.16–2.79
Telimaa et al., 1988	7	17	6	14	0.94	0.23–3.83
Odds ratio and 95% CI					0.75	0.40–1.38

Note: Chi-square = 0.6, *P* = 0.4398. Breslow-Day test for homogeneity: chi-square = 0.54, 3 df, *P* = 0.9098.
Abbreviation: CI, confidence interval.

TABLE 11.—Ovulation Suppression Treatment for Endometriosis-Associated Infertility in Danazol-Controlled Randomized Clinical Trials

Authors	Exper.		Control		Odds Ratio	95% CI
	Preg.	Total	Preg.	Total		
Fedele et al., 1989a	6	20	7	19	0.74	0.20–2.76
Fedele et al., 1988b	13	30	12	32	1.27	0.46–3.48
Henzl et al., 1988	42	104	16	45	1.22	0.60–2.50
Dmowski et al., 1989	8	18	5	8	0.50	0.10–2.56
Shaw et al., 1992	33	113	13	54	1.29	0.63–2.66
Noble & Letc, 1979	4	10	7	12	0.50	0.10–2.56
Odds ratio and 95% CI					1.07	0.71–1.61

Note: Chi-square = 0.05, P = 0.817. Breslow-Day test for homogeneity: chi-square = 2.18, 5 df, P = 0.70.
Abbreviation: CI, confidence interval.

Description of Data

Level of evidence	RCTs
Publication dates	1979–1992
Number of studies	9[106–114]
Number of patients	620
Outcome evaluated	pregnancy
Treatment effect	odds ratio

The combined data from trials comparing danazol, gestrinone and MPA with placebo show no evidence of a treatment effect (Table 10). The combined data from trials comparing gestrinone, GnRHa and oral contraceptive with danazol as an active control also show no evidence of a treatment effect (Table 11). The aggregate pregnancy rates were 41% during placebo therapy, and 41%, 40%, 36%, 35% and 28% after MPA, oral contraceptives, GnRHa, danazol, and gestrinone treatment, respectively.

Laparoscopic Ablation of Endometriosis

Selection of data: Six cohort studies that were assembled in a recent meta-analysis comprise the data for this section.

Description of Data

Level of evidence	cohort studies
Publication dates	1979–1992
Number of studies	6[115–120]
Number of patients	1,073
Outcome evaluated	pregnancy
Treatment effect	odds ratio

The combined data from cohort studies comparing laparoscopic ablation therapy with ovulation suppression or no therapy show significant evidence of a treatment effect (Table 12). The aggregate number of patients and pregnancy rates were 439 of 677 (65%) in the ablation group vs. 154 of 396 (39%) in the controls. Although a pregnancy rate of 65% for any

TABLE 12.—Laparoscopic Ablation for Endometriosis-Associated Infertility

Authors	Laparoscopy		Control		Odds	95% CI
	Preg.	Total	Obs	Total	Ratio	
Levinson, 1989	44	83	9	21	1.50	0.58–3.88
Paulson et al., 1991	236	315	76	157	3.26	2.17–4.88
Nowroozi et al., 1987	42	69	10	54	5.59	2.73–11.46
Fayez et al., 1988	60	82	20	76	6.44	3.46–12.00
Chong et al., 1990	37	83	23	47	0.84	0.41–1.72
Seiler et al., 1986	20	45	16	41	1.25	0.53–2.92
Odds ratio and 95% CI					2.85	2.20–3.69

Note: Breslow-Day test for homogeneity: chi-square = 30.3, 5 df, $P < 0.001$.
Abbreviation: CI, confidence interval.

infertility treatment is extremely encouraging, numerous methodological problems suggest that clinical practice should not be altered until the results of randomized trials become available.

Surgical Treatment for Endometriosis

Evaluations of surgical treatment for endometriosis consist mainly of retrospective case series or cohort comparisons. Severity of disease is the key determinant of whether patients are given surgical treatment and of the type of surgical treatment given. Tubal obstruction, ovarian endometriomas, extensive adhesions, and cul-de-sac obliteration are indications for surgery. Such patients comprise a minority of those with endometriosis-associated infertility.[121]

Male Infertility

DIAGNOSIS

The role played by the male factor in a couple's infertility was shown in an investigation of a large number of male partners (Table 13). These men took part in a WHO multicenter clinical study that used a standardized investigation scheme.[25] Half of the men had normal semen parameters (no demonstrable cause group), and in one fourth no etiologic factor could be identified, although semen measurements were abnormal (idiopathic abnormal semen group). Varicocele was the most common abnormality found on examination (observed in 18% of the men), but it was only considered an etiologic factor when associated with abnormal semen measurements. This combination occurred in 12% of the men. However, the role of varicocele in male infertility is still unclear.[122] The distribution of diagnoses occurring in a European infertility clinic is shown in Table 14.

Assessment of male fertility is based on history, physical examination including imaging techniques, semen analysis, and other ancillary investigations.

History and Examination

The male partner of an infertile couple should be evaluated by history and physical examination. Recently, WHO published a scheme that sets

TABLE 13.—Distribution of Male Diagnoses (Percent of Men) Among
Infertile Couples (Based on 7,057 Men With Complete Diagnoses
From the WHO Standardized Investigation of the Infertile Couple)

No demonstrable cause*	48.5
Sexual factors	1.7
Infectious factors	6.6
Congenital factors	2.1
Varicocele†	12.3
Other acquired factors	2.6
Endocrine disturbances	0.6
Immunological factors	3.1
Idiopathic abnormal semen‡	26.4
—oligozoospermia	12
—asthenozoospermia	4
—teratozoospermia	7
—other abnormality	3
Total	103.9

* Normal semen quality, normal sexual and ejaculatory function. All other diagnoses require abnormal semen quality.

† Varicocele in the presence of abnormal semen quality. Varicoceles with normal semen are classified as No Demonstrable Cause.

‡ Classification of semen abnormalities based on a hierarchical system that considers semen factors in the sequence: sperm concentration, motility, morphology, viability, and then seminal fluid characteristics.

(Courtesy of Farley TMM, Belsey EM: The prevalence and aetiology of infertility, in *Biological Components of Fertility. The Proceedings of the African Population Conference.* Dakar, Senegal, November 1988. International Union for the Scientific Study of Population, Liege, Belgium, Vol. 1, 1988, pp 2.1.15–2.1.30.)

out the minimum requirements for this examination.[25] Note should be made of any physical and, in particular, any genital abnormality, such as maldescended testes, absent vas deferens, phimosis, or hypospadia. A varicocele should be evaluated by Valsalva maneuver and documented by Doppler and/or ultrasonography. Estimation of testicular volume and consistency give good indications of sperm production, and objective volume measurement such as ultrasound or orchidometry must be used. Ultra-

TABLE 14.—Percentage Distribution of Diagnoses From 7,802
Consecutive Patients Attending an Infertility Clinic

Idiopathic infertility	31.7
Varicocele	16.6
Endocrine hypogonadism	8.9
Infections	9.0
Maldescended testes	8.5
Ejaculatory/erectile dysfunction	5.7
General diseases	5.0
Sperm antibodies	4.2
Testicular tumors*	2.3
Obstruction	1.5
Remainder	6.6

* Including patients attending for cryopreservation of sperm because of malignancies.

(Courtesy of Behre HM, Kliesch S, Meschede D, et al: Hypogonadismus and Infertilitat des Mannes, in Gerok W, Hartmann F, Pfrcundschuh M, et al (eds): *Klinik der Gegenwart.* Urban und Schwarzenberg, Munchen 2:1–73, 1994.)

TABLE 15.—Results of Scrotal Sonography for 650 Patients Consecutively by Attending an Infertility Clinic

	No.	%
Normal	360	55
Varicocele	141	22
Hydrocele	43	7
Epididymal pathology	43	7
Spermatocele	40	6
Testicular pathology		
inhomogeneity	26	4
cyst	7	1
tumor*	4	0.6

* Freshly diagnosed.

(Courtesy of Nashan D, Behre HM, Grunert J-H, et al: Diagnostic value of scrotal sonography in infertile men: Report on 658 cases. *Andrologia* 22:387–395, 1990.)

sonography of the scrotal organs should be performed routinely because patients with infertility show a high rate of abnormalities that may otherwise remain undiscovered (Table 15)[123]; in particular, testicular tumors can be diagnosed at an early stage before they become clinically evident. It should be remembered that some men with infertility, e.g., maldescended testis or gonadal dysgenesis, are at increased risk for testicular malignancy, and appropriate investigations should be undertaken for any man with painful testes, palpable abnormality within the body of the testis, or abnormal semen cytology.

Semen Analysis

Since 1980, WHO has published 3 editions of a "Laboratory Manual for the Examination of Human Semen and Sperm-Cervical Mucus Interaction"[13] that have been translated into several languages. This laboratory manual must be used for semen analysis as it provides the basis for standardization of techniques and quality control. The manual provides normal values (Table 16) as well as nomenclature for normal and pathologic findings (Table 17).

These values help to identify patients who should not experience difficulty in inducing pregnancy. However, unless there is azoospermia, the predictive value of subnormal semen variables is limited. No functional test has been established that can unequivocally predict the fertilizing capacity of sperm. Nor has videocinematographic computer-assisted semen analysis (CASA) proven to be more predictive than classical semen analysis. Quality control, which is not yet routinely applied in most andrology laboratories, should improve the value of semen analysis.[124] Various schemes for internal and external quality control are being explored on a trial basis.[125–127]

Azoospermia

When there is azoospermia, obstruction or ejaculatory dysfunction should be distinguished from damage to spermatogenesis (primary or

---

TABLE 16.—Normal Values of Semen Variables

Standard tests	
Volume	2.0 mL or more
pH	7.2–8.0
Sperm concentration	20×10^6 spermatozoa/mL or more
Total sperm count	40×10^6 spermatozoa per ejaculate or more
Motility	50% or more with forward progression (categories 'a' and 'b') or 25% or more with rapid progression (category 'a') within 60 minutes of ejaculation
Morphology	30% or more with normal forms*
Vitality	75% or more live, i.e., excluding dye
White blood cells	Fewer than 1×10^6/mL
Immunobead test	Fewer than 20% spermatozoa with adherent particles
MAR test	Fewer than 10% spermatozoa with adherent particles
Optional tests	
a-Glucosidase (neutral)	20 mU or more per ejaculate
Zinc (total)	2.4 µmol or more per ejaculate
Citric acid (total)	52 µmol or more per ejaculate
Acid phosphatase (total)	200 U or more per ejaculate
Fructose (total)	13 µmol or more per ejaculate

* Although no clinical studies have been completed, experience in a number of centers suggests that the percentage of normal forms should be adjusted downward when more strict criteria are applied. An empirical reference value is suggested to be 30% or more with normal forms.

(World Health Organization: *WHO Laboratory Manual for the Examination of Human Semen and Sperm-Cervical Mucus Interaction*, ed 3. Cambridge University Press, 1992, pp 44–45.)

---

secondary hypogonadism). This differential diagnosis is often obvious if careful note is made of testicular and epididymal size and consistency, of whether both vasa deferentia are palpable, and if the volume of the ejaculate is reported. Small firm testes (less than 10 mL on each side) with normal ejaculate volume (greater than 2 mL) are indicative of damaged spermatogenesis. Such damage may be confirmed by elevated serum FSH or by testicular biopsy. In general, however, testicular biopsy is not needed if the serum FSH is above the upper limit of normal established in a fertile control group.[128] Very small hard testes, gynecomastia, and small or normal

---

TABLE 17.—Nomenclature for Normal and Pathologic Findings in Semen Analysis

Normozoospermia	Normal ejaculate (as defined in Table 16)
Oligozoospermia	Sperm concentration fewer than 20×10^6/mL
Asthenozoospermia	Fewer than 50% spermatozoa with forward progression (categories 'a' and 'b') or fewer than 25% spermatozoa with category 'a' movement
Teratozoospermia	Fewer than 30% spermatozoa with normal morphology
Oligoasthenotertozoospermia	Signifies disturbance of all three variables (combinations of only two prefixes may also be used)
Azoospermia	No spermatozoa in the ejaculate
Aspermia	No ejaculate

(World Health Organization: *WHO Laboratory Manual for the Examination of Human Semen and Sperm-Cervical Mucus Interaction*, ed 3. Cambridge University Press, 1992, pp 44–45.)

---

ejaculate volume indicate the possibility of Klinefelter's syndrome (XXY), which must be confirmed by chromosome analysis. Severe oligoastheno-teratozoospermia or azoospermia may be caused by deletions in the genes on the long arm of the Y chromosome (e.g., azoospermia factor), and these deletions can be diagnosed by molecular genetics techniques. Normal-sized testes of normal consistency with normal semen volume, normal serum FSH, and low seminal glucosidase levels indicate obstruction, usually in the epididymis, but also congenital bilateral absence of the vas deferens (CBAVD). Because CBAVD is associated with a high incidence of mutations in the cystic fibrosis gene, the patients and their wives should be investigated for such mutations to assess the risk of producing a child with cystic fibrosis before applying direct intracytoplasmic sperm injection (ICSI). Small ejaculate volume and low fructose concentrations in semen with normal testes may be associated with absent or dysfunctioning seminal vesicles. Most men with retrograde ejaculation are not azoospermic, and there is usually a small droplet of antegrade ejaculate rich in sperm.

Accessory Gland Infection

The role of infection in male infertility is controversial.[129] Most clinicians will accept the diagnosis if there are more than 1×10^6 leukocytes in the ejaculate, especially when associated with a heavy growth of a single bacterial strain on semen culture. Unfortunately, it is difficult to distinguish leukocytes from immature germ cells without special stains (e.g., peroxidase stain),[13] and often the ejaculate is contaminated by bacteria. Other indications of the infection are a history of STD or symptoms such as urethral discharge and perineal pain or dysuria. The many and varied criteria in the literature for male accessory gland infection indicate our current lack of understanding of this condition.

Immotility

When all spermatozoa in the ejaculate are immotile, the differential diagnosis is between artefactual immotility and other causes. The first step in further investigation is to ask the man to produce additional samples, preferably near the laboratory. He should avoid use of lubricating jelly or soap when masturbating to produce the sample. Possible causes of true sperm immotility include infections, defects in the axonemata and dynein arms of the sperm tail, antisperm antibodies, excessive superoxide production by seminal leukocytes, and "hostile seminal plasma."[130] Structural defects in the sperm tails may be associated with similar defects in the cilia of the airways, and repeated colds and bronchial infections may be indicative of these defects.[131]

PREVENTION

It is extremely difficult to obtain convincing evidence concerning measures that would prevent male infertility. Because STD is the largest single preventable cause worldwide, it is obvious that major efforts should be applied to its prevention and cure. In the preantibiotics era, both gonococcal and "unspecific" bilateral epididymitis caused infertility in about 4 of 10 cases.[132] Similar figures on postinfection infertility in males are still reported from some developing countries. Although STD agents account for the majority of cases of acute epididymitis, this complication is far less common than salpingitis in the female, is almost always unilateral, and is treatable with good results.[129, 132]

Concerning the impact of uncomplicated STDs on male fertility, published results are conflicting, probably because the "grey-zone" between sterility and normal fertility may be very wide in the male.[73, 129] This makes it difficult to demarcate the precise effects of infection on the different sperm parameters as well as on fertility.

In some countries there are programs to identify teenagers with varicocele, with the hope that early treatment may prevent later infertility. There is considerable controversy about the role of varicocele in male infertilty, and preventive varicocele ligation for the asymptomatic teenager cannot be recommended at the present time. A survey of published data suggested that there might be a "secular trend" toward lower sperm counts and quality during the past 50 years.[133] This report received much publicity. However, a recent reanalysis of the same publications using different statistical procedures concluded that such a decline does not exist; in fact, there may have been a slight increase in sperm counts during the past 20 years.[134] In the same vein, environmental estrogens were claimed as causes of declining male fertility.[135] However, a recent study of the fertility of male offspring of mothers treated in 1951–1952 with the synthethic estrogen diethylstilbestrol in high doses to maintain a threatened pregnancy shows that the fertility of these men is not compromised when compared with the placebo-treated control group.[136] Although environmental factors cannot be excluded as causes of male infertility, no "secular trend" in sperm counts appears to exist. Nevertheless, toxic effects from environmental agents, as known from factory workers exposed to very high doses of such compounds, can cause infertility and should be eliminated wherever possible. No additional practical preventive measures can be recommended to date.[137]

Cryopreservation of semen can be offered to men before chemotherapy or radiotherapy for malignancy if it is likely to damage spermatogenesis or before removal of both testes for medical reasons. This is appropriate for men with testicular tumors, Hodgkin's disease, leukemia, and tumors afflicting men of reproductive age. Even adolescent boys with malignancies can be considered as candidates for cryopreservation.[138] Today it appears reasonable to offer cryostorage irrespective of sperm quantity or quality, because continuing advances such as ICSI may enable such samples to be used to fertilize ova in vitro in the future.

UNTREATED PROGNOSIS

The long-term prognosis for the untreated couple is of great interest to the counseling physician. Included among 2,198 couples reported by Collins et al.[105] were 741 men whose partners had normal tubal patency and ovulatory function and did not have endometriosis. The clinical data and the semen analysis were evaluated with respect to the occurrence of live births independently of treatment. Of the factors analyzed, the most important for good prognoses were: duration of infertility less than 3 years, secondary infertility, female age younger than 30 years, and male income greater than the 75th percentile. Sperm counts below 5×10^6/mL and motility below 20% had relatively marginal effects, and male age was of no importance. The clinical data could predict with 61% accuracy which couples would first achieve pregnancy. In a retrospective analysis, Bostofte et al.[139] identified the following as the best prognostic parameters: the man's age (reflecting his wife's age), the percentage of morphologically normal sperm, and sperm motility. These two studies, as examples of many others, highlight the wide range of parameters and constellations that have been found to predict fertility. In clinical practice, these models should not be considered exclusive; the information obtained from the diagnostic workup should rather form the basis for counseling and guiding the couple. The effect of psychological support to the patient/couple in achieving a pregnancy is largely underestimated, but does in fact exist, as the positive effects of placebo treatments indicate. Finally, the best treatment of a man's infertility remains optimization of the female's reproductive functions.[140]

TREATMENT

If there are no obvious correctable male factors the physician's initial advice will depend on the "trying time" (duration of involuntary infertility) and the age of the female partner.[141] When the female partner is younger than 23 years of age, it is reasonable to wait for at least 2 years before proceeding to such involved and expensive treatments as IVF or ICSI, even if the man's sperm concentration is less than 5×10^6 per mL.

Azoospermia with secondary hypogonadism caused by either hypothalamic failure (idiopathic hypothalamic hypogonadism or Kallmann's syndrome) or pituitary insufficiency may respond to gonadotropin treatment (hMG/hCG) or pulsatile GnRH treatment (in the case of hypothalamic failure). The efficacy of this treatment in achieving sperm quality sufficient to induce a pregnancy is high.[142] However, the number of these patients is small in relation to the general infertility clientele.

When there are infections, the female partner must also be treated. General health advice (e.g., obesity) should be given and any severe systemic diseases (e.g., insulin-dependent diabetes, renal insufficiency) should be treated as well as possible. The effectiveness of treatment of varicocele is controversial. Although surgical ligation and more recently radiologic embolization have been performed for over 50 years, these treatments have never been definitively evaluated with respect to pregnancy rates.[143] Only recently have some properly controlled studies emerged, but these cause further controversy. One study (as part of a WHO multicenter trial) suggests a positive effect of varicocele treatment on pregnancy rates,[144] whereas another strictly controlled study indicates that counseling varicocele patients and their wives may be as effective as occlusion of the spermatic vein for the treatment of varicocele.[145] The important differences between the 2 studies are the different criteria for patient inclusion and the fact that the patients in the Madgar study who were not operated on were left alone for one year, whereas the patients not treated for varicocele in the Nieschlag study were seen, investigated, and counseled every 3 months. A large nonrandomized retrospective study also failed to show benefits from varicocele treatment.[9] There is some evidence that response to treatment may take up to 2 years, and couples should be counseled in the light of all this information.

Obstructive azoospermia may be further investigated with appropriate imaging techniques, and for some cases microsurgical anastomosis is appropriate. When this is not technically possible or when anastomosis fails, consideration may be given to sperm aspiration from the epididymis and ICSI.

Disorders of ejaculation may be treated in various ways, including teaching the couple artificial insemination homologous techniques to use at home, recovery of sperm from urine for artificial insemination, electro-ejaculation, and penile and urethral surgery.

The WHO clinical study, quoted earlier, identified one quarter of the male partners who had idiopathic abnormal semen for whom various empirical treatments had been tried, including testosterone, hMG/hCG, clomiphene, tamoxifen, kallikrein, and, more recently, FSH. None of these treatments has been demonstrated in controlled studies to show benefits.[140, 146–148]

One effect of reduced sperm numbers is to reduce chances of sperm-egg interaction. This may be partly compensated for by inducing multiple ovulations in the female partner. The consensus is that assisted procreation techniques improve the prognosis through aspecific mechanisms (induction of multiple ovulation, selection of sperm, facilitated migration of spermatozoa). Nevertheless, there are still insufficient data available about the relative efficiency of the various strategies.[149–152]

Various methods for increasing the likelihood of fertilization in vitro include partial zona dissection (PZD), subzonal insertion (SUZI), and direct ICSI. Of these, the direct injection of sperm into the cytoplasm of the oocyte seems to be the most promising technique.[153–155] There is no consensus as yet concerning inclusion or exclusion criteria for the various techniques of assisted procreation. It is clear, however, that minimal requirements have to be fulfilled for ICSI. Single sperm, regardless of their shape, can be used successfully for ICSI provided they are vital.[156] In the light of increasing numbers of genetic causes of infertility, genetic counseling of the couples and targeted searches for abnormalities by molecular techniques appear to be advisable.[157] As for IVF and other procedures of medically assisted procreation, a careful analysis of the occurrence of congenital malformations and a prospective follow-up of children born after ICSI is necessary before application of this novel procedure becomes widespread. The high success rate of ICSI in rich countries obviates the need for donor insemination.

At all stages during management of fertility problems, couples should be given realistic information about the costs of treatments and the chances of live birth so they may make appropriate choices.

RESULTS

Just Waiting

A recent comprehensive overview has led to the conclusion that few conventional treatments for male infertility confer any benefit as measured by improved fertility.[148] In this context, conventional therapy did not include donor insemination and various applications of IVF. The authors of the overview found no evidence of efficacy with respect to fertility in studies of bromocriptine or androgens. They also found no published support from strictly randomized trials for the use of antiestrogen therapy or intrauterine insemination (IUI) with prepared semen from the husband. Antiestrogen therapy and IUI are, nevertheless, widely used in an attempt to treat male factor infertility. Therefore, this section will summarize the randomized clinical trials of antiestrogen therapy and the trials of IUI vs. timed intercourse or intracervical insemination that were included in the comprehensive overview.[148]

Antiestrogen Therapy

Selection of data: In a recent overview of treatments for male infertility that included 8 reported trials of antiestrogens in which pregnancy was an outcome measure, only 4 were considered by the authors to have been truly randomized parallel studies.[148]

Description of Data

Level of evidence	RCTs
Publication date	1980–1988
Number of studies	4[146, 147, 158, 159]
Number of patients	282
Outcome evaluated	pregnancy
Treatment effect	pregnancy rate

The aggregate pregnancy rates were 18% in the treated and 15% in the control groups (Table 18). Antiestrogen therapy in the form of clomiphene or tamoxifen appears to have little value as a treatment to improve fertility.

TABLE 18.—Clomiphene vs. Vitamin C or Placebo for Male Infertility

Authors	Clomiphene		Control		Odds	95% CI
	Preg.	Total.	Preg	Total	Ratio	
Abel et al., 1982	15	93	10	86	1.45	0.62–3.37
Ronnberg, 1980	1	14	1	15	1.07	0.06–18.10
Török, 1985	9	27	5	27	2.13	0.64–7.12
Sokol et al., 1988	1	11	4	9	0.17	0.02–1.21
Odds ratio and 95% CI					1.27	0.67–2.41

Note: Breslow-Day test for homogeneity: chi-square = 5.12, 3 df, P = 0.16.
Abbreviation: CI, confidence interval.

Intrauterine Insemination of Husband's Sperm "Prepared"

Selection of data: In a recent overview of treatments for male infertility that included 8 reported trials of IUI in which pregnancy was an outcome measure, only 1 was considered by the authors to have been a truly randomized parallel study.[148] A crossover design was the main shortcoming in the other trials; therefore, all of the studies are included here. For one study, the latest report from the same center has been substituted.[151, 160] Any study reported only in an abstract form was excluded. Another study based on a latin square design was also excluded.[161]

Description of data

Level of evidence	RCTs
Publication date	1987–1990
Number of studies	6[150, 151, 162–165]
Number of cycles	2,051
Outcome evaluated	pregnancy
Treatment effect	pregnancy rate per cycle

The pregnancy rate per cycle was 29 of 1,195 cycles (2.4%) in cycles of insemination and 18 of 856 (2.1%) in control cycles (Table 19). The typical odds ratio suggests a nonsignificant 42% increase in fertility, but the baseline rate in these couples is so low that it calls into question any value from the treatment. Trials included in the Treatment section in unexplained infertility below, however, indicate that there may be value in using ovulation stimulation therapy together with IUI.

In Vitro Fertilization Treatments

Selection of data: In vitro fertilization treatment is applied for a wide range of diagnostic conditions for which previous treatment has failed. In general the diagnosis does not influence the success rate in a material way unless there is a male factor (Table 19).

TABLE 19.—Intrauterine Insemination vs. Control Treatment (Coitus or Intracervical Insemination) for Male Infertility

Authors	IUI		Control		Odds Ratio	95% CI
	Pregnancies observed	Total cycles	Pregnancies observed	Total cycles		
Hughes et al., 1987	0	33	0	32	0.97	0.06–15.84
te Velde et al., 1989	3	109	2	88	1.21	0.20–7.20
Ho et al., 1989	0	114	1	123	0.15	0.00–7.36
Glazener et al., 1987	2	221	3	249	0.75	0.13–4.39
Friedman et al., 1989	0	45	2	43	0.13	0.01–2.05
Kirby et al., 1991	24	373	10	321	2.04	1.02–4.06
Odds ratio and 95% CI					1.42	0.80–2.51

Note: Breslow-Day test for homogeneity: chi-square = 8.73, 5 df, $P = 0.19$.
Abbreviation: CI, confidence interval.

Description of Data

Level of evidence	Registry results
Publication date	1994
Number of studies	1[103]
Number of cycles	29,404
Outcome evaluated	term delivery
Treatment effect	term delivery per cycle

Given that IVF is usually a final treatment after other methods have failed, even when there is male subfertility, IVF may be a successful therapy (see Table 9). Which of the IVF procedures is the most effective? This question has been addressed in RCTs. The European trial of unexplained infertility and two other trials with broader inclusion criteria found no advantage for gamete intrafallopian transfer (GIFT) over IVF.[166–168] In 3 trials of zygote intrafallopian transfer (ZIFT) vs. IVF in patients with unselected diagnoses, the pregnancy rates were lower with ZIFT.[167, 169, 170] The evidence appears to favor IVF among the IVF procedures. The exception may be in cases of severe male factor infertility, in which ICSI is a useful adjunct.

Unexplained Infertility

DIAGNOSIS

Unexplained infertility is a term applied to an infertile couple whose standard investigations (semen analysis, tubal patency, and laboratory assessment of ovulation) yield normal results. It is not established that additional investigations contribute to effective diagnosis. Assuming that the diagnostic test must be reliable for identifying conditions that can be shown during follow-up studies to impair fertility, decisions should be based on the cumulative results of such studies. With respect to luteal-phase defect, delays in histologic maturation of the endometrium do exist, and an endometrial cause of infertility would be plausible. The question is whether delayed endometrial maturation is correlated with fertility; such a correlation would be required to conclude that an abnormal test result from an endometrial biopsy represents an endometrial cause of infertility. At this time, no association has been established between fertility and the luteal-phase defect defined by histological or hormonal evaluation.[8, 171]

With respect to the postcoital test, in a review of the available studies of the correlation between postcoital test results and pregnancy, it was concluded that this test "lacks validity as a test for infertility."[2] A recent prospective study[172] came to the same conclusion. This conclusion does not question whether cervical dysfunction is a possible cause of infertility; it questions whether the postcoital test is an accurate diagnostic test for the detection of cervical dysfunction. Another diagnostic test, the zona free hamster egg penetration test, has only marginal ability to discriminate between fertile and infertile men.[7, 173] Immunologic causes as an isolated factor have not been shown to alter fertility prognosis, and, in particular, unexplained infertility does not appear to be caused by the presence of antisperm antibodies in serum.[6] Follow-up studies are needed to evaluate the relatively infrequent occurrence of very high titers of IgG or IgA on motile sperm and the correlation with the results of the sperm–cervical mucus contact test.

UNTREATED PROGNOSIS

Achievement of pregnancy in apparently normal couples with infertility can be delayed for a variety of reasons. First, some couples are apparently normal, but they have below-average fecundity. Second, an additional group of couples have below-average fecundity because the female partner is older than 30 years of age. In one study of 1,773 couples, 219 (12%) fell into this category.[174] Female age is the major variable contributing to unexplained infertility. Other apparently normal couples are truly subfertile, either because of older age of the female partner or because of the presence of latent, undetectable defects in the prerequisites for successful conception. Latent defects in the female partner could explain differing success rates in donor insemination programs according to the husband's diagnosis.[175] The unexplained group probably includes couples with true sterility, in whom the latent defect is irremediable (e.g., the sperm's inability to fertilize the partner's eggs). It is very difficult to quote data in support of various aspects of the prognosis for patients with unexplained infertility, either treated or untreated, for many reasons. One of these reasons is "publication bias," with which studies having inconclusive findings may remain unpublished. Other reasons include the retrospective nature of many studies, most of which suffer from lack of randomization and other shortcomings of the experimental design. Nevertheless 4 studies have been published in which rates of conception over time were calculated in a group of couples with a normal diagnostic infertility evaluation. The results of these 4 studies show that without treatment, 15% to 60% of the couples studied conceived by 1 year and 40% to 80% conceived by 3 years.[176–179]

The following are factors that affect prognosis that can be mentioned with some confidence: The effect of duration of infertility on the prognosis for pregnancy is powerful and clinically important. With increasing duration of infertility there is a gradual decline in the calculated prognosis for an individual couple (Table 20). After 3 years of infertility, the pregnancy rate without treatment decreases by 2% for every month (24% for every additional year) of infertility. When the duration of infertility has been brief, the prognosis is relatively good. There seems to be no correlation with the age of the male, but for women who have been trying to conceive for more than 3 years, advancing age over 30 decreases the possibility of success. Other factors influencing the prognosis are a history of a previous pregnancy and the frequency of coitus, which is a factor in a few cases.

Pregnancy rates with unexplained infertility are higher in couples with a history of prior conception than in those with primary infertility. The pregnancy rate with secondary infertility, defined as a previous pregnancy in the present relationship, was nearly double the pregnancy rate with primary infertility.[180]

TABLE 20.—Cumulative Pregnancy Rates (%) in the First Year After Registration Among Untreated Couples With Unexplained Infertility

Duration of infertility	No.	Age of the female partner			
		19–25	26–30	31–35	35+
Primary Infertility					
1–2 yrs	109	52.3 (13.9)	41.3 (7.2)	29.8 (8.9)	32.3 (15.4)
2–3 yrs	62	33.2 (12.3)	21.3 (9.5)	12.1 (8.0)	18.2 (16.5)
3–5 yrs	50	28.6 (24.2)	31.8 (10.0)	7.1 (6.9)	0
5+ yrs	36	no cases	28.2 (14.0)	5.3 (5.1)	0
Subtotal	257	41.2 (8.9)	33.7 (4.8)	16.4 (4.3)	17.1 (7.9)
Secondary Infertility					
1–2 yrs	44	60.0 (21.9)	71.4 (12.1)	50.9 (12.7)	50.0 (17.7)
2–3 yrs	13	no cases	60.0 (21.9)	66.7 (27.2)	60.0 (21.9)
3–5 yrs	18	50.0 (35.4)	66.7 (27.2)	0	66.7 (27.2)
5+ yrs	8	no cases	0	33.3 (27.2)	0
Subtotal	83	57.1 (18.7)	65.7 (10.0)	35.9 (8.7)	45.0 (11.1)
Total	340	44.4 (8.2)	39.8 (4.5)	22.0 (4.1)	30.2 (7.0)

Note: Standard error in parentheses.

(Reprinted from Collins JA, Rowe TC: Age of the female partner as a prognostic factor in prolonged unexplained infertility: A prospective study. *Fertil Steril* 52:15–20, 1989. Reprinted with permission of the publisher, the American Society for Reproductive Medicine [formerly the American Fertility Society].)

TREATMENT

Treatment is more effective when the treatment protocol is based on a pathophysiologic rationale and the hypothesis based on that rationale has been proven in randomized clinical trials. With unexplained infertility, however, no biological defect is known; thus, only empirical strategies are applicable. In addition, there have been relatively few well-designed studies of effectiveness.

Published data exist to suggest that danazol therapy and bromocriptine therapy have no effect on the fertility of couples with unexplained infertility.[181] Also, although psychological factors have been considered to play a part in unexplained infertility, there is no evidence that such factors are causative, and there are no controlled trials showing that psychological or educational counseling is effective. The empirical use of clomiphene has been evaluated in 4 comparative trials,[171, 182–184] but only 1 of these evaluated clomiphene alone without co-intervention.[171] The combined results suggest that ovarian stimulation with clomiphene can double the spontaneous pregnancy rate. The treatment effect was not significant among couples with a duration of infertility less than 3 years.[171] Induction of superovulation with hMG yields more follicles than with clomiphene, but additional controlled studies are needed[185, 186] to determine whether fecundity is higher with hMG than with clomiphene. If results are not achieved with ovarian stimulation alone, ovarian stimulation in conjunction with insemination procedures may be indicated. Intrauterine insemination and intraperitoneal insemination (IPI) appear to significantly improve the results (0.1–0.2 monthly fecundability rate).[166, 187] If inseminations with prepared spermatozoa do not yield pregnancy in 6 months (the average reported duration of treatment is 2–3 months), then IVF or one of its variants, done by an established center can be used with good results. A word of caution was expressed by the group about the possible complications of ovarian stimulation. Great care must be taken to minimize hyperstimulation resulting in higher-order multiple gestations.

RESULTS

Clomiphene

Selection of data: Four randomized clinical trials, which featured differences in dosage and co-interventions (IUI, ovulatory hCG, or luteal hCG).

Description of Data

Level of evidence	randomized clinical trials
Publication dates	1985–1990
Number of studies	4[171, 182-184]
Number of patients	363
Outcome evaluated	pregnancy
Treatment effect	odds ratio

The aggregate of the pregnancy rates in these trials was 2.8% (21 of 747) in placebo cycles and 6.8% (50 of 738) in clomiphene cycles (Table 21). The typical odds ratio for pregnancy rate per cycle was 2.1 (95% CI, 1.3–3.6). The Breslow-Day test for heterogeneity was 2.34 ($P = 0.51$), revealing no statistically significant heterogeneity, but there were clearly important clinical differences in the study populations.

Despite these clinical differences, a consistent clomiphene effect was observed. Odds ratios in these studies were not associated with dose. In one randomized trial, the greatest relative increase in conception rates occurred when clomiphene was given to women who had been infertile for more than 3 years.[171] There is no evidence to support use of this treatment beyond 6 cycles.

IUI With or Without Ovarian Stimulation

Selection of data: Thirteen randomized clinical trials addressed the use of IUI with or without hMG or clomiphene as augmentation therapy.[151, 161, 162, 164, 166, 184, 188-194] The data from these studies were assembled to estimate the independent effects of hMG, clomiphene, and IUI therapy among such patients.

TABLE 21.—Clomiphene Treatment for Unexplained Infertility: Odds Ratios for Pregnancy Rates

Authors	Odds ratio (95% CI)	Number of patients
Deaton et al., 1990	3.0 (0.8–12.6)	67
Fisch et al., 1989	2.4 (0.7–9.2)	148
Glazener et al., 1990	1.7 (0.8–3.4)	118
Harrison et al., 1985	7.1 (0.5–999)	30
Odds ratio	2.1 (1.3–3.6)	363

Abbreviation: CI, confidence interval.

TABLE 22.—Aggregate Pregnancy Rates in Trials of Intrauterine Insemination With and Without Ovarian Stimulation

Ovulation stimulation	Intrauterine insemination			Timed intercourse			Odds ratio (95% CI)
	Cycles	Pregnancies		Cycles	Pregnancies		
		No.	(%)		No.	(%)	
No stimulation	1,102	61	(5)	963	25	(3)	2.09 (1.35–3.22)
Clomiphene	249	27	(11)	54	5	(9)	1.18 (0.45–3.07)
Gonadotropin	625	90	(14)	331	21	(6)	2.19 (1.45–3.32)

Abbreviation: CI, confidence interval.

This heterogeneous grouping of trials was necessary because the majority lacked untreated control groups. The use of active control treatments, which have not themselves been shown to be effective, is a shortcoming in many infertility trials. The common element in this analysis was IUI treatment. In all trials, either IUI treatment was compared with timed intercourse or IUI treatment was the active control treatment. The use of clomiphene and hMG varied among the trials.

A logistic regression analysis on pregnancy (yes, no) as the dependent variable included indicator variables for IUI, report, and diagnosis (tubal defect, endometriosis, ovulation defect, and seminal defect as defined by WHO standards), with unexplained infertility as the reference category. Further indicator variables were included for ovulation stimulation [none (reference group), clomiphene, gonadotropin]. An interaction variable for hMG and IUI treatment together was also included in the analysis. The logistic regression analysis was adjusted in this way for study center, diagnosis group, type of ovulation stimulation, and whether IUI treatment was used. With this analysis, it was possible to estimate the independent effects of each therapeutic modality while adjusting for diagnostic group. The nature of the published information did not allow adjustment for the duration of infertility or age of the female partner.

The unadjusted aggregate results are shown in Table 22. The pregnancy rate per cycle was 3% in cycles of observation with timed intercourse, 6% in hMG cycles, and 14% in cycles of hMG and IUI. From the logistic regression analysis, the effects of IUI and hMG treatment are similar: each treatment significantly increases the likelihood of conception by approximately two times (Table 23).

The clomiphene treatment effect also was significant although slightly lower (adjusted odds ratio, 1.7; 95% CI, 1.1–2.7). The interaction term for hMG and IUI was not significant. The presence of a seminal defect significantly reduced the likelihood of conception by nearly one half. A diagnosis of endometriosis tended to reduce the likelihood of conception, but this diagnosis was not significant and did not enter the final model.

TABLE 23.—Likelihood of Conception With Intrauterine Insemination or Ovulation Stimulation Based on a Meta-Analysis of 13 Trials

	Adjusted likelihood of pregnancy (95% CI)
Intrauterine insemination	2.10 (1.52, 2.91)
Clomiphene	1.72 (1.10, 2.70)
Gonadotropin	2.01 (1.45, 2.79)
Seminal defect	0.55 (0.40, 0.77)

Note: Logistic regression analysis that included indicator variables for study, diagnosis group, stimulation, and insemination type. The point estimates represent the independent effect of the given treatment or diagnostic factor. With multiple treatments (e.g., gonadotropins and intrauterine insemination) the point estimates can be multiplied (e.g., 2.10 × 2.01). The baseline pregnancy rate is the untreated rate in Table 22 (25 of 963) (3% per cycle).

Abbreviation: CI, confidence interval.

Assisted Procreation

PATIENTS

Patients requiring assisted reproductive technology (ART) to alleviate involuntary childlessness have been infertile for variable periods, usually at least 1–2 years. The time when ART has to be started depends on the age of the female patient; before 30 years of age, the waiting period can be longer than it is after 35 years of age because the declining fecundity of women with increasing age may influence the outcome of all forms of ART.[195] In many couples treated by ART, other forms of treatment have been tried before, such as controlled ovarian stimulation and timed intercourse or artificial insemination with washed and selected husband spermatozoa.

Couples requiring ART treatment may be infertile for different reasons. Some of them have only female factors, some of them show only male factors, and in quite a number of infertile couples, there may be a factor causing infertility or subfertility in both partners. Couples requiring ART include female patients with tubal infertility resulting from the presence of extensive adhesions after pelvic inflammatory disease, tubes removed after ectopic pregnancy, failed microsurgery for adhesions, or reversal of tubal ligation. In vitro fertilization was initially developed to circumvent severe tubal infertility. Other female causes of infertility or unexplained infertility may require ART if other types of treatment have been unsuccessful.

Most causes of male infertility are of unknown idiopathic origin. They are diagnosed by alterations of the semen parameters assessed in carefully conducted repeated semen analyses. Conventional semen parameters include volume, concentration of spermatozoa, motility characteristics, and morphology assessment after fixation and coloration. There is a wide range of semen abnormalities in the different semen parameters, ranging from limited deviation from the reference values established to achieve natural conception to complete absence of spermatozoa in the ejaculate. The strategy of treatment will of course depend on the severity of the semen impairment.

Azoospermia may be caused by obstruction in the excretory ducts or by reduced or absent spermogenesis or spermatogenesis. Until recently, azoospermic patients could only be helped by artificial insemination with donor sperm. Now, many of these couples can be helped by IVF in combination with ICSI.[196]

TREATMENTS

The standard procedure of ART consists of IVF after controlled ovarian stimulation of the ovaries by one of several different protocols. Currently, the most commonly used regimen is a combination of GnRH analogues and hMG and hCG.[197] Cumulus-oocyte complexes are retrieved by vaginal ultrasound-guided needles. The cumulus-oocyte complexes are inseminated a few hours later with progressively motile spermatozoa at a concentration of 100,000 to 200,000 spermatozoa/mL. Oocytes and spermatozoa are kept in bicarbonate-buffered culture medium at 37°C in an atmosphere of 5% CO_2, 5% O_2 and 90% N_2, or in 5% CO_2 in air. After 16–18 hours of in vitro incubation, normal fertilization is assessed by looking for 2 distinct or fragmented polar bodies. After in vitro culture, further embryo cleavage of the normally fertilized oocytes is assessed on the second day after insemination of the cumulus-oocyte complexes.[198] The number of blastomeres and the presence of anucleate fragments are assessed under the inverted microscope at 200× or 400× magnification. There are different morphological scoring systems for the cleaved embryos, such as excellent-quality embryos without anucleate fragments, good-quality embryos with 1% to 20% of the volume filled with anucleate fragments, fair-quality embryos with 21% to 50% of the volume filled with anucleate fragments, and poor-quality embryos with more than 50% fragmentation.[198] A uterine embryo transfer is usually carried out on the second day after insemination and for most patients (under age 40 years) it may be recommended to limit the number of transferred embryos to 2 or 3 embryos to avoid the occurrence of multiple pregnancies.[198] Especially for patients younger than 37 years with a large cohort of morphologically excellent- and good-quality embryos, the number of replaced embryos must be limited to 2. For patients 40 years and older and patients with repeated failures of implantation after embryo transfer, one may consider placing 4 and even more embryos. Extra 2-pronuclear oocytes or cleaved embryos may be cryopreserved for eventual later use. The most widely used cryopreservation protocol uses 1,2-propanediol as cryoprotectant, but other cryoprotectants may also be used, such as dimethylsulfoxide for cleavage-stage embryos and glycerol for blastocysts.

Two related ART procedures can also be used instead of conventional IVF and uterine embryo replacement. These are GIFT and ZIFT or pronucleate stage oocyte transfer (PROST). Both procedures can only be applied when the female patient has at least one healthy fallopian tube. Tubal replacement therapy of early cleavage-stage embryos can also be performed. In most circumstances, the tubal replacement of oocytes and spermatozoa, of 2-pronuclear oocytes or cleaved embryos is carried out by direct access to the oviducts via the uterine cervix. Both ZIFT and PROST have as a drawback that 2 successive invasive operations are required: oocyte retrieval and tubal placement.

Standard IVF treatment is certainly also useful for couples with male infertility, but it is less successful and there may be very limited or no fertilization after insemination with spermatozoa from a semen sample with impaired semen parameters.[199] Furthermore, a certain number of couples are not accepted for IVF when there are no spermatozoa in the ejaculate or when, after sperm treatment, the number of morphologically normal and progressively motile spermatozoa is below a certain threshold number, such as 500,000. Several procedures for assisting the fertilization process have been developed in experimental models and are also applied clinically. These include zona drilling (ZD) with acid-Tyrode's, partial zona dissection (PZD),[200] and subzonal insemination (SUZI).[201] In ZD and PZD, a hole is made in the zona pellucida by chemical or mechanical means and the oocytes are then inseminated with motile spermatozoa, as in standard IVF. In SUZI, a few spermatozoa (3–20) are introduced by micromanipulation into the perivitelline space between the zona pellucida and the plasma membrane of the oocyte. Very moderate successes have been obtained with these procedures in terms of normal fertilization, which never exceeded 20% to 25% of the microinjected oocytes, further embryo cleavage, implantation of transferred embryos, pregnancy, and delivery. Quite a number of couples could not be helped by PZD or SUZI. In 1992, the first delivery after the transfer of an embryo obtained after microinjection of a single spermatozoon into the cytoplasm of fertilizable metaphase-II oocytes occurred. It soon became clear that ICSI[153–155, 196] was much more efficient than PZD or SUZI; the number of normally fertilized oocytes was significantly higher after ICSI and more embryos were available for transfer or freezing. High implantation rates were achieved and by now ICSI is the sole currently used procedure of assisted fertilization.

Outcome

The results of ART are summarized regularly in national and international surveys.[202, 203] The results of ICSI with ejaculated, epididymal and testicular spermatozoa in terms of fertilization, embryo cleavage, and implantation rate after transfer are similar to the results of standard IVF treatment in infertile couples with nonandrologic infertility. Table 24 summarizes the results of four years of ICSI (1991–1994) as collected by the ESHRE Task Force on ICSI.

Patient counseling is an essential part of all forms of ART. If ICSI has to be applied to alleviate the couple's infertility, the patients should be informed about the recency of the ICSI procedure and about its many unknown aspects. It might be recommended to ask the couples to have prenatal karyotypes and to participate in a prospective follow-up study of children born after ICSI. Although the results of about 500 prenatal karyotypes and the prospective follow-up of 750 children do not indicate any increase in abnormal fetal karyotypes or major congenital malformations, it is important to continue this careful follow-up of the children in different centers practicing ICSI.

TABLE 24.—Survey (1991–1994) of European Society of Human Reproduction (ESHRE) Task Force on Intracytoplasmic Sperm Injection (ICSI)

	Ejaculated	Epididymal	Testicular
Number of cycles	13,178	539	193
Oocytes injected	111,291	5,744	2,057
% intact after ICSI	90.3	91.9	89.6
% of intact oocytes with 2PN	58.5	50.4	50.9
% transferred or frozen embryos	69.2	61.4	71.9
% embryo transfers	91.1	93.3	87.6
% positive hCG/cycle	28.7	34.9	33.2

Abbreviations: 2PN, 2-pronuclear; *hCG*, human chorionic gonadotropin.

Risks for Pregnancies Induced by ART

Specific risks for the pregnancies originated by ART are linked to the elevated maternal age and to the frequently occurring multiple gestations. In fact, the quality of the conception decreases with maternal age, which is the cause of the double abortion rate observed in women after 40 years of age.[204] Similarly, the higher frequency of chromosomal abnormalities in pregnancies in women after the fourth decade is well known.[205]

Paternal age also plays a role in causing autosomal dominant mutations expressed as macroscopic malformations, such as achondroplasia, Apert syndrome, and retinoblastomas.[206] Apart from the quality of the conceptus, increased maternal age is more likely to be associated with such obstetric complications as toxemia, gestational diabetes, and hypertension.[207] The risk of having a fetus with low birth weight is also double in mothers around 40 years of age. The impaired fetal growth is presumably caused by the placental hypoperfusion by the myometrial arteries. Between the third and fourth decades, these vessels show a consistent increase in sclerotic processes.[208] Because of the above events, the perinatal mortality rises from 9.5 in women aged 30–34 years to 17 per 1,000 births in women older than 40 years of age.[209] Maternal mortality also increases. In a recent study from France, maternal mortality in women aged 40–44 years was 6 times that of women aged 25–29 years.[210] Interestingly, there is a threefold increase of cesarean sections in ART-originated pregnancies.

Ovum donation rules out the problem related to "old" oocytes, but it does not protect against the increased incidence of pregnancy complications.[211] The perinatal death rate in twin pregnancy is elevated, being 3–11 times higher than in single pregnancies,[212] and twin pregnancy is a frequent outcome of ART-induced pregnancy. Multiple gestation also increases maternal complications during pregnancy, such as preeclampsia, hydramnios varicosities, and anemia.[212] The above data clearly indicate the potential risks associated with the use of ART. Nevertheless, this increase in risk appears to be manageable in the context of modern obstetric care.[209]

Counseling and the Emotional Impact of Infertility

Infertility generates a variety of emotional responses in individual men and women and couples. At one extreme, a minority take their childlessness in stride, and at the other extreme are those who are profoundly affected by the infertile state. The majority of patients have levels of distress that will vary in intensity depending on their socioeconomic background, stage of investigation or treatment, duration of infertility, age, religious affiliations, and whether they are female or male.[213] The infertility represents a threat to attainment of one of life's goals and may greatly tax the couple's strategies for coping with stress.[214, 215] Feelings of helplessness and desperation are common.[214] Sexual function may be significantly affected, and great stress can be placed on the relationship. In other cases, the experience of infertility strengthens the ties between partners.[213] Infertile couples also speak of their isolation and helplessness and the lack of control.[213, 216, 217]

THE ROLE OF INFERTILITY CLINICIANS

Couples respond in different ways to continuing childlessness, to the procedures used in the investigation and treatment of infertility, and to the apparent failure of management when childlessness persists.[218] Physicians and other clinical staff can help couples to understand the sources of anxiety and stress that arise from the infertile state.

Infertility treatment choices are more difficult than other clinical decisions, because frequently the level of evidence is scarce, and there may be high costs and unwanted adverse effects. Also, each couple has distinctive family and cultural values and characteristic approaches to risk taking that will help to shape their final choices about treatment. Furthermore, the difficulty is often compounded by the lack of a specific defect and the need to fall back on empiric therapy. Thus, although treatment planning usually dominates clinical consultations, infertility treatment will be more in tune with the wishes of the couple if the discussion proceeds further to address additional questions. Would any further diagnostic tests be useful? What is the baseline prognosis without treatment? For each treatment choice, what is the rationale and what are the expected benefits, unwanted side effects, costs, and time involved? Last, but far from least important, what is the couple's timetable?

This comprehensive approach is aimed to help each couple develop a therapy plan that will take into account the lives they are leading at present and provide them over the long term with the feeling that they have explored all options that they would consider to be reasonable. The process is time-consuming, but that is typical of clinical decisions in long-standing disorders, in which psychosocial and economic factors strongly influence the choices that will be made by individuals. In the case of infertility, the importance of families and children also modifies the approach that will be taken in each case. Although few physicians have formal training in counseling, the requirements needed for helping infertile couples are consistent with generally accepted clinical skills. The essential task is to take the time needed. Couples with prolonged infertility frequently change physicians during the course of management, in the hope that any new approach might increase their chances of conception. Changing physicians may also reflect dissatisfaction with the time taken by the physician and other members of the clinical team to deal with the personal issues.

Extra time is needed, especially during the first visit, at the time of diagnosis, when treatment choices are made, and after treatment failures. At the first visit, both partners should be seen together. If necessary, individual appointments can be arranged later. Before the clinical data-gathering begins, it is usually helpful to inform the couple that they will be in control of the eventual management decisions. It is also useful to ask a simple question such as "What would you like us to do for you?" to establish the needs of each individual couple. The investigative strategy must be discussed with the couple, and decisions whether to proceed with a given test or treatment option must be left to them. In this way, control is maintained by the couple. As the investigation proceeds, ample time must be available to answer the inevitable questions that arise and to permit patients to express their hurt and confusion. In many clinics, these services are provided by the nursing staff.

THE ROLE OF OTHER PROFESSIONALS

It can easily be predicted that psychosocial disturbances may occur that are not amenable to ordinary clinical management. Couples often feel despair when they hear an honest prognosis. Many couples are despondent after the completion of therapy, especially short-term intensive therapy such as IVF, without success. Thus, couples who are under observation in infertility clinics with or without treatment have a real need for continuing support and counseling.

Many clinics provide the services of counselors trained in the behavioral sciences. In some clinics, attendance for counseling is mandatory; in others, counseling is mandatory only for certain procedures such as IVF or donor insemination. In a few centers, counseling is offered only to patients for whom a need is perceived by the physician or the patients. Professional counseling is provided in different ways, but infertile couples need access to knowledgeable counseling. Competent counseling may come from backgrounds in social work, psychology, nursing, or from interested psychiatrists. For infertile couples, counseling has more value if the professional involved has a knowledge of the clinical and biological bases, of infertility.

A main task for such counselors is to help couples face the uncertainty about whether they will have continuing childlessness. Counseling is also of key importance when infertile women experience pregnancy loss, with its resulting depression. Provision of accurate information, empathetic support, and vesting control in the couple are essential to such counseling.

Although only 10% to 15% of infertile couples discontinue therapy without success, counseling can be an important adjunct to resolving infertility.[105] Providing support and helping couples to believe that they have indeed made their very best effort may be the foundations of ultimate resolution. Such couples must be helped to believe not that they have "given up" (a very negative statement in our society), but rather that they have done their utmost and that they may now give themselves permission to let go.

References

1. Hargreave TB, Elton RA: Fecundability rates from an infertile male population. *Br J Urol* 58:194–197, 1986.
2. Griffith CS, Grimes DA: The validity of the postcoital test. *Am J Obstet Gynecol* 162:616–620, 1990.
3. Hughes EG, Fedorkow DM, Collins JA: A quantitative overview of controlled trials in endometriosis-associated infertility. *Fertil Steril* 59:963–970, 1993.
4. Eggert-Kruse W, Leinhos G, Gerhard I, et al: Prognostic value of in vitro sperm penetration into hormonally standardized human cervical mucus. *Fertil Steril* 51:317–323, 1989.

5. Taylor PJ, Lewinthal D, Leader A, et al: A comparison of Dextran 70 with carbon dioxide as the distention medium for hysteroscopy in patients with infertility or requesting reversal of a prior tubal sterilization. *Fertil Steril* 47:861–863, 1987.
6. Kremer J, Jager S: The significance of antisperm antibodies for sperm-cervical mucus interaction. *Hum Reprod* 7:781–784, 1992.
7. Gwatkin RBL, Collins JA, Jarrell JF, et al: The value of semen analysis and sperm function assays in predicting pregnancy among infertile couples. *Fertil Steril* 53:693–699, 1990.
8. Wentz AC, Kossoy LR, Parker RA: The impact of luteal phase inadequacy in an infertile population. *Am J Obstet Gynecol* 162:937–945, 1990.
9. Baker HWG, Burger HG, de Kretser DM, et al: Testicular vein ligation and fertility in men with varicoceles. *BMJ* 291:1678–1680, 1985.
10. Dunphy BC, Scudamore I, Cooke ID: Falloposcopy, a technological gimmick or a clinical tool? *J Soc Obstet Gynecol Can* 15:25–32, 1993.
11. Landgren BM, Undén A-L, Diczfalusy E: Hormonal profiles of the cycle in 68 normally menstruating women. *Acta Endocrinol* 94:89–98, 1980.
12. Crosignani PG, Collins J, Cooke ID, et al: Unexplained infertility. *Hum Reprod* 8:977–980, 1993.
13. World Health Organization: WHO laboratory manual for the examination of human semen and sperm-cervical mucus interaction, ed 3. Cambridge, England, Cambridge University Press, 1992, pp 44–45.
14. Wilcox LS, Mosher WD: Use of infertility services in the United States. *Obstet Gynecol* 82:122–127, 1993.
15. Collins JA, Burrows EA, Willan AR: The prognosis for live birth among untreated infertile couples. *Fertil Steril* 64:22–28, 1995.
16. Eimers JM, te Velde ER, Gerritse R, et al: The prediction of the chance to conceive in subfertile couples. *Fertil Steril* 61:44–52, 1994.
17. Chalmers TC, Celano P, Sacks H, et al: Bias in treatment assignment in controlled clinical trials. *N Engl J Med* 309:1358–1361, 1983.
18. U.S. Preventive Services Task Force: Appendix A Task Force ratings, in Fisher M, Eckart C (eds): *Guide to Clinical Preventive Services: An Assessment of the Effectiveness of 169 Interventions.* Baltimore, Williams & Wilkins, 1989, p 387–396.
19. Cook DJ, Guyatt GH, Laupacis A, et al: Rules of evidence and clinical recommendations on the use of antithrombotic agents. *Chest* 102: 3058–3115, 1992.
20. Pasquali R, Antenucci D, Casimirri F, et al: Clinical and hormonal characteristics of obese amenorrheic hyperandrogenic women before and after weight loss. *J Clin Endocrinol Metab* 68:173–179, 1989.
21. Frisch RE: Fatness, menarche and female fertility. *Perspect Biol Med* 28:611–633, 1985.
22. Lenton EA, Sulaiman R, Sobowale O, et al: The human menstrual cycle: Plasma concentrations of prolactin, LH, FSH, oestradiol and progesterone in conceiving and non-conceiving women. *J Reprod Fertil* 65:131–139, 1982.
23. Blackwell RE: Hyperprolactinemia: Evaluation and management, in Moghissi KS (ed): *Endocrinol Metab Clin North Am* 21(1):105–124, 1992.
24. Keye WR Jr, Chang RJ, Wilson CB, et al: Prolactin-secreting pituitary adenomas in women. III. Frequency and diagnosis in amenorrhea-galactorrhea. *JAMA* 244:1329–1333, 1980.
25. Rowe PJ, Comhaire FH, Hargreave TB, et al: WHO Manual for the Standardized Investigation of the Infertile Couple. Cambridge, England, Cambridge University Press, 1993.
26. Steinkampf MP: Ultrasonography in infertility management, in Behrman SJ, Patton GW Jr, Holz G (eds): *Progress in Infertility.* Boston, Little Brown, 1994, pp 339–369.
27. Baird DT: Amenorrhoea, anovulation and dysfunctional uterine bleeding, in De-Groot LJ (ed): *Endocrinology.* New York, WB Saunders, 1995, pp 2059–2079.
28. Layman LC, Reindollar RH: The genetics of hypogonadism, in Layman LC (ed): *Infertil Reprod Med Clin North Am* 1:53–68, 1994.

29. Moult PJA, Rees H, Besser GM: Pulsatile gonadotrophin secretion in hyperprolactinemic amenorrhoea and the response to bromocriptine therapy. *Clin Endocrinol (Oxf)* 16:153–162, 1982.
30. Filicori M, Flamigni C, Cognigni G, et al: Increased insulin secretion in patients with multifollicular and polycystic ovaries and its impact on ovulation induction. *Fertil Steril* 62:279–285, 1994.
31. Crosignani PG, Ferrari C, Liuzzi A, et al: Treatment of hyperprolactinemic states with different drugs: A study with bromocriptine, metergoline, and lisuride. *Fertil Steril* 37:61–66, 1982.
32. Vermesh M, Fossum GT, Kletzy OA: Vaginal bromocriptine: Pharmacology and effect on serum prolactin in normal women. *Obstet Gynecol* 72:693–698, 1988.
33. Ferrari C, Crosignani PG: Review. Medical treatment of hyperprolactinaemic disorders. *Hum Reprod* 1:507–514, 1986.
34. Webster J, Piscitelli G, Polli A, et al: A comparison of cabergoline and bromocriptine in the treatment of hyperprolactinemic amenorrhea. *N Engl J Med* 331:904–909, 1994.
35. Diamant YZ, Yarkoni S, Evron S: Combined clomiphene-bromocriptine treatment in anovulatory, oligomenorrheic and hyperprolactinemic women resistant to separate clomiphene or bromocriptine regimens. *Infertility* 3:11–16, 1980.
36. Weil C: The safety of bromocriptine in hyperprolactinemic female infertility: A literature review. *Curr Med Res Opin* 10:172–195, 1986.
37. Filicori M, Flamigni C, Meriggiola MC, et al: Ovulation induction with pulsatile gonadotropin-releasing hormone: Technical modalities and clinical perspectives. *Fertil Steril* 56:1–13, 1991.
38. Salat-Baroux J, Antoine JM: Accidental hyperstimulation during ovulation induction. *Baillieres Clin Obstet Gynaecol* 4:627–638, 1990.
39. Couzinet B, Lestrat N, Brailly S, et al: Stimulation of ovarian follicular maturation with pure follicle-stimulating hormone in women with gonadotropin deficiency. *J Clin Endocrinol Metab* 66:552–556, 1988.
40. Rebar RW, Connolly HV: Clinical features of young women with hypergonadotropic amenorrhea. *Fertil Steril* 53:804–810, 1990.
41. Jones SG, de Morales-Ruehsen M: A new syndrome of amenorrhoea in association with hypergonadism and apparently normal ovarian follicular apparatus. *Am J Obstet Gynecol* 104:597–600, 1969.
42. Adams J, Franks S, Polson DW, et al: Multifollicular ovaries: Clinical and endocrine features and response to pulsatile gonadotropin-releasing hormone. *Lancet* 2:1375–1379, 1985.
43. Hammond MG, Halme JK, Talbert LM: Factors affecting the pregnancy rate in clomiphene citrate induction of ovulation. *Obstet Gynecol* 62:196–202, 1983.
44. Borenstein R, Shoham Z, Yemini M, et al: Tamoxifen treatment in women with failure of clomiphene citrate therapy. *Aust N Z J Obstet Gynaecol* 29:173–175, 1989.
45. Daly DC, Walters CA, Soto-Albors CE, et al: A randomized study of dexamethasone in ovulation induction with clomiphene citrate. *Fertil Steril* 41:844–848, 1984.
46. Yong EL, Glasier A, Hillier H, et al: Effect of cyclofenil on hormonal dynamics, follicular development and cervical mucus in normal and oligomenorrheic women. *Hum Reprod* 7:39–43, 1992.
47. Gysler M, March CM, Mishell DR Jr, et al: A decade's experience with an individualization clomiphene treatment regimen including its effect on the postcoital test. *Fertil Steril* 37:161–167, 1982.
48. Bateman BG, Nunley WC Jr, Kolp LA: Exogenous estrogen therapy for treatment of clomiphene-induced cervical mucus abnormalities: Is it effective? *Fertil Steril* 54:577–579, 1990.
49. Hamilton-Farley D, Kiddy D, Watson H, et al: Low-dose gonadotrophin therapy for induction of ovulation in 100 women with polycystic ovary syndrome. *Hum Reprod* 6:1095–1099, 1991.

50. Jones D: Report of the meeting on infertility. Edinburgh. *Br J Obstet Gynaecol* 102:73–76, 1994.
51. Fauser BC, Donderwinkel P, Schoot DC: The step-down principle in gonadotrophin treatment and the role of GnRH analogues. *Baillieres Clin Obstet Gynaecol* 7:309–330, 1993.
52. Armar NA, Lachelin GC: Laparoscopic ovarian diathermy: An effective treatment for anti oestrogen resistant anovulatory infertility in women with PCOS. *Br J Obstet Gynaecol* 100:161–164, 1993.
53. Donesky BW, Adashi EY: Surgically induced ovulation in the polycystic ovary syndrome: Wedge resection revisited in the age of laparoscopy. *Fertil Steril* 63:439–463, 1995.
54. Dabirashrafi H, Mohamad K, Behjatnia Y, et al: Adhesion formation after ovarian electrocoagulation on patients with PCO syndrome. *Fertil Steril* 55:1200–1201, 1991.
55. Tang LCH, Sung ML, Ma HK: Hyperprolactinaemic amenorrhoea in Hong Kong. *Aust N Z J Obstet Gynaecol* 23:165–169, 1983.
56. Al-Suleiman SA, Najashi S, Rahman J, et al: Outcome of treatment with bromocriptine in patients with hyperprolactinaemia. *Aust N Z J Obstet Gynaecol* 29:176–179, 1989.
57. Connaughton JF, Garcia CR, Wallach EE: Induction of ovulation with cisclomiphene and a placebo. *Obstet Gynecol* 43:697–701, 1974.
58. Cudmore DW, Tupper WRC: Induction of ovulation with clomiphene citrate. *Fertil Steril* 17:363–373, 1996.
59. Garcia CR, Freeman EW, Rickels K, et al: Behavioral and emotional factors and treatment responses in a study of anovulatory infertile women. *Fertil Steril* 44:478–483, 1985.
60. Johnson JE, Cohen MR, Goldferb AF, et al: The efficacy of clomiphene citrate for induction of ovulation. *Int J Fertil* 11:265–270, 1996.
61. Caspi E, Levin S, Bukovsky I, et al: Induction of pregnancy with human gonadotropins after clomiphene failure in menstruating ovulatory infertility patients. *Isr J Med Sci* 10:249–255, 1974.
62. Ellis JD, Williamson JG: Factors influencing the pregnancy and complication rates with human gonadotrophin therapy. *Br J Obstet Gynaecol* 82:52–57, 1975.
63. Lunenfeld B, Serr DM, Mashiach S, et al: Therapy with gonadotrophins: Where are we today? Analysis of 2890 menotropin treatment cycles in 914 patients, in Insler V, Bettendorf G (eds): *Advances in Diagnosis and Treatment of Infertility.* New York, Elsevier North Holland, 1981, p 27–31.
64. Fluker MR, Urman B, Mackinnon M, et al: Exogenous gonadotrophin therapy in World Health Organization Groups I and II ovulatory disorders. *Obstet Gynecol* 83:189–196, 1994.
65. Martin KA, Hall JE, Adams JM, et al: Comparison of exogenous gonadotropons and pulsatile gonadotropin-releasing hormone for induction of ovulation in hypogonadotropic amenorrhea. *J Clin Endocrinol Metab* 77:125–129, 1993.
66. Navot D, Bergh PA, Laufer N: Ovarian hyperstimulation syndrome in novel reproductive technologies: Prevention and treatment. *Fertil Steril* 58:249–261, 1992.
67. Whittemore AS, Harris R, Itnyre J, and the Collaborative Ovarian Cancer Group: Characteristics relating to ovarian cancer risk: Collaborative analysis of 12 US case-control studies. II. Invasive epithelial ovarian cancers in white women. *Am J Epidemiol* 136:1184–1203, 1992.
68. Rossing MA, Daling JR, Weiss NS, et al: Ovarian tumors in a cohort of infertile women. *N Engl J Med* 331:771–776, 1994.
69. Stamm WE, Holmes KK: *Chlamydia trachomatis* infection of the adult, in Holmes KK, Mårdh P-A, Sparling PF, et al (eds): *Sexually Transmitted Diseases,* ed 2, New York, McGraw Hill, 1990, pp 181–194.
70. Mårdh P-A: An overview of infectious agents in acute salpingitis, their biology, and recent advances in methods of detection. *Am J Obstet Gynecol* 138:933–951, 1980.

71. Weström L, Wolner-Hanssen P: Pathogenesis of pelvic inflammatory disease (review). *Genitourin Med* 69:9–17, 1993.
72. Holtz F: Klinische Studien uber die nicht tuberkulose Salpingooophoritis. *Acta Obstet Gynaecol Scand* 10 (Suppl 1), 1930.
73. Weström L: Sexually transmitted diseases and infertility. *Sex Transm Dis* 21:S32–S37, 1994.
74. Weström L: Effect of pelvic inflammatory disease on fertility. *Am J Obstet Gynecol* 121:707–713, 1975.
75. Weström L, Berger GS: Consequences of pelvic inflammatory disease, in Berger GS, Weström L (eds): *Pelvic Inflammatory Disease*. New York, Raven Press, 1992, pp 101–114.
76. Svensson L, Mårdh P-A, Weström L: Infertility after acute salpingitis with special reference to *Chlamydia trachomatis*. *Fertil Steril* 40:322–329, 1983.
77. Johansson E, Forslin L, Moi H, et al: Gonorrhoea, chlamydia, and urethritis in partners to women with acute salpingitis [in Swedish]. *Lakartidningen* 85:2974–2976, 1988.
78. Weström L: Effect of pelvic inflammatory disease on fertility. *Venereology* 4:150–153, 1995.
79. Hills SD, Joesoef R, Marchbanks PA, et al: Delayed care for pelvic inflammatory disease as a risk factor for impaired fertility. *Am J Obstet Gynecol* 168:1503–1509, 1993.
80. Wolner-Hanssen P: Oral contraceptive use modifies the manifestations of pelvic inflammatory disease. *Br J Obstet Gynaecol* 93:619–624, 1986.
81. Wolner-Hanssen P, Kiviat NK, Holmes KK: Atypical pelvic inflammatory disease: Subacute, chronic or subclinical upper genital tract infection in women, in Holmes KK, Mårdh P-A, Sparling PF, et al (eds): *Sexually Transmitted Diseases*, ed 2, New York, McGraw Hill, 1990, pp 615–620.
82. Osser S, Persson K, Liedholm P: Tubal infertility and silent salpingitis. *Hum Reprod* 4:280–284, 1989.
83. DeCherney AH: Infertility: General principles of evaluation, in Kase NG, Weingold AB, Lucas WE, et al (eds): *Principles and Practice of Clinical Gynecology*, New York, J Wiley & Sons, 1983, pp 425–436.
84. Swart P, Mol BWJ, van der Veen F, et al: The accuracy of hysterosalpingography in the diagnosis of tubal pathology: A meta-analysis. *Fertil Steril* 64:486–491, 1995.
85. Adelusi B, Al-Nuaim L, Makanjuola D, et al: Accuracy of hysterosalpingography and laparoscopic hydrotubation in diagnosis of tubal patency. *Fertil Steril* 63:1016–1020, 1995.
86. DeCherney AH, Kort H, Barney JB, et al: Increased pregnancy rate with oil-soluble hysterosalpingography dye. *Fertil Steril* 33:407–410, 1980.
87. The American Fertility Society: The American Fertility Society classification of adnexal adhesions, distal tubal occlusion, tubal occlusion secondary to tubal ligation, tubal pregnancies, Mullerian anomalies and intrauterine adhesions. *Fertil Steril* 49:944–955, 1988.
88. Winston RML, Margara RA: Microsurgical salpingostomy is not an obsolete procedure. *Br J Obstet Gynaecol* 98:637–642, 1991.
89. Boer-Meisel ME, te Velde ER, Habbema JDF, et al: Predicting the pregnancy outcome in patients treated for hydrosalpinx: A prospective study. *Fertil Steril* 45:23–29, 1986.
90. De Bruyne F, Puttemans P, Boeckx W, et al: The clinical value of salpingoscopy in tubal infertility. *Fertil Steril* 51:339–340, 1989.
91. Novy M, Thurmond A, Patton P, et al: Diagnosis of cornual obstruction. *Hum Reprod* 10:1156–1159, 1988.
92. Kerin J, Daykhovsky L, Segalowitz J, et al: Falloposcopy: A microendoscopic technique for visual exploration of the human fallopian tube from the uterotubal ostium to the fimbria using a transvaginal approach. *Fertil Steril* 54:390–400, 1990.

93. Dlugi AM, Reddy S, Saleh WA, et al: Pregnancy rates after operative endoscopic treatment of total (neosalpingostomy) or near total (salpingostomy) distal tubal occlusion. *Fertil Steril* 62:913–920, 1994.

94. Reiss H: Management of tubal infertility in the 1990s. *Br J Obstet Gynaecol* 98:619–623, 1991.

95. Lavy G, Diamond MP, DeCherney AH: Ectopic pregnancy: Its relationship to tubal reconstructive surgery. *Fertil Steril* 47:543–556, 1987.

96. Canis M, Mage G, Pouly JL, et al: Laparoscopic distal tuboplasty: Report of 87 cases and a 4-year experience. *Fertil Steril* 56:616–621, 1991.

97. Motta ELA, Nelson J, Batzofin J, et al: Selective salpingography with an insemination catheter in the treatment of women with cornual Fallopian tube obstruction. *Hum Reprod* 10:1156–1159, 1995.

98. Marana R, Quagliarello J: Distal tubal occlusion: Microsurgery versus in vitro fertilization—A review. *Int J Fertil* 33:107–115, 1988.

99. Holst N, Maltau JM, Forsdahl F, et al: Handling of tubal infertility after introduction of in vitro fertilization: Changes and consequences. *Fertil Steril* 55:140–143, 1991.

100. Haan G: Effects and costs of in-vitro fertilization. *Int J Technol Assess Health Care* 7:585–593, 1991.

101. Thurmond AS: Pregnancies after selective salpingography and tubal recanalization. *Radiology* 190:11–13, 1994.

102. Gleicher N, Confino E, Corfman RS, et al: The multicentre transcervical balloon tuboplasty study: Conclusions and comparison to alternative technologies. *Hum Reprod* 8:1264–1271, 1993.

103. Society for Assisted Reproductive Technology, The American Fertility Society: Assisted reproductive technology in the United States and Canada: 1992 results generated from The American Fertility Society/Society for Assisted Reproductive Technology Registry. *Fertil Steril* 62:1121–1128, 1994.

104. International Working Group for Registers on Assisted Reproduction: World Collaborative Report 1993. Montepellier, International Federation of Fertility Societies, 1995, pp 1–43.

105. Collins JA, Burrows EA, Willan AR: Occupation and the follow-up of infertile couples. *Fertil Steril* 60:477–485, 1993.

106. Thomas EJ, Cooke ID: Successful treatment of asymptomatic endometriosis: Does it benefit infertile women? *BMJ* 294:1117–1119, 1987.

107. Bayer SR, Seibel MM, Saffan DS, et al: Efficacy of danazol treatment for minimal endometriosis in fertile women: A prospective randomized study. *J Reprod Med* 33:179–183, 1988.

108. Telimaa S: Danazol and medroxyprogesterone acetate inefficacious in the treatment of infertility in endometriosis. *Fertil Steril* 50:872–875, 1988.

109. Fedele L, Bianchi S, Viezzoli T, et al: Gestrinone versus danazol in the treatment of endometriosis. *Fertil Steril* 51:781–785, 1989.

110. Fedele L, Bianchi S, Arcaini L, et al: Buserelin versus danazol in the treatment of endometriosis-associated infertility. *Am J Obstet Gynecol* 161:871–876, 1989.

111. Henzl MR, Corson SL, Moghissi K, et al: Administration of nasal nafarelin as compared with oral danazol for endometriosis: A multicenter double-blind comparative clinical trial. *N Engl J Med* 318:485–489, 1988.

112. Dmowski WP, Radwanska E, Binor Z, et al: Ovarian suppression induced with buserelin or danazol in the management of endometriosis: A randomized, comparative study. *Fertil Steril* 51:395–400, 1989.

113. Shaw RW, and the Zoladex Endometriosis Study Team: An open randomized comparative study of the effect of goserelin depot and danazol in the treatment of endometriosis. *Fertil Steril* 58:265–272, 1992.

114. Noble A, Letchworth A: Medical treatment of endometriosis: A comparative trial. *Postgrad Med J* 55:37–39, 1979.

115. Levinson CJ: Endometriosis therapy: Rationale for expectant or minimal therapy in minimal/mild cases (AFSI). Proceedings of the Second World Congress of Gynecologic Endoscopy (Abstract), 1989.

116. Paulson JD, Asmar P, Saffan DS: Mild and moderate endometriosis. Comparison of treatment modalities for infertile couples. *J Reprod Med* 36:151–155, 1991.
117. Nowroozi K, Chase JS, Check JH, et al: The importance of laparoscopic coagulation of mild endometriosis in infertile women. *Int J Fertil* 32:442–444, 1987.
118. Fayez J, Collazo LM, Vernon C: Comparison of different modalities of treatment for minimal and mild endometriosis. *Am J Obstet Gynecol* 159:927–932, 1988.
119. Chong AP, Keene ME, Thornton NL: Comparison of three modes of treatment for infertility patients with minimal pelvic endometriosis. *Fertil Steril* 53:407–410, 1990.
120. Seiler JC, Gidwani G, Ballard L: Laparoscopic cauterization of endometriosis for fertility: A controlled study. *Fertil Steril* 46:1098–1100, 1986.
121. Adamson GD, Pasta DJ: Surgical treatment of endometriosis-associated infertility: Meta-analysis compared with survival analysis. *Am J Obstet Gynecol* 171:1488–1505, 1994.
122. Hargreave TB: Varicocele: A clinical enigma. Review article. *Br J Urol* 72:401–408, 1993.
123. Nashan D, Behre HM, Grunert J-H, et al: Diagnostic value of scrotal sonography in infertile men: Report on 658 cases. *Andrologia* 22:387–395, 1990.
124. Barratt CLR: On the accuracy and clinical value of semen laboratory tests. *Hum Reprod* 10:250–252, 1995.
125. Neuwinger J, Behre HM, Nieschlag E: External quality control in the andrology laboratory: An experimental multicenter trial. *Fertil Steril* 54:308–314, 1990.
126. Cooper TG, Neuwinger J, Bahrs S, et al: Internal quality control of semen analysis. *Fertil Steril* 58:172–178, 1992.
127. Clements S, Cooke ID, Barratt CLR: Implementing comprehensive quality control in the andrology laboratory. *Hum Reprod* 10:2096–2106, 1995.
128. Bergmann M, Behre HM, Nieschlag E: Serum FSH and testicular morphology in male infertility. *Clin Endocrinol* 40:133–136, 1994.
129. Purvis K, Christiansen E: Infection in the male reproductive tract. Impact, diagnosis and treatment in relation to male infertility (review). *Int J Androl* 16:1–14, 1993.
130. Gagnon C: *Controls of Sperm Motility: Biological and Clinical Aspects.* Boca Raton, Fla, CRC Press, 1990.
131. Neugebauer D-Ch, Neuwinger J, Jockenhövel F, et al: "9+0" axoneme in spermatozoa and some nasal cilia of a patient with totally immotile spermatozoa associated with thickened sheath and short midpiece. *Hum Reprod* 5:981–986, 1990.
132. Berger RE: Acute epididymitis, in Holmes KK, Mårdh P-A, Sparling PF, et al (eds): *Sexually Transmitted Diseases*, ed 2, New York, McGraw Hill, 1990, pp 641–652.
133. Carlsen E, Giwercman A, Keiding N, et al: Evidence for decreasing quality of semen during past 50 years. *BMJ* 305:609–613, 1992.
134. Olsen GW, Bodner KM, Ramlow JM, et al: Have sperm counts been reduced 50 percent in 50 years? A statistical model revisited. *Fertil Steril* 63:887–893, 1995.
135. Sharpe RM, Skakkebaek NE: Are oestrogens involved in falling sperm counts and disorders of the male reproductive tract? *Lancet* 341:1392–1395, 1993.
136. Wilcox AJ, Baird DD, Weinberg CR, et al: Fertility in men exposed prenatally to diethylstilbestrol. *N Engl J Med* 332:1411–1416, 1995.
137. Bonde JP, Giwercman A: Occupational hazards to male fecundity. *Reprod Med Rev* 4:59–73, 1995.
138. Kliesch S, Behre HM, Jürgens H, et al: Cryopreservation of semen from adolescent patients with malignancies. *Med Pediatr Oncol* 26:20–27, 1995.
139. Bostofte E, Bagger P, Michael A, et al: Fertility prognosis for infertile men: Results of follow-up study of semen in infertile men from two different populations evaluated by the Cox regression model. *Fertil Steril* 54:1100–1106, 1990.
140. Nieschlag E: Current therapy: Care for the infertile male (review). *Clin Endocrinol* 38:123–133, 1993.
141. The ESHRE Capri Workshop Group: Male sterility and subfertility: Guidelines for management. *Hum Reprod* 9:1260–1264, 1994.

142. Kliesch S, Behre HM, Nieschlag E: High efficacy of gonadotropin or pulsatile GnRH treatment in hypogonadotropic hypogonadal men. *Eur J Endocrinol* 131:347–354, 1994.

143. Schlesinger MH, Wilets IF, Nagler HM: Treatment outcome after varicocelectomy: A critical analysis. *Urol Clin North Am* 21:517–529, 1994.

144. Madgar I, Weissenberg R, Lunenfeld B, et al: Controlled trial of high spermatic vein ligation for varicocele in infertile men. *Fertil Steril* 63:120–124, 1995.

145. Nieschlag E, Hertle L, Fischedick AR, et al: Treatment of varicocele: Counselling as effective as occlusion of the vena spermatica. *Hum Reprod* 10:347–353, 1995.

146. Sokol RZ, Steiner BS, Bustillo M, et al: A controlled comparison of the efficacy of clomiphene citrate in male infertility. *Fertil Steril* 49:865–870, 1988.

147. Abel B, Carswell G, Elton RA, et al: Randomized trial of clomiphene citrate treatment and vitamin C for male infertility. *Br J Urol* 54:780–784, 1982.

148. O'Donovan PA, Vandekerckhove P, Lilford RJ, et al: Treatment of male infertility: Is it effective? Review and meta-analyses of published randomized controlled trials. *Hum Reprod* 8:1209–1222, 1993.

149. Friedman A, Haas S, Kredentser J, et al: A controlled trial of intrauterine insemination for cervical factor and male factor: A preliminary report. *Int J Fertil* 34:199–203, 1989.

150. Hughes EG, Collins JP, Garner PR: Homologous artificial insemination for oligoasthenospermia: A randomized controlled study comparing intracervical and intrauterine techniques. *Fertil Steril* 48:278–281, 1987.

151. Kirby CA, Flaherty SP, Godfrey BM, et al: A prospective trial of intrauterine insemination of motile spermatozoa versus timed intercourse. *Fertil Steril* 56:102–107, 1991.

152. Crosignani PG, Walters DE: Clinical pregnancy and male subfertility: The ESHRE Multicentre Trial on the treatment of male subfertility. *Hum Reprod* 9:1112–1118, 1994.

153. Van Steirteghem A, Liu J, Joris H, et al: Higher success rate by intracytoplasmic sperm injection than by subzonal insemination. Report of a second series of 300 consecutive treatment cycles. *Hum Reprod* 8:1055–1060, 1993.

154. Van Steirteghem A, Nagy Z, Joris H, et al: High fertilization and implantation rates after intracytoplasmic sperm injection. *Hum Reprod* 8:1061–1066, 1993.

155. Van Steirteghem A, Liu J, Nagy Z, et al: Use of assisted fertilization. *Hum Reprod* 8:1784–1785, 1993.

156. Nagy ZP, Liu J, Joris H, et al: The result of intracytoplasmic sperm injection is not related to any of the three basic sperm parameters. *Hum Reprod* 10:1123–1129, 1995.

157. Meschede D, De Geyter Ch, Nieschlag E, et al: Genetic risk in micromanipulative assisted reproduction. *Hum Reprod* 10:2880–2886, 1995.

158. Ronnberg L: The effect of clomiphene citrate on different sperm parameters and serum hormone levels in preselected infertile men: A controlled double-blind crossover study. *Int J Androl* 3:479–486, 1980.

159. Török L: Treatment of oligozoospermia with tamoxifen (open and controlled studies). *Andrologia* 17:497–501, 1985.

160. Kerin JF, Kirby C, Peek J, et al: Improved conception rate after intrauterine insemination of washed spermatozoa from men with poor quality semen. *Lancet* 1:533–535, 1984.

161. Martinez AR, Bernardus RE, Voorhorst FJ, et al: Intrauterine insemination does and clomiphene citrate does not improve fecundity in couples with infertility due to male or idiopathic factors: A prospective, randomized, controlled study. *Fertil Steril* 53:847–853, 1990.

162. Ho PC, Poon IML, Chan SYW, et al: Intrauterine insemination is not useful in oligoasthenospermia. *Fertil Steril* 51:682–684, 1989.

163. Glazener CMA, Coulson C, Lambert PA, et al: The value of artificial insemination with husband's semen in infertility due to failure of postcoital sperm-mucus penetration—Controlled trial of treatment. *Br J Obstet Gynaecol* 94:774–778, 1987.

164. te Velde ER, van Kooy RJ, Waterreus JJH: Intrauterine insemination of washed husband's spermatozoa: A controlled study. *Fertil Steril* 51:182–185, 1989.
165. Friedman AJ, Juneau-Norcross M, Sedensky B, et al: Life table analysis of intrauterine insemination pregnancy rates for couples with cervical factor, male factor, and idiopathic infertility. *Fertil Steril* 55:1005–1007, 1991.
166. Crosignani PG, Walters DE, Soliani A: The ESHRE multicentre trial on the treatment of unexplained infertility: A preliminary report. *Hum Reprod* 6:953–958, 1991.
167. Tanbo T, Dale PO, Abyholm T: Assisted fertilization in infertile women with patent Fallopian tubes. A comparison of in-vitro fertilization, gamete intra-Fallopian transfer and tubal embryo stage transfer. *Hum Reprod* 5:266–270, 1990.
168. Leeton J, Rogers P, Caro C, et al: A controlled study between the use of gamete intrafallopian transfer (GIFT) and in vitro fertilization and embryo transfer in the management of idiopathic and male infertility. *Fertil Steril* 48:605–607, 1987.
169. Fluker MR, Zouves CG, Bebbington MW: A prospective randomized comparison of zygote intrafallopian transfer and in vitro fertilization embryo transfer for nontubal factor infertility. *Fertil Steril* 60:515–519, 1993.
170. Tournaye H, Devroey P, Camus M, et al: Zygote intrafallopian transfer or in vitro fertilization and embryo transfer for the treatment of male-factor infertility: A prospective randomized trial. *Fertil Steril* 58:344–350, 1992.
171. Glazener CMA, Coulson C, Lambert PA, et al: Clomiphene treatment for women with unexplained infertility: Placebo-controlled study of hormonal responses and conception rates. *Gynecol Endocrinol* 4:75–83, 1990.
172. Glatstein IZ, Best CL, Palumbo A, et al: The reproducibility of the postcoital test: A prospective study. *Obstet Gynecol* 85:396–400, 1995.
173. Mao C, Grimes DA: The sperm penetration assay: Can it discriminate between fertile and infertile men? *Am J Obstet Gynecol* 159:279–286, 1988.
174. Hargreave T: In the management of male infertility, in Hargreave T, Teoh Eng Soon PG (eds): Publishing Singapore, Hong Kong, New Dehli, Auckland, Boston, pp 7–18.
175. Edvinsson A, Forssman L, Milsom I, et al: Factors in the infertile couple influencing the success of artificial insemination with donor semen. *Fertil Steril* 53:81–87, 1990.
176. Barnea ER, Holford TR, McInnes DRA: Long-term prognosis of infertile couples with normal basic investigations: A life-table analysis. *Obstet Gynecol* 66:24–26, 1985.
177. Hull MGR: Review. Infertility treatment: Relative effectiveness of conventional and assisted conception methods. *Hum Reprod* 7:785–796, 1992.
178. Rousseau S, Lord J, Lepage Y, et al: The expectancy of pregnancy for "normal" infertile couples. *Fertil Steril* 40:768–772, 1983.
179. Templeton AA, Penney GC: The incidence, characteristics, and prognosis of patients whose infertility is unexplained. *Fertil Steril* 37:175–182, 1982.
180. Collins JA, Rowe TC: Age of the female partner as a prognostic factor in prolonged unexplained infertility: A prospective study. *Fertil Steril* 52:15–20, 1989.
181. Collins JA, Crosignani PG: Unexplained infertility: A review of diagnosis, prognosis, treatment efficacy and management. *Int J Gynaecol Obstet* 39:267–275, 1992.
182. Harrison RF, O'Moore RR: The use of clomiphene citrate with and without human chorionic gonadotropin. *Ir Med J* 76:273–274, 1983.
183. Fisch P, Casper RF, Brown SE, et al: Unexplained infertility: Evaluation of treatment with clomiphene citrate and human chorionic gonadotropin. *Fertil Steril* 51:828–833, 1989.
184. Deaton JL, Gibson M, Blackmer KM, et al: A randomized, controlled trial of clomiphene citrate and intrauterine insemination in couples with unexplained infertility or surgically corrected endometriosis. *Fertil Steril* 54:1083–1088, 1990.
185. Welner S, Decherney AH, Polan ML: Human menopausal gonadotropins: A justifiable therapy in ovulatory women with long-standing idiopathic infertility. *Am J Obstet Gynecol* 158:111–117, 1988.

186. Simon A, Avidan B, Mordel N, et al: The value of menotrophin treatment for unexplained infertility prior to an in-vitro fertilization attempt. *Hum Reprod* 6:222–226, 1991.

187. Hull MGR, Fahy U, Abiuzeid MI, et al: Expectations of assisted conception for infertility. *BMJ* 304:1465–1469, 1992.

188. Arici A, Byrd W, Bradshaw K, et al: Evaluation of clomiphene citrate and human chorionic gonadotropin treatment: A prospective, randomized, crossover study during intrauterine insemination cycles. *Fertil Steril* 61:314–318, 1994.

189. Evans JH, Wells C, Gregory L, et al: A comparison of intrauterine insemination, intraperitoneal insemination, and natural intercourse in superovulated women. *Fertil Steril* 56:1183–1187, 1991.

190. Ho PC, So WK, Chan YF, et al: Intrauterine insemination after ovarian stimulation as a treatment for subfertility because of subnormal semen: A prospective randomized controlled trial. *Fertil Steril* 58:995–999, 1992.

191. Karlstrom PO, Bergh T, Lundkvist O: A prospective randomized trial of artificial insemination versus intercourse in cycles stimulated with human menopausal gonadotropin or clomiphene citrate. *Fertil Steril* 59:554–559, 1993.

192. Martinez AR, Bernardus RE, Voorhorst FJ, et al: Pregnancy rates after timed intercourse or intrauterine insemination after human menopausal gonadotropin stimulation of normal ovulatory cycles: A controlled study. *Fertil Steril* 55:258–265, 1991.

193. Nulsen JC, Walsh S, Dumez S, et al: A randomized and longitudinal study of human menopausal gonadotropin with intrauterine insemination in the treatment of infertility. *Obstet Gynecol* 82:780–786, 1993.

194. Zikopoulos K, West CP, Thong PW, et al: Homologous intra-uterine insemination has no advantage over timed natural intercourse when used in combination with ovulation induction for the treatment of unexplained infertility. *Hum Reprod* 8:563–567, 1993.

195. Scott RT, Opsahl MS, Leonardi MR, et al: Life table analysis of pregnancy rates in a general infertility population relative to ovarian reserve and patient age. *Hum Reprod* 10:1706–1710, 1995.

196. Van Steirteghem A, Tournaye H, Van der Elst J, et al: Intracytoplasmic sperm injection three years after the birth of the first ICSI child. *Hum Reprod* 10:2517–2528, 1995.

197. Daya S, Gunby J, Hughes E, et al: Follicle-stimulating hormone versus human menopausal gonadotropin for in vitro fertilization cycles: A meta-analysis. *Fertil Steril* 64:347–354, 1995.

198. Staessen C, Van den Abbeel E, Janssenswillen C, et al: Controlled comparison of Earle's balanced salt solution with Ménézo B2 medium for human in-vitro fertilization performance. *Hum Reprod* 9:1915–1919, 1994.

199. Tournaye H, Devroey P, Camus M, et al: Comparison of in-vitro fertilization in male and tubal infertility: A 3 year survey. *Hum Reprod* 7:218–222, 1992.

200. Malter HE, Cohen J: Partial zona dissection of the human oocyte: A nontraumatic method using micromanipulation to assist zona pellucida penetration. *Fertil Steril* 57:139–148, 1989.

201. Ng SG, Bongso A, Ratnam SS: Microinjection of human oocytes: A technique for severe oligoasthenoteratozoospermia. *Fertil Steril* 56:1117–1123, 1991.

202. Anonymous: French in vitro fertilization registry. 1994 report. *Contracept Fertil Sex* 23:490–493, 1995.

203. Society for Assisted Reproductive Technology, American Society for Reproductive Medicine: Assisted reproductive technology in the United States and Canada: 1993 results generated from the American Society for Reproductive Medicine/Society for Assisted Reproductive Technology Registry. *Fertil Steril* 64:13–21, 1995.

204. Warburton D, Kline J, Stein Z: Cytogenetic abnormalities in spontaneous abortions of recognized conceptions, in Willey HA (ed): *Perinatal Genetics: Diagnosis and Treatment*. New York, Academic Press, 1990, pp 133–141.

205. Lansac J: Debate. Delayed parenting. Is delayed childbearing a good thing? *Hum Reprod* 10:1033–1036, 1995.

206. Auroux M: Evolution de la fertilité masculine en function de l'âge et risque pour la progéniture. *Contracept Fertil Sex* 19:945–949, 1991.
207. Berkowitz GS, Skovron ML, Lapinski RH, et al: Delayed childbearing and the outcome of pregnancy. *N Engl J Med* 322:659–664, 1990.
208. Aldous M, Edmonson M: Maternal age at first child birth and risk of low birth weight and preterm delivery in Washington state. *JAMA* 270:2574–2577, 1993.
209. Bowman MC, Saunders DM: Rates of aneuploid in oocytes of older women: Are equivocal findings of concern for postmenopausal embryo recipients? *Hum Reprod* 9:1200–1201, 1994.
210. Bouvier-Colle MH, Varnoux N, Costes P: Mortalité maternelle en France. *J Gynecol Obstet Biol Reprod* 20:885–891, 1991.
211. Sauer MV, Paulson RJ, Lobo RA: Pregnancy after age 50: Application of oocyte donation to women after natural menopause (see comments). *Lancet* 341:344–345, 1993.
212. Garcia PM, Gall AA: Multiple pregnancy, in Scoot JR, DiSaia PJ, Hammond CB, et al: (eds): *Danforth's Obstetrics and Gynecology*, ed 6. Philadelphia, J.B. Lippincott Company, 1990, pp 381–401.
213. Daniluk JC: Infertility: Intrapersonal and interpersonal impact. *Fertil Steril* 49:982–990, 1988.
214. Frank DI: Counseling the infertile couple. *J Psych Nurs* 22(5):17–23, 1984.
215. Seibel M, Taymor M: Emotional aspects of infertility. *Fertil Steril* 37:137–146, 1982.
216. Lalos A, Lalos O, Jacobsson L, et al: A psychosocial characterization of infertile couples before surgical treatment of the female. *J Psychosom Obstet Gynaecol* 4:83–87, 1985.
217. Link PW, Darling CA: Couples undergoing treatment for infertility: Dimensions of life satisfaction. *J Sex Marital Ther* 12:46–59, 1986.
218. Mahlstedt PP: The psychological component of infertility. *Fertil Steril* 43:335–346, 1985.

1 Reproductive Endocrinology

Ultrasonographical and Hormonal Description of the Normal Ovulatory Menstrual Cycle
Bakos O, Lundkvist Ö, Wide L, Bergh T (Uppsala Univ, Sweden)
Acta Obstet Gynecol Scand 73:790–796, 1994   1–1

Introduction.—Most ultrasonographic studies of the normal menstrual cycle in healthy women have used abdominal techniques. The availability of transvaginal techniques and other technical improvements allow more detailed examination of the internal genital organs. Transvaginal ultrasonography was used to study the morphological changes in the ovaries and uterus during normal menstrual cycles. The findings were than correlated with the endocrine events occurring in the same cycles.

Methods.—The subjects were 23 healthy women with normal menstrual cycles and a normal body mass index. None of the women were using any type of contraception or hormonal therapy. The investigators performed transvaginal ultrasonography using dynamically focused, phased-array ultrasound equipment. The initial examination was performed on days 5–7 of the menstrual cycle. Each woman underwent 8–10 scans covering the follicular, periovulatory, and luteal phases. Hormonal investigations were also performed throughout the menstrual cycle. Day 0 was defined as the day of the midcycle luteinizing hormone (LH) surge.

Findings.—Serum estradiol (E_2) concentrations peaked at day 0, with 5–6 days between the first observable E_2 rise and the E_2 peak. Serum progesterone levels began to increase on day 0 and peaked at day +6. The follicular diameter changed significantly throughout the follicular phase; the mean diameter of the dominant follicle on day 0 was 21.5 mm (Fig 1). During the follicular phase, the diameter of the dominant follicle and the serum E_2 concentration correlated well. There was wide variation in follicular diameter on the day of the LH peak.

No persistent pattern was noted in ovarian volume during the luteal phase, and the diameters of the corpora lutea did not correlate with serum progesterone values. The endometrium appeared as a thin echogenic line during the menstrual period. Endometrial thickness increased steadily from day -7 to -6, with the texture changing from 1 to 3 echogenic lines

1

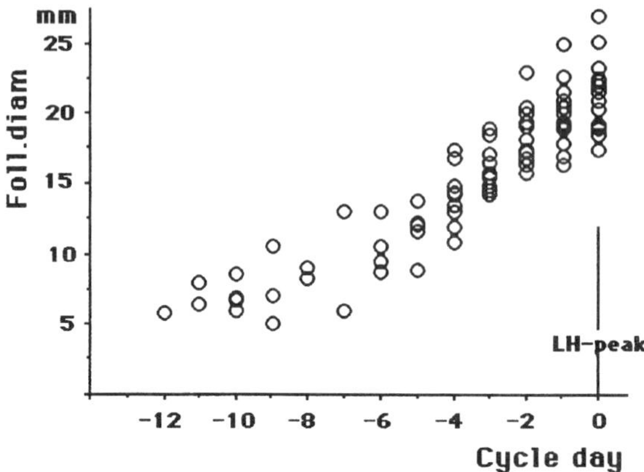

FIGURE 1.—The growth of the dominant follicle during the follicular phase of a spontaneous ovulatory cycle in 16 healthy women. (Courtesy of Bakos O, Lundkvist Ö, Wide L, et al: Ultrasonographical and hormonal description of the normal ovulatory menstrual cycle. *Acta Obstet Gynecol Scand* 73:790–796, Copyright 1994, Munksgaard International Publishers Ltd., Copenhagen, Denmark.)

(Fig 3). The endometrial volume was 1.6 mL in the early follicular phase, 4.8 mL in the late follicular phase, 6.5 mL in the early luteal phase, and 5.9 mL in the late luteal phase. Uterine volume increased from 55 mL in the early follicular phase to 150 mL in the late luteal phase. Good correlation was noted between serum E_2 levels and endometrial thickness. Sonographically measurable fluid was seen in the pouch of Douglas in half of the observations made in the days after ovulation.

Conclusion.—The information presented will be useful in understanding the physiologic changes that occur in the menstrual cycle and in monitoring therapy to induce ovulation.

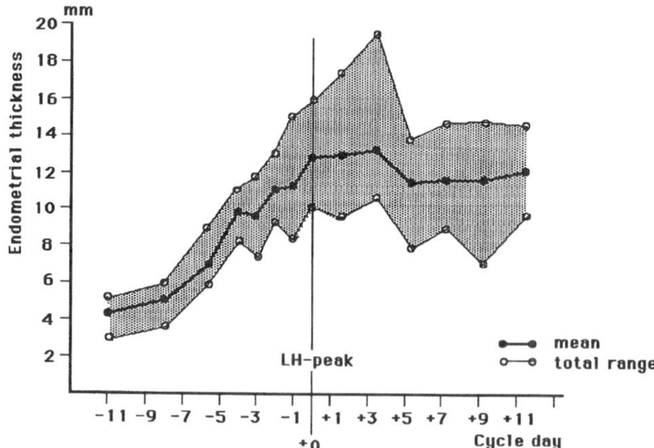

FIGURE 3.—The endometrial thickness in millimeters measured by transvaginal ultrasound, presented as the mean and the total range, in 16 women during an ovulatory cycle. Each point on the curve represents a minimum of 6 observations. (Courtesy of Bakos O, Lundkvist Ö, Wide L, et al: Ultrasonographical and hormonal description of the normal ovulatory menstrual cycle. *Acta Obstet Gynecol Scand* 73:790–796, Copyright 1994, Munksgaard International Publishers Ltd., Copenhagen, Denmark.)

▶ This unique study correlates endocrinologic changes in the normal menstrual cycle with morphological changes as measured by transvaginal ultrasonography. The data obtained are of use when monitoring the effect of exogenous gonadotropins in women undergoing ovarian stimulation for assisted reproductive techniques. The data may also be useful in determining the cause of infertility of some couples with so-called unexplained infertility. If these morphological changes do not correlate with their endocrinologic changes, infertility may occur as a result.

D.R. Mishell, Jr., M.D.

Timing of Sexual Intercourse in Relation to Ovulation: Effects on the Probability of Conception, Survival of the Pregnancy, and Sex of the Baby

Wilcox AJ, Weinberg CR, Baird DD (Natl Inst of Environmental Health Sciences, Research Triangle Park, NC)
N Engl J Med 333:1517–1521, 1995   1–2

Objective.—It is agreed that conception must take place near the time of ovulation, but the precise timing and duration of fertility remain uncertain. For this reason, the timing of intercourse was monitored in 221 healthy women who were planning to conceive.

Methods.—Daily first morning urine specimens were collected from the time the participants stopped using birth control and were analyzed for estrogen and progesterone metabolites. Specimens were collected up to week 8 of clinical pregnancy or for up to 6 months. A total of 625 ovulatory cycles in 217 women were available for analysis.

Findings.—Without exception, conception was associated with at least 1 episode of intercourse in the 6-day period ending on the day of ovulation. None of 31 cycles lacking intercourse during this time resulted in conception. When intercourse took place only once during the 6-day period, it most commonly was on the day of ovulation. The chance of conception decreased substantially with intercourse less often than every other day during the 6-day period. Only 6% of conceptions were definitively related to fertilization by sperm that were 3 or more days old. No particular pattern of intercourse could be related to infant gender.

Implications.—The fertile period of the cycle lasts approximately 6 days and ends on the day of ovulation. The findings do not support limiting the frequency of intercourse to achieve pregnancy. Deliberately timing intercourse for the day of ovulation will not aid sex selection.

▶ The results of this study provide additional data for confirming the long-standing belief that the length of time after vaginal insemination whereby spermatozoa can fertilize the human ovum is much longer than the length of time after ovulation during which the human egg is capable of being fertilized by spermatozoa. In this study, if sexual intercourse occurred on the estimated day of ovulation or 1 or 2 days before ovulation, the conception rate was about 35%. If insemination occurred 3–5 days before ovulation, the conception rate varied from 8% to 13%. If vaginal insemination occurred more than 5 days before ovulation or on any day after the day of ovulation, pregnancy did not occur.

Thus, these data provide additional evidence to substantiate the current practice with subfertile couples seeking to become pregnant of using tests that measure urinary luteinizing hormone, which peaks before ovulation, to determine the optimal time for sexual intercourse or intrauterine insemination. For couples who wish to use natural methods of family planning to avoid pregnancy, once ovulation has occurred, as documented by a substantial rise in basal body temperature, sexual intercourse can be undertaken without the likelihood of conception occurring.

D.R. Mishell, Jr., M.D.

Variability of Day 3 Follicle-Stimulating Hormone Levels in Eumenorrheic Women
Brown JR, Liu H-C, Sewitch KF, Rosenwaks Z, Berkeley AS (New York Hosp–Cornell Med Ctr)
J Reprod Med 40:620–624, 1995   1–3

Objective.—The variability of early follicular (cycle day 3) concentrations of follicle-stimulating hormone (FSH) and estradiol (E_2) was studied prospectively in 48 women 22–48 years of age who had regular menstrual cycles lasting 21–35 days.

Methods.—Sera were sampled on cycle day 3 for up to 10 cycles, and in 1 cycle consecutive samples were drawn on cycle days 2, 3, and 4. Day 3 results were available for an average of 4½ cycles per subject. Both FSH and E_2 were estimated by radioimmunoassay. All women were studied within a 1-year period.

Findings.—Women aged 40 years and older had higher average day 3 FSH levels than younger participants. In women less than 40 years of age, most day 3 FSH values were less than 15 mIU/mL, and nearly all estimates were less than 20 mIU/mL. Levels were more evenly distributed in older women. Of 33 younger women having multiple day 3 estimates, 5 had subsequent levels of 20 mIU/mL or higher. Older women were likelier to have multiple day 3 FSH values exceeding 25 mIU/mL. There was no clear age trend for E_2 levels except for relatively high levels in the 2 women aged 45 years and older, who also had markedly increased FSH levels. Follicle-stimulating hormone levels varied less than E_2 levels on cycle day 3, and also when consecutive day 2–4 samples were analyzed.

Implications.—In women less than 40 years of age, an FSH value of less than 20 mIU/mL on cycle day 3 is highly predictive that subsequent values obtained within a year also will be normal. Estimates of FSH values made on cycle day 2 or 4 are acceptably reliable, but E_2 estimates are more variable.

▶ Elevation of FSH levels on day 3 of the menstrual cycle is associated with an extremely low pregnancy rate when in vitro fertilization is performed in that cycle. Thus, an elevated day 3 FSH value has been shown to indicate that the ova released from the ovary, even if fertilized, are unlikely to result in an ongoing pregnancy. For this reason, many clinicians, including myself, measure FSH levels on day 3 of the cycle as part of the initial infertility examination, especially if the woman is older than 35 years of age. If the day 3 FSH value remains elevated in subsequent cycles, the chances of producing a viable pregnancy with any type of infertility treatment (including controlled ovarian hyperstimulation and intrauterine insemination or an assisted reproductive technique) are extremely unlikely, and the couple should be counseled accordingly. The results of this study indicate that if initially normal, serial day 3 FSH levels should be obtained in several cycles if the infertile woman is over age 40 years and that values on day 2 or 4 of the cycle are usually similar to those on day 3.

D.R. Mishell, Jr., M.D.

Onapristone (ZK 98.299): A Potential Antiprogestin for Endometrial Contraception
Katkam RR, Gopalkrishnan K, Chwalisz K, Schillinger E, Puri CP (Inst for Research in Reproduction, Bombay, India; Research Labs of Schering Ag, Berlin)
Am J Obstet Gynecol 173:779–787, 1995   1–4

Background.—Antiprogestin drugs such as mifepristone, onapristone, and HRP 2000 are promising new methods of birth control. The effects of 2 low-dose onapristone regimens on fertility in bonnet monkeys were investigated for 4–7 consecutive cycles.

Methods.—Four monkeys were given 2.5 mg/day of onapristone subcutaneously, 5 were given 5 mg of onapristone, and 5 were given vehicle only. Three animals served as controls. Treatment was begun on day 5 of the first cycle. Thereafter, onapristone was administered every third day for 4–7 consecutive cycles. The females were placed with male monkeys during the periovulatory period.

Findings.—All 5 vehicle-treated monkeys became pregnant, compared with 1 of the 9 onapristone-treated monkeys. Four monkeys given 2.5 mg of onapristone for 17 cycles and 4 given 5 mg for 21 cycles did not conceive. The mean menstrual cycle length was not significantly affected by treatment. However, 1 monkey had a shortened cycle, and another 2 had prolonged cycles. The mean duration of menses was also not affected significantly, although it was reduced in some cycles. In addition, bleeding was slight in some cycles. Ovulation occurred in 30 of 45 treatment cycles. Prolonged treatment suppressed luteal activity in some ovulatory cycles. The duration of the follicular and luteal phases was not affected significantly in the ovulatory cycles, however. A delayed increase in serum estradiol levels was apparent in anovulatory cycles, suggesting that folliculogenesis was partially inhibited. Endometrial growth and development was retarded and rendered out of phase in the treated monkeys. The endometrial glands had partially regressed in the monkeys given the 5-mg dose. In addition, their secretory activity was blocked, and stromal compaction was observed. Onapristone did not significantly affect serum cortisol levels.

Conclusion.—Low-dose onapristone throughout the menstrual cycle prevents pregnancy without disturbing the menstrual cycle or ovulation in most cycles. During prolonged treatment, however, some monkeys had anovulation and luteal insufficiency. The contraceptive effect of onapristone in the ovulatory cycles appears to be associated mainly with the retardation of endometrial development, resulting in the inhibition of endometrial receptivity. Thus, a dose or treatment regimen of onapristone that will inhibit endometrial receptivity and prevent implantation without affecting the menstrual cycle, even on prolonged treatment, could be identified.

▶ Here we see onapristone, a relatively pure antiprogestin that has a potential role as a contraceptive agent because it is able to alter the endometrium. Low doses like those used in this study are able to do this in the monkey model and, clearly, a dose will be found that will have the same effect in women. For example, with RU486, it has been shown that doses as low as 1 mg can affect endometrial morphology, whereas much larger doses (7,100 mg) are needed for abortifacient action.

The mechanism of action is retardation of endometrial progestin effects such that the embryo is unable to implant. However, there are other potential effects of this antiprogestin action as well as that on tubal motility. As shown in Figure 2 in the original article, larger doses such as 5 mg can result in anovulation. This is clearly a dose-related phenomenon.

The one failure in the study was at the 5-mg dose. However, the article explains that it was probable that the monkey had short menstrual cycles and that the 5-mg dose was started too late for it to have an effect. Therefore, chronic exposure, even at a low dose, is what is required. It is of interest that because these agents can retard the endometrium therapeutically, we might be able to use them in the future to oppose the enhancement of endometrial development that occurs with hyperstimulation, as with in vitro fertilization. So it may be possible to use small doses to manipulate endometrial development for infertility treatment.

R.A. Lobo, M.D.

Immunogenetic Study of Couples With Recurrent Spontaneous Abortions

Belingard V, Hedon B, Eliaou J-F, Seignalet J, Clot J, Viala J-L (Montpellier Univ 1, France)

Eur J Obstet Gynecol Reprod Biol 60:53–60, 1995   1–5

Background.—The cause of recurrent spontaneous abortion (RSA) is unknown in 23% of cases. The immunologic hypothesis suggests that genetic disparity is necessary for maternal tolerance of the fetus. This disparity would be measured via the HLA system, especially at the highly polymorphic DRB1 locus. The HLA status of couples seen with RSA was examined at the Regional Hospital of Montpellier.

Subjects.—This study included white couples with a history of at least 3 spontaneous abortions. There were 7 couples with primary unexplained RSA, 18 couples with either RSA of known cause or secondary RSA, and 21 couples with at least 2 children and no history of spontaneous abortion.

Methods.—Microlymphocytotoxicity was performed to type HLA-A and HLA-B molecules from both partners. The HLA-DR molecules were typed by a reverse dot-blot technique.

Results.—There were no significant differences among the 3 groups in number of couples without shared HLA alleles. There were no differences in allelic frequencies between these 3 groups.

Conclusion.—Decreased genetic disparity at the HLA locus does not appear to be a factor in unexplained RSA, nor does any particular HLA type appear to be associated with RSA. Therefore, the immunologic hypothesis was not confirmed. HLA typing is not necessary for screening of couples with RSA.

▶ There have been at least 24 published studies that have analyzed the extent of HLA sharing among couples with a history of RSA of undetermined cause. Most of these studies have included a group of fertile couples as controls, and most have found that there is no greater incidence of sharing of HLA-A and HLA-B alleles between couples with RSA and controls. However, the majority of studies found a greater frequency of sharing of HLA-DR alleles between couples with RSA compared with controls.

The results of this study—which used a specific molecular biology technique—did not indicate that there was a greater frequency of HLA-DR sharing among the couples with a history of RSA. It is unlikely that HLA sharing among couples is an immunologic cause of abortion. HLA screening is an expensive diagnostic test and should not be performed as part of the routine diagnostic evaluation of couples with a history of RSA.

D.R. Mishell, Jr., M.D.

Reproductive Failure and the Major Histocompatibility Complex

Jin K, Ho H-N, Speed TP, Gill TJ III (Univ of Pittsburgh, Pa; Natl Taiwan Univ, Taipei; Univ of California, Berkeley)
Am J Hum Genet 56:1456–1467, 1995   1–6

Objectives.—The shared-allele test was used to analyze the distribution of HLA alleles in 123 couples with recurrent spontaneous abortion (RSA) and 76 with unexplained infertility to precisely identify the region of the major histocompatibility complex (MHC) involved in these reproductive abnormalities. HLA sharing was related to the outcome of in vitro fertilization (IVF) in the couples with unexplained infertility.

Methods.—The shared-allele test avoids the problem of rare alleles at HLA loci and also provides substantially more analytic power than the simple χ^2 test. Both a corrected homogeneity test and a bootstrap approach were used to compare allele frequencies at the HLA-A, -B, -DR, and -DQ loci to those in 51 normally fertile couples. All research subjects were from an ethnically homogeneous population of Taiwan Chinese.

Findings.—No difference was found between the patient groups and controls in the frequency of HLA alleles. There was, however, a significant excess of HLA-DR sharing in couples with RSA. Those with unexplained infertility who failed to conceive after IVF exhibited excessive HLA-DQ sharing.

Implications.—Genes in different regions of the MHC influence different aspects of reproductive function. Sharing of HLA antigens is not in itself the basic cause of these defects. The fact that the involved segment of the MHC also contains genes related to autoimmune disorders may explain clinical associations between these conditions and abnormal reproductive function.

▶ It is possible that certain recessive genes or the HLA-DR are a cause of RSA. If both members of the couple have these recessive genes, then pregnancies will terminate in abortion. As the authors state, sharing of HLAs does not necessarily indicate that there is an immunologic cause for the recurrent abortions, and immunotherapy is not indicated if HLA-DR sharing is present.

D.R. Mishell, Jr., M.D.

A Contribution to the Classification of Cases of Non-Classic 21-Hydroxylase-Deficient Congenital Adrenal Hyperplasia

Phocas I, Chryssikopoulos A, Sarandakou A, Rizos D, Trakakis E (Athens Univ, Greece)
Gynecol Endocrinol 9:229–238, 1995   1–7

Objective.—An endocrinologic study was undertaken in an attempt to distinguish patients with the nonclassic form of 21α-hydroxylase–deficient congenital adrenal hyperplasia (CAH) and heterozygous carriers from other individuals with hyperandrogenemia. Forty-five young women with symptoms of polycystic ovary syndrome (PCOS) were studied, together with 21 family members, 12 of whom were men. Progesterone, 17-hydroxyprogesterone (17-OHP), and cortisol were measured after adrenocorticotropic hormone (ACTH) injection.

Findings.—Cluster analysis distinguished 4 groups consisting, respectively, of 3, 11, 36, and 16 individuals. The proportion of patients having elevated levels of 17-OHP decreased from 100% in group I to 0% in group IV. The proportion of patients with high plasma cortisol levels increased in the same direction. Hyperprolactinemia was most prevalent in group IV patients. All 3 group I subjects had skin changes, obesity, and premature pubarche, and the single female in this group was amenorrheic. Obesity and clinical signs of hyperandrogenemia were more variable in the other groups. The response of 17-OHP to ACTH injection was more marked and occurred more rapidly in groups III and IV than in the other subjects. HLA typing showed that group I patients were 21α-hydroxylase–deficient; group II patients had a homozygous haplotype; group III patients were heterozygous; and group IV patients did not have 21α-hydroxylase deficiency.

Conclusion.—Women with hirsutism and/or menstrual irregularity should undergo ACTH stimulation testing so that nonclassic CAH caused by 21α-hydroxylase deficiency can be recognized.

▶ When the onset of symptoms of hyperandrogenism and menstrual irregularity occurs during a woman's early postadolescent years, the cause can be PCOS, idiopathic hirsutism, or late-onset 21α-hydroxylase deficiency, also called nonclassic congenital adrenal hyperplasia. Late-onset CAH is an autosomal recessive disorder whose frequency and severity vary among ethnic groups. Because the treatment and genetic counseling of individuals with late-onset CAH differ from those with PCOS or other causes of hyperandrogenism, it is important to establish the diagnosis.

The results of this study indicate that with ACTH testing it is possible to differentiate patients with the severe, mild, and minimal forms of late-onset CAH from hyperandrogenic individuals without this metabolic disorder. It is important to note that some individuals with minimal forms of late-onset CAH have normal blood levels of 17-OHP. Thus, the finding of normal levels of this hormone does not rule out the existence of this genetic disorder.

D.R. Mishell, Jr., M.D.

A Comparison of the Effects of Human and Ovine Corticotropin-Releasing Hormone on the Pituitary-Adrenal Axis

Trainer PJ, Faria M, Newell-Price J, Browne P, Kopelman P, Coy DH, Besser GM, Grossman AB (St Bartholomew's Hosp, London; Royal London Hosp; Tulane Univ, New Orleans, La)
J Clin Endocrinol Metab 80:412–417, 1995   1–8

Background.—Corticotropin-releasing hormone (CRH) can accurately distinguish between the causes of adrenocorticotropic hormone (ACTH)-dependent Cushing's syndrome. The first studies of CRH were performed with the ovine sequence, but now the human sequence peptide is more widely available. There is some evidence that the ovine sequence may be more useful in the differential diagnosis of Cushing's syndrome. The clinical efficacy of ovine and human sequence CRH were compared.

Methods.—Three groups of subjects were studied: 10 normal volunteers, 10 patients with simple obesity, and 13 patients with pituitary-dependent Cushing's disease or adrenal-dependent Cushing's syndrome. All subjects were studied twice in random order. An IV bolus of CRH, 100 µg, was given through an in-dwelling forearm cannula at 9:30 A.M. For the next 2 hours, ACTH and cortisol were measured every 15 minutes.

Results.—In normal subjects, ovine CRH yielded a greater peak ACTH, peak incremental ACTH, and mean area under the curve after CRH treatment. The cortisol response to CRH was no different between the 2 sequences (Fig 1). In the obese patients, neither the ACTH nor cortisol response to the 2 preparations was any different. There were no differences for either cortisol or ACTH between the obese and normal groups.

Both types of CRH yielded greater responses for ACTH and cortisol in Cushing's disease patients than in the other 2 groups, with no difference between ovine and human CRH. With human CRH, all 10 patients with Cushing's disease showed a significant cortisol response, defined as an increase of more than 4 times the assay's coefficient of variation. With ovine CRH, this was the case for 8 of 10 patients. Neither sequence altered the serum cortisol level in the 3 patients with adrenal tumors. Plasma ACTH was undetectable at all times in this group.

Conclusion.—Ovine sequence CRH appears to yield more prolonged and greater increases in ACTH secretion, and possibly cortisol secretion, than human sequence CRH. However, the 2 preparations are comparable in terms of making the diagnosis or differential diagnosis of Cushing's syndrome. The CRH test is also useful in distinguishing between Cushing's disease and simple obesity.

▶ This reproductive endocrinologist may not have had the opportunity to use CRH for testing purposes. The original studies were carried out with ovine CRH, and now that human CRH is available, it is useful to compare these 2 agents. As shown in the figure, there is a greater stimulatory response with the ovine product compared with the native human peptide. This is explained by the longer clearance of the ovine preparation. It is

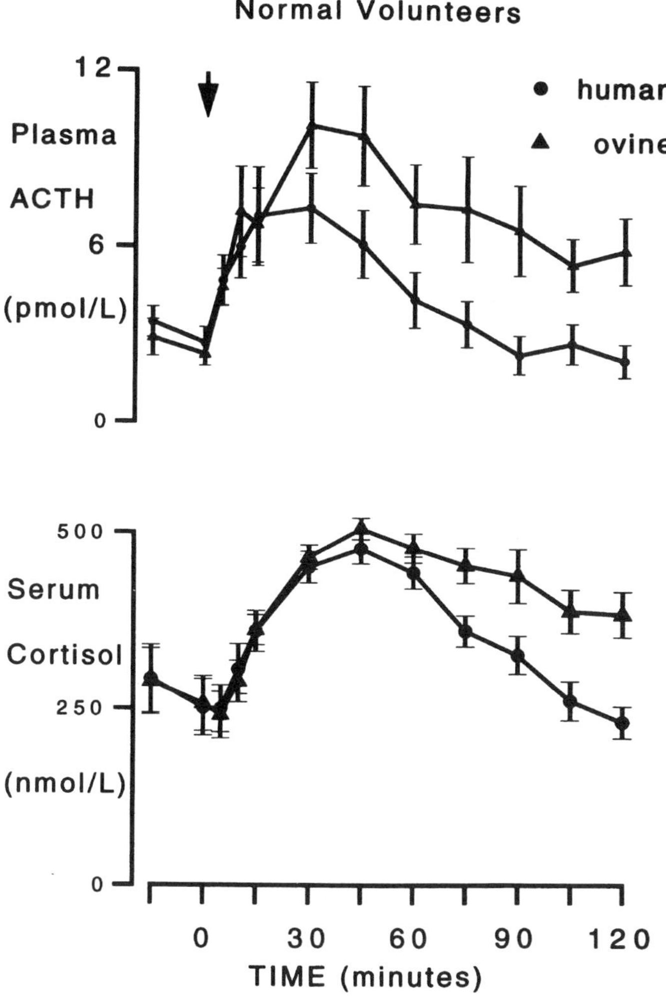

FIGURE 1.—The plasma adrenocorticotropic hormone (*ACTH*) (**top section**) and serum cortisol (**bottom section**) responses to an IV bolus of 100 μg of human or ovine corticotropin-releasing hormone (*arrow*) in 10 normal volunteers. The mean ± standard error of the mean are shown. (Courtesy of Trainer PJ, Faria M, Newell-Price J, et al: A comparison of the effects of human and ovine corticotropin-releasing hormone on the pituitary-adrenal axis. *J Clin Endocrinol Metab* 80:412–417, Copyright 1995, The Endocrine Society.)

generally longer acting and, therefore, elicits a greater response. However, as pointed out in this report, the diagnostic accuracy of the 2 preparations is similar and when used to diagnose patients with Cushing's syndrome, there does not seem to be a difference between the 2 preparations.

The ovine CRH preparation has some advantages in other areas, for example, when stimulation of adrenal androgens for diagnostic and research purposes is needed. A similar analogy can be made in terms of CRH testing in comparison with ACTH testing for adrenal androgen responses. In the doses used, ACTH (normally 0.25 mg of cosyntropin) elicits a much greater response than CRH testing, which in general elicits only a physiologic response of ACTH under normal circumstances. Thus, again, even though ACTH and CRH have equal diagnostic accuracy in terms of diagnosing disorders such as congenital adrenal hyperplasia, the use of CRH provides a more physiologic stimulus; whereas it would not lead to a missed diagnosis with a true enzyme deficiency, it may not uncover subtle enzymatic defects, such as those that may occur in adult patients with elevations of androgens.

R.A. Lobo, M.D.

Comparative Study of Tranexamic Acid and Norethisterone in the Treatment of Ovulatory Menorrhagia

Preston JT, Cameron IT, Adams EJ, Smith SK (Univ of Cambridge, England; Univ of Glasgow, Scotland)
Br J Obstet Gynaecol 102:401–406, 1995   1–9

Background.—About 9% to 14% of women of reproductive age have menorrhagia (> 80 mL of menstrual blood loss per cycle). The efficacy and safety of norethisterone and tranexamic acid therapy for menorrhagia were compared in a randomized, double-blind, placebo-controlled, prospective clinical study.

Methods.—The 103 women with heavy periods recruited into the study were supplied with sanitary protection and were told how to collect menstrual blood loss. To be included in the treatment phase, women had to have an average menstrual loss over 2 cycles of > 80 mL/cycle and to be ovulating (mid-luteal phase serum progesterone > 9 nmol/L). The alkaline hematin method was used to measure menstrual blood loss. Women acted as their own controls in the first placebo-treated cycles. Women who met the study criteria were treated for 2 cycles with either 5 mg of norethisterone twice a day on days 19 to 26 or 1 g of tranexamic acid 4 times a day on days 1 to 4.

Results.—Forty-two of the 46 women included in the treatment phase completed both treatment cycles. Patients treated with tranexamic acid had an average decrease in menstrual blood loss of 45% (*P* < 0.0001). Patients treated with norethisterone had an average increase of menstrual blood loss of 20% (*P* = 0.26). Mean menstrual blood losses of < 80 mL/cycle were achieved by 14 of 25 women in the tranexamic acid–treated group and 2 of 21 women in the norethisterone-treated group. The only significant biochemical difference between the 2 groups was a reduction in transferrin concentration in the tranexamic acid group. Although the effect of treatment on general health did not differ between the 2 groups, the group receiving tranexamic acid had less flooding or leakage and fewer limitations on their social and sexual activities. Common symptoms included dysmenorrhea (in 80% of women treated with tranexamic acid and 85% of women treated with norethisterone), headache (32% with tranexamic acid and 48% with norethisterone), and gastrointestinal symptoms (12% with tranexamic acid and 33% with norethisterone).

Conclusion.—Tranexamic acid (1 g 4 times a day for the first 4 days of menstruation) is safe and effective for the treatment of ovulatory menorrhagia. Norethisterone (5 mg twice a day administered in the late luteal phase) is not effective therapy for ovulatory menorrhagia.

▶ There is a tremendous amount of confusion regarding the treatment for ovulatory dysfunctional uterine bleeding, which is the reason this paper was abstracted. Ovulatory dysfunctional uterine bleeding occurs in patients who have normal luteal function but have excessive blood loss (menorrhagia), usually defined as > 80 mL at the time of menses. The defects that have been uncovered relate to abnormalities in prostacyclin production whereby elevated levels lead to vasodilation and inadequate platelet function. However, other causes are certainly possible as well. There is established dogma that progestins are generally beneficial for this entity. However, as pointed out in this paper, the way in which they are prescribed and the type of progestin used significantly alter the response.

This placebo-controlled trial was carried out with objective measures of blood. We do not tend to use antifibrinolytic agents in this country, but this study and several Scandinavian studies have shown efficacy for this approach when administered during the days of menstrual bleeding. Similarly, the antiprostaglandins have also been found to reduce blood loss by 40% to 50% when given during the menstrual cycle. However, the progestins when administered in this regimen, i.e., during the luteal phase, between days 19 and 26, do not show efficacy, and in this study there was a trend toward increasing blood loss, even though a large dose (10 mg per day) was used. Ten milligrams of norethindrone has tremendous potency; it lowers high-density lipoprotein cholesterol and has an adverse effect on lipoprotein metabolism. This dose, which is administered only during the luteal phase when serum progesterone levels are quite adequate, could not be expected to have a beneficial effect on the endometrium. This kind of regimen, whether with norethindrone, or with other types of progestins, should be avoided.

Other studies that have shown benefit in terms of progestin use for ovulatory dysfunctional uterine bleeding used a progestin regimen similar to that of oral contraceptives for approximately 21 days. Thus, in such a regimen, 5 mg would be administered daily between days 5 and 26 of the menstrual cycle. The use of an oral contraceptive has been shown also to reduce blood loss by about 40%. Using a progestin for 8 days, as suggested in this paper, against the backdrop of normal endogenous progesterone would not be expected to be beneficial.

R.A. Lobo, M.D.

Impaired Action of Thyroid Hormone Associated With Smoking in Women With Hypothyroidism

Müller B, Zulewski H, Huber P, Ratcliffe JG, Staub J-J (Univ Hosp, Basel, Switzerland; Queen Elizabeth Med Centre, Birmingham, England)
N Engl J Med 333:964–969, 1995   1–10

Purpose.—There are conflicting reports regarding the effects of smoking on thyroid function. Furthermore, the possible effects of smoking on the peripheral actions of thyroid hormone are unknown. Women with and without hypothyroidism were studied to determine the effects of smoking on serum concentrations of thyrotropin and thyroid hormone and on thyroid hormone action.

Methods.—The study included 138 normal women and 135 women with primary hypothyroidism. In the hypothyroid group, 84 women had subclinical and 51 had overt hypothyroidism. The women were classified as cigarette smokers or nonsmokers; 23% of the women were smokers. All subjects underwent assessment of thyroid function, including measurements of serum thyrotropin, free thyroxine, and triiodothyronine. Assessments of peripheral thyroid hormone action included a clinical score, measurement of ankle-reflex time, and measurement of serum lipids and creatine kinase. Sixty hypothyroid women were studied again while receiving thyroxine therapy.

Results.—Smokers with subclinical hypothyroidism had a serum thyrotropin concentration of 21 mU/L, compared with 13 mU/mL for nonsmokers in the same group. The smokers also had a 30% higher ratio of serum triiodothyronine to serum free thyroxine, a 16% higher serum total cholesterol level, and a 28% higher low-density lipoprotein (LDL) cholesterol level.

In the overt hypothyroidism group, smoking status made no significant difference in the serum thyrotropin, free thyroxine, and triiodothyronine level. The smokers had a greater degree of hypothyroidism, as assessed by clinical score. The smokers also had 25% higher serum concentrations of total and LDL cholesterol, a 25% longer ankle-reflex time, and a 236% higher serum concentration of creatine kinase.

In the women with overt hypothyroidism, a higher "dose" of cigarette smoking was linked to higher serum concentrations of total and LDL cholesterol and serum creatine kinase. In the subclinical hypothyroidism group, there were dose-response relationships between smoking and serum total and LDL cholesterol levels. Thyroxine treatment normalized all metabolic effects in smokers (Fig 1).

Conclusion.—Cigarette smoking has dose-dependent influences on the metabolic effects of hypothyroidism. It has adverse effects on both the secretion and action of thyroid hormones. Smoking may play a role in the high reported incidence of subclinical hypothyroidism, and may aggravate its peripheral biochemical effects. Smoking may also worsen the signs, symptoms, and biochemical effects of overt hypothyroidism.

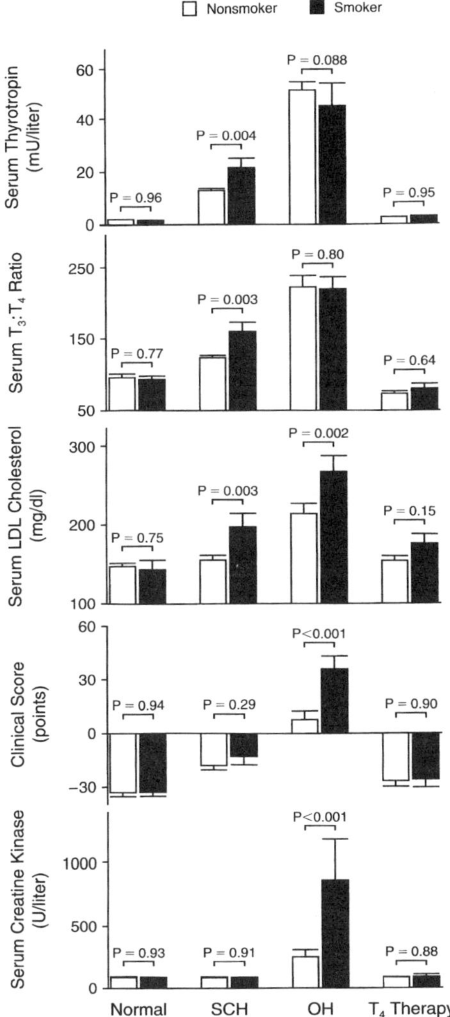

FIGURE 1.—Influence of cigarette smoking on thyroid function and results of tests of thyroid hormone action in normal women and women with subclinical or overt hypothyroidism. *P* values were derived by 1-way analyses of variance. Boxes represent means and bars represent standard errors. *Abbreviations: LDL,* low-density lipoprotein cholesterol; *SCH,* subclinical hypothyroidism; *OH,* overt hypothyroidism; *T₃,* triiodothyronine; and *T₄,* free thyroxine. To convert values for serum LDL cholesterol to millimoles per liter, multiply by 0.026. (Reprinted by permission of *The New England Journal of Medicine,* Müller B, Zulewski H, Huber P, et al: Impaired action of thyroid hormone associated with smoking in women with hypothyroidism. *N Engl J Med* 333:964–969, Copyright 1995, Massachusetts Medical Society.)

▶ Add thyroid function to a long list of problems associated with smoking. This paper demonstrates nicely that smoking interferes with both the secretion and action of thyroid hormone. Of interest was the finding that subclinical hypothyroidism could be significantly exaggerated by the presence of smoking and that the relationship was dose related. Total cholesterol and LDL cholesterol were dramatically increased in smokers with altered thyroid function. In close evaluation of the dosage data, it appears that the majority of findings occur in women who smoke between 1 and 2 packs per day. Thus, women who smoke 1 pack or less do not have the dramatic effects of smoking on thyroid function.

In a way, smoking can be viewed as a stress test for abberant thyroid function. Therefore, women seen with thyroid dysfunction, or who are evaluated and found to have thyroid dysfunction, should be questioned as to whether they are smokers. It may then be important, as well, to test smokers for thyroid function, particularly those women who smoke 2 packs or more per day. In addition, because thyroxine therapy was effective in eliminating the metabolic effects, a strong argument can be made, as the authors point out, for the treatment of even subclinical hypothyroidism in women who smoke.

R.A. Lobo, M.D.

A Double-Blind Trial of Oral Progesterone, Alprazolam, and Placebo in Treatment of Severe Premenstrual Syndrome
Freeman EW, Rickels K, Sondheimer SJ, Polansky M (Univ of Pennsylvania, Philadelphia; Hahnemann Univ, Philadelphia)
JAMA 274:51–57, 1995   1–11

Introduction.—Severe premenstrual syndrome (PMS)—a premenstrual dysphoric syndrome in which the core symptom is dysphoric mood—is a significant health problem that has been little studied until recently. Research has shown the metabolites of progesterone potentiate γ-aminobutyric acid (GABA) transmission, suggesting that progesterone metabolism and GABA-ergic transmission may have an anxiolytic effect. Differences in doses or absorption might make this effect more evident after oral progesterone administration. The effectiveness of alprazolam, an anxiolytic and antipanic medication, in patients with PMS has not been sufficiently studied. A randomized, double-blind trial was performed to compare the effectiveness of placebo, progesterone, and alprazolam in women with PMS.

Methods.—One hundred eighty-five women with PMS were screened and randomized. All had had regular menstrual cycles and PMS for at least 6 months. On daily symptom reports, all women had a daily symptom report score of at least 70 and a premenstrual symptom score at least 50% higher than the postmenstrual score. They also had moderate-to-severe functional impairment, no current major mental disorder, and prospective confirmation of symptom status by daily ratings. The patients were assigned to receive oral micronized progesterone, alprazolam, or placebo premenstrually—from day 18 to the first day of menses—for at least 3 cycles. Dosages were flexible, starting with a daily dose of 1,200 mg of oral micronized progesterone, 1 mg of alprazolam, or 4 placebo capsules in divided doses 4 times per day. By the third cycle, mean dosages were 1,760 mg/day for progesterone, 1.5 mg/day for alprazolam, and 6.7 capsules for placebo.

Results.—One hundred seventy patients were available for analysis, of whom 81% completed 3 cycles of treatment. Adverse effects were reported by 74% of patients—including 88% of the progesterone group, 79% of the alprazolam group, and 55% of the placebo group—but there were no serious side effects. Fatigue/sedation was the most commonly reported side effect. Cycle length was unchanged.

Symptom scores improved to a greater degree in the alprazolam group than in the progesterone or placebo group. Alprazolam was superior to the other treatments on end-point analysis. Patients in the alprazolam group had significantly greater improvement than those in the progesterone group at 2 months, and greater improvement than either progesterone or placebo at 3 months (Figure). Alprazolam was preferred for the symptoms of mental function, pain, and mood, but not for the physical symptoms of breast tenderness and swelling, which improved with progesterone. Clinician and patient ratings both favored progesterone. Symptom scores improved by at least 50% from baseline in 37% of the alprazolam group, 29% of the progesterone group, and 30% of the placebo group.

Conclusion.—For women with PMS, alprazolam appears to be more effective than oral progesterone or placebo. The effects on mental function, mood, and pain are better with alprazolam, whereas the physical

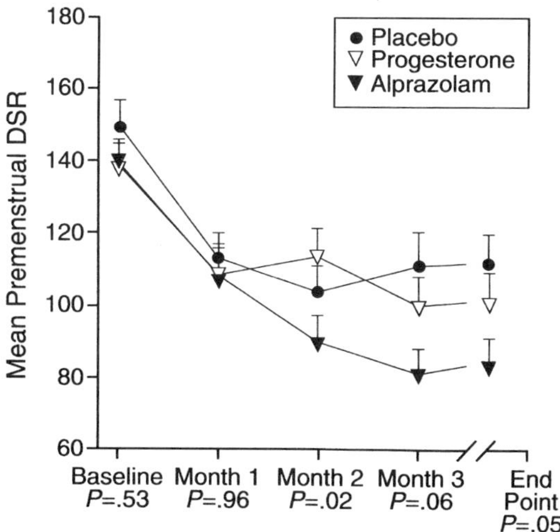

FIGURE.—Premenstrual daily symptom report (*DSR*) scores at baseline and during 3 months of treatment. Repeated measures analysis of covariance by treatment group with average baseline scores as the covariate resulted in main effect of group, $P = 0.04$. Significant pairwise comparisons ($P < 0.05$) were as follows: alprazolam vs. progesterone at month 2 and alprazolam vs. placebo at month 3 and at end point. Values are raw means of premenstrual DSR scores with standard errors. At baseline, $n = 170$; at month 3, $n = 138$; and at end point, $n = 170$. (Courtesy of Freeman EW, Rickels K, Sondheimer SJ, et al: A double-blind trial of oral progesterone, alprazolam, and placebo in treatment of severe premenstrual syndrome. *JAMA* 274:51–57, Copyright 1995, American Medical Association.)

symptoms respond better to progesterone. Alprazolam administration can be restricted to the luteal phase, with a low risk of dependence in women with clearly diagnosed PMS.

Fluoxetine in the Treatment of Premenstrual Dysphoria

Steiner M, for the Canadian Fluoxetine/Premenstrual Dysphoria Collaborative Study Group (McMaster Univ, Hamilton, Ontario, Canada)
N Engl J Med 332:1529–1534, 1995   1–12

Background.—Premenstrual syndrome (PMS), characterized by a cluster of symptoms (most commonly, tension, irritability, and dysphoria) occurring in the late luteal phase, is reported to affect 3% to 8% of women in the United States during their reproductive years. No cause has been identified, and no treatment has been consistently effective. The syndrome shares some features with depression and anxiety states, which have been linked to serotonin dysregulation. Because fluoxetine therapy inhibits the reuptake of serotonin, it was hypothesized that it would be effective in treating PMS. This hypothesis was tested in a multicenter, randomized, double-blind, placebo-controlled trial.

Methods.—A total of 313 women aged 18–45 years and diagnosed with late–luteal-phase dysphoric disorder participated in the study, and 180 completed it. The women were given placebo for 2 menstrual cycles for a washout period, then were randomly assigned to treatment with placebo or either a 20-mg or a 60-mg dose of fluoxetine per day for 6 menstrual

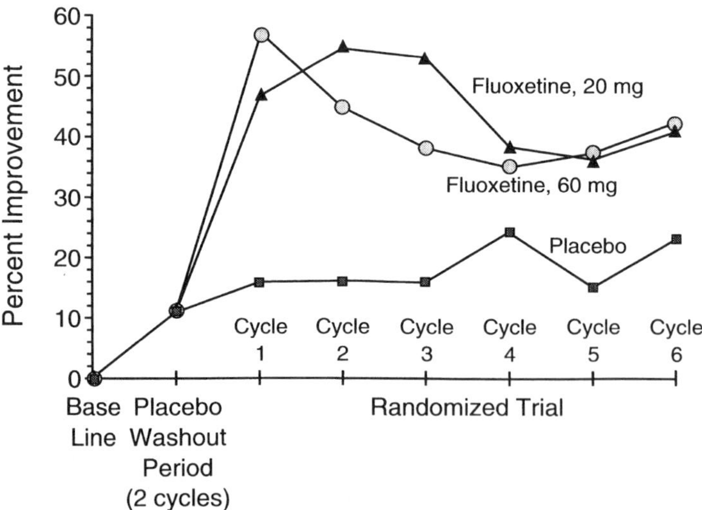

FIGURE 1.—Percentage improvement in the total luteal-phase scores of the visual analogue scale for the 180 women who completed the protocol (*P* < 0.001). (Reprinted by permission of *The New England Journal of Medicine,* Steiner M, for the Canadian Fluoxetine/Premenstrual Dysphoria Collaborative Study Group: Fluoxetine in the treatment of premenstrual dysphoria. *N Engl J Med* 332:1529–1534, Copyright 1995, Massachusetts Medical Society.)

cycles. Symptoms of tension, irritability, and dysphoria were measured with visual analogue scales at baseline, during the follicular and late luteal phases of each cycle, and at the end of the study. The frequency of side effects was noted.

Results.—Either dose of fluoxetine was significantly more effective than placebo in reducing tension, irritability, and dysphoria as early as the first cycle of treatment. Visual analogue scores were reduced by 50% during the luteal phase of the first treatment cycle in 46 of the 96 women given 20 mg of fluoxetine, in 49 of the 86 women given 60 mg of fluoxetine, and in only 21 of the 95 women given placebo (Fig 1). The rates of response remained consistent throughout the trial. The most common side effects were insomnia, nausea, tremor, fatigue, dizziness, anorexia, somnolence, sweating, visual disturbance, dry mouth, minor cardiovascular symptoms, and yawning. Their frequency was dose related.

Conclusion.—Fluoxetine, taken at doses of 20 mg or 60 mg per day, was significantly more effective than placebo in relieving symptoms associated with PMS. The 2 doses were equally effective, but significantly more adverse side effects were experienced by women taking the larger dose.

▶ Premenstrual syndrome, which is a difficult disorder to treat, is extremely common and appears more frequently in women as they get older. One of the most useful treatments to be developed in the past few years is the use of the gonadotropin-releasing hormone analogue with add-back therapy. However, this is an expensive and difficult regimen and is considered almost a last resort in treating patients with severe symptoms. These 2 papers suggest altered approaches in which different types of agents affecting the CNS may be used to an advantage.

The paper by Freeman et al. (Abstract 1–11) reports on a placebo-controlled trial with varying doses of either oral micronized progesterone or alprazolam. Of interest here is that the doses were quite large and adjusting the dose regimen was possible in this study. The authors commented that a single capsule of 300 mg of micronized progesterone has been shown not to have behavioral effects. However, with the multiple doses used, sedation was quite likely. Indeed, although progesterone has been shown to be only marginally efficacious in PMS and fairly comparable to placebo, I have assumed these findings to result from the sedative properties of the high doses of progesterone.

An interesting finding in the study is that all these doses were only used during the luteal phase, starting on day 18 of the menstrual cycle through day 2 of the following cycle. This is an attractive regimen which potentially avoids a chronic—perhaps a habituating—dose of medication. Of interest, although alprazolam was generally accepted and shown to be beneficial, it did not have any effect on physical symptoms. Premenstrual syndrome obviously is a constellation of many different symptoms, and some people have considered physical symptomatology in the overall syndrome. Nevertheless, physical symptom relief would not be expected for alprazolam because it primarily has a CNS effect.

The figure in the report by Freeman illustrates nicely that there is a substantial improvement compared with placebo.

Whereas the focus of the paper by Freeman et al. was concerned with the antianxiolytic aspects of the symptom complex, perhaps involving GABA receptors, the paper by Steiner et al. (Abstract 1–12) points to the theory of the serotonin pathway in the etiology of PMS. In this second paper, fluoxetine was used. After a prolonged washout period, patients were randomized to 2 doses of fluoxetine compared with placebo and the 20-mg and 60-mg doses of fluoxetine were found to be comparable in this study. Unlike the study using alprazolam, fluoxetine was not prescribed only during the luteal phase of menstrual cycle. However, there are data at hand that suggest that luteal phase treatment may also be effective under these circumstances. Thus, these 2 recent reports investigating drugs for treating CNS symptomatology through different mechanisms offer some hope for patients with severe PMS and give options other than requiring the use of gonadotropin-releasing hormone agonist therapy.

R.A. Lobo, M.D.

Leuprolide and Estrogen *Versus* Oral Contraceptive Pills for the Treatment of Hirsutism: A Prospective Randomized Study
Azziz R, Ochoa TM, Bradley EL Jr, Potter HD, Boots LR (Univ of Alabama, Birmingham)
J Clin Endocrinol Metab 80:3406–3411, 1995   1–13

Background.—Hyperandrogenic women who receive a long-acting gonadotropin-releasing hormone (GnRH) analogue experience the suppression of androgen and gonadotropin production. Most randomized studies of women with hirsutism have compared a GnRH analogue with and without adjuvant hormonal treatment. The expense of GnRH analogue treatment and the potential side effects make it appropriate to compare this treatment with other accepted measures.

Study Design.—Seventeen otherwise healthy hirsute women of reproductive age were randomized to receive either a GnRH analogue combined with estrogen replacement therapy or an oral contraceptive (OC) for 6 months. One group received 3.75 mg of leuprolide IM each month; 0.625 mg of conjugated estrogen; and 10 mg of medroxyprogesterone acetate on days 1–12 of each month. The comparison group received 1 mg of ethynodiol diacetate combined with 35 μg of ethinyl estradiol. Treatment began 3–8 days after a spontaneous cycle or progestin-induced bleed.

Assessment.—The rate of hair growth was documented by photographing the cheek/chin region and also by plucking hairs from this area. The diameter of plucked hairs was estimated and hair density determined from photos of cheek hair.

Results.—The leuprolide-treated patients were heavier than were patients given OC therapy and had a greater rate of hair growth at the outset.

Gonadotropin levels at most intervals declined significantly only in the leuprolide group. The percentage decrease in free testosterone decreased significantly in both groups, but more markedly in the OC recipients. Subjectively, hirsutism decreased significantly only in the leuprolide-treated patients (Fig 2). A majority of these patients but only 2 of those given OC therapy noted improved hair growth and texture. Objectively, neither group had significant changes in average facial hair density or outer hair diameter, but women given leuprolide had a decreased hair growth rate.

Conclusion.—A combination of leuprolide and cyclical estrogen replacement therapy appears to be more effective than OC therapy in women with hirsutism. Side effects are minimal, but cost remains a consideration.

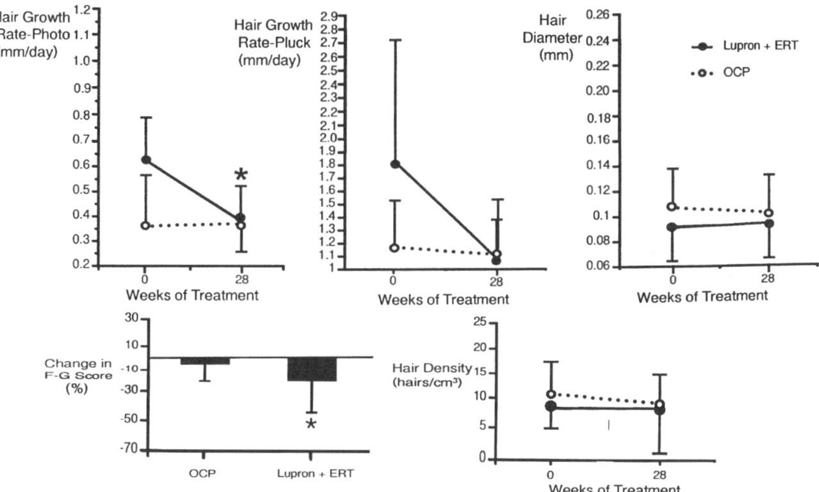

FIGURE 2.—Mean (±SD) facial hair growth rate (determined either photographically or in plucked hairs), hair diameter or hair density, and percent change in the F-G score before (week 0) and after 6 months of treatment (week 28) with either leuprolide plus cyclic estrogen-progestin (Lupron + ERT; *closed circles*; $n = 9$) or an OCP (*open circles*; $n = 8$). The *asterisk* denotes a significant difference between the measurements obtained at weeks 28 and 0 ($P < 0.05$). Furthermore, at week 0, leuprolide + ERT-treated patients had a greater rate of hair growth determined photographically ($P < 0.02$) than OCP-treated patients. (Courtesy of Azziz R, Ochoa TM, Bradley EL Jr, et al: Leuprolide and estrogen *versus* oral contraceptive pills for the treatment of hirsutism: A prospective randomized study. *J Clin Endocrinol Metab* 80:3406–3411, Copyright 1995, The Endocrine Society.)

Comparison of a Gonadotropin-Releasing Hormone Agonist and a Low Dose Oral Contraceptive Given Alone or Together in the Treatment of Hirsutism

Heiner JS, Greendale GA, Kawakami AK, Lapolt PS, Fisher M, Young D, Judd HL (Univ of California, Los Angeles; Syntex Labs Inc, Palo Alto, Calif)
J Clin Endocrinol Metab 80:3412–3418, 1995   1–14

Rationale.—Hirsutism is often a distressing problem for hyperandrogenic women. Ongoing treatment with a gonadotropin-releasing hormone (GnRH) agonist suppresses hair growth but may produce hypoestrogenic side effects such as hot flashes and bone loss. Oral contraceptives (OCs) also suppress ovarian androgen production, suggesting that a combination of these agents might prove clinically effective and, at the same time, eliminate hypoestrogenic side effects.

Study Plan.—Sixty-four women 18–45 years of age who had at least moderate hirsutism were entered into a 6-month double-masked trial and randomized to receive 400 µg of nafaralin (NAF) by intranasal spray twice a day; norethindrome/ethinyl estradiol (NOR); both treatments together; or placebo. An appropriate placebo was included in each of the single-treatment regimens.

Results.—Follicle-stimulating hormone was significantly suppressed only in patients given combined treatment. Total testosterone levels decreased significantly in women given combined treatment and those given NAF alone. Only women given NOR had a significant rise in levels of sex hormone–binding globulin. Other androgens declined most markedly in patients given combined treatment. Hair growth was suppressed most evidently in the combined treatment group. Significant hot flashes occurred only in women given NAF alone.

Conclusion.—These preliminary findings suggest that hirsutism is most effectively and safely treated by combining a GnRH agonist with an OC.

▶ These 2 papers are of interest because there are few well-conducted randomized and controlled trials on the treatment of hirsutism. In the report by Azziz et al. (Abstract 1–13) the effects of OCs were compared with leuprolide acetate with estrogen treatment. In the second report (Abstract 1–14), use of an OC (NOR) NAF, NOR + NAF, and placebo was compared. The major variable is whether OCs are additionally beneficial to the GnRH analogue treatment of patients with hirsutism.

What comes out in both of these papers is that hirsutism is difficult to assess, both subjectively and objectively. Clearly, in the first report, it was suggested that leuprolide acetate was more beneficial for the treatment of hirsutism than were OCs. I do not believe that there are major differences in the types of OCs used in these 2 studies. However, even though this was a randomized study, the groups were different. The leuprolide group tended to have more severe symptoms and a greater rate of change. This is drawn out in Figure 2, in which the groups appear to be different, although again the effects of treatment are more pronounced in the leuprolide group. The free testosterone concentrations are more greatly affected by OCs because ethinyl estradiol in the OCs has a more potent effect on sex hormone–binding globulin than does supplemental estrogen as is used in postmenopausal replacement. The second paper has similar conclusions in that it shows that GnRH analogue treatment is efficacious, although here nasal nafarelin was used. Although the addition of OCs to the regimen may be of additional benefit, the data suggesting this point are not clear in this report. Figure 4 in the article from which Abstract 1–14 was taken is illustrative of the difficulty in the assessment of hirsutism, particularly with subjective methods, such as the Ferriman-Gallwey score. The effects are noted to jump around between the different regimens, showing the baseline and point variability for this measurement.

The conclusions of these papers are that the GnRH agonist, in general, has greater efficacy in the treatment of hirsutism than do OCs and that the addition of some form of estrogen (either postmenopausal regimens or OCs) may be of additional benefit. It is important to note, however, that GnRH agonist therapy is expensive and difficult and has not been approved by the Food and Drug Administration (FDA). Indeed, there is no treatment that has been officially approved by the FDA for the treatment of hirsutism.

R.A. Lobo, M.D.

Quantitative Analysis of Androgen Receptor Messenger Ribonucleic Acid Developing Leydig Cells and Sertoli Cells by *In Situ* Hybridization

Shan L-X, Zhu L-J, Bardin CW, Hardy MP (The Population Council, New York)
Endocrinology 136:3856–3862, 1995   1–15

Background.—Testosterone is produced by Leydig cells in the adult male to maintain spermatogenesis by Sertoli cells. Androgen receptors (ARs) have been detected in prepubertal rat Leydig cells, suggesting a role for testosterone in Leydig cell differentiation. To examine this role for androgen in the development of the Leydig cells, AR messenger RNA (mRNA) was localized and quantitated in the rat during sexual development.

Methods.—In situ hybridization was used to measure AR mRNA in sections of rat testes on day 21 post partum, when Leydig cells are progenitors; on day 35, when they are immature (during puberty); and on day 90, when they are functional (sexual maturity).

Results.—Testicular AR mRNA could be detected in Leydig cells, pericytes, peritubular myoid cells and Sertoli cells. Levels of Leydig and Sertoli cell AR mRNA were significantly altered during development (Fig 3). Leydig cell AR mRNA was intermediate on day 21, highest on day 35, and lowest on day 90. Sertoli cell AR mRNA was lowest on day 21, intermediate on day 35, and highest on day 90. In other words, in Leydig cells the highest level of AR mRNA was present during puberty, whereas in Sertoli cells, the highest level of AR mRNA was present after sexual maturity.

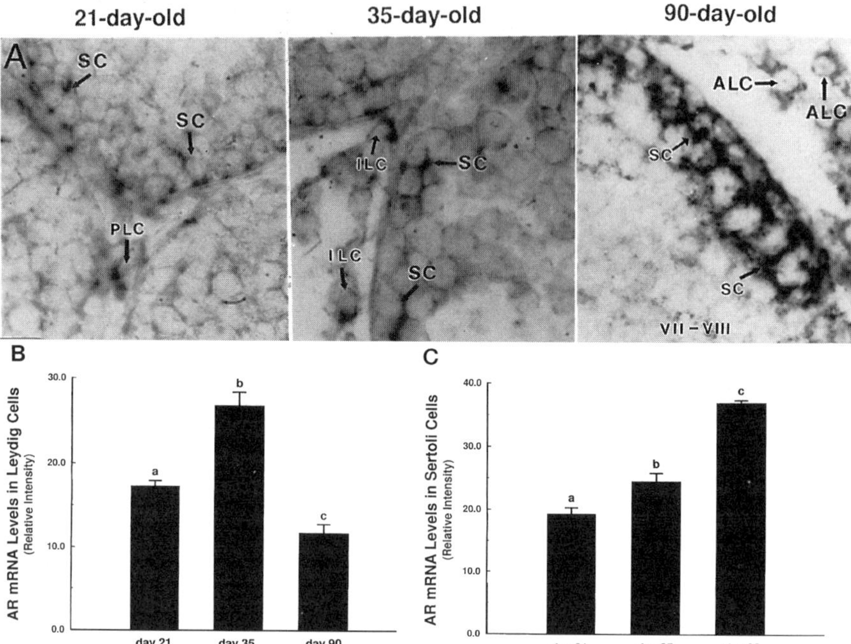

FIGURE 3.—Developmental trends of androgen receptor messenger RNA (AR mRNA) in Leydig cells and Sertoli cells. **A,** magnification, ×150. The level of AR mRNA staining in the cytoplasm of Leydig cell progenitors (*left*), immature Leydig cells (*middle*), and adult Leydig cells (*right*) was measured by image analysis. **B,** the relative signal intensities for AR mRNA are plotted (mean ± standard error of the mean). **C,** the relative signal intensities for AR mRNA in Sertoli cells are plotted. Groups with different letter codes were significantly different ($P < 0.05$). *Abbreviations: SC,* Sertoli cells; *PLC,* Leydig cell progenitors; *ILC,* immature Leydig cells; and *ALC,* adult Leydig cells. (Courtesy of Shan L-X, Zhu L-J, Bardin CW, et al: Quantitative analysis of androgen receptor messenger ribonucleic acid developing Leydig cells and Sertoli cells by *in situ* hybridization. *Endocrinology* 136:3856–3862, Copyright 1995, The Endocrine Society.)

Conclusion.—The presence of AR mRNA in Leydig cells, with maximal levels during puberty, is consistent with an important role for androgen in Leydig cell differentiation during puberty.

▶ Androgen receptors are expressed in specific testicular cell types. These include Leydig cells, pericytes, peritubular myoid cells, and Sertoli cells. To date, ARs have not been definitively identified in germ cells. Previous data published by Hardy and co-workers suggest that androgens facilitate the differentiation of Leydig cell progenitors into immature Leydig cells. The finding in the present study that AR mRNA levels are highest during puberty suggests that androgen stimulation is involved in Leydig cell differentiation.

R.Z. Sokol, M.D.

Nested Polymerase Chain Reaction Study of 53 Cases With Turner's Syndrome: Is Cytogenetically Undetected Y Mosaicism Common?
Binder G, Koch A, Wajs E, Ranke MB (Univ Children's Hosp, Tübingen, Germany)
J Clin Endocrinol Metab 80:3532–3536, 1995   1–16

Introduction.—Reportedly, 50% to 60% of women with Turner's syndrome, a form of gonadal dysgenesis characterized by primary amenorrhea and sexual infantilism, have the 45,X karyotype. The remaining patients have either structural changes in one of the X chromosomes or—more often—mosaicism. It is estimated that 5% of those affected have mosaicism with a cell line containing a Y chromosome.

Objective and Methods.—The nested polymerase chain reaction (PCR) technique was used to screen for a number of genetic abnormalities in 53 patients with Turner's syndrome, excluding those with an apparent Y chromosome or unidentifiable marker chromosome. The average patient age was 12 years. Patients were screened for sex-determining region (SRY) located on the distal short arm of chromosome Y; the testis-specific protein, Y-encoded (TSPY) gene on the proximal short arm; and the DYZ3 repeat at the Y centromere. Genomic DNA from blood leukocytes was amplified in 2 rounds of PCR, a method sensitive enough to detect 0.0001% male DNA on a female background.

Findings.—Thirty of the 53 girls (57%) had the 45,X karyotype, whereas 23 (43%) had mosaicism and/or had structural changes in 1 X chromosome. No patient was positive for Y-specific loci after the initial round of PCR but, after the second round, 2 cases were positive for SRY mapping to the distal short arm of chromosome Y. One of these subjects had a 45,X karyotype, and in the other it was 46,Xi(Xq). No subject was positive for the TSPY gene on the proximal short arm or the centromeric DYZ3 repeat.

Conclusion.—Low-level Y mosaicism is very infrequent in females with Turner's syndrome, and routine testing is not warranted.

▶ It was determined many years ago that low-level mosaicism is common in cases of Turner's syndrome. The presence of a small piece of the Y chromosome can be allusive, yet increase the risk of a gonadoblastoma to develop in a patient with streak gonads. The knowledge of the low frequency of Y mosaicism in patients with gonadal potential is of interest. A previous study using Southern blot PCR had determined that there was a fairly high prevalence of Y mosaicism in patients with Turner's syndrome. Therefore, this study was carried out, using more sensitive methods to determine whether the Y chromosome is present in patients with Turner's syndrome.

It is clear that probing SRY is the most sensitive method as compared with other probes for the Y chromosome. Yet, even with this method, after 2 rounds of PCR, 2 of 53 patients were positive. Thus, the presence of Y appears to be extremely uncommon in patients with conventional Turner's syndrome, and unless there are symptoms or signs of some androgenization, patients may not need to undergo an exhaustive search for Y. Figure 3 in the original article merely points out the nested PCR results showing the greater sensitivity of SRY in picking up an abnormality (lanes 3 and 4). These lanes were negative for the other Y probes.

R.A. Lobo, M.D.

Menstrual Disturbance and Hypersecretion of Progesterone in Women With Congenital Adrenal Hyperplasia Due to 21-Hydroxylase Deficiency

Holmes-Walker DJ, Conway GS, Honour JW, Rumsby G, Jacobs HS (Univ College, London)
Clin Endocrinol 43:291–296, 1995

1–17

Purpose.—Women with congenital adrenal hyperplasia (CAH) may have menstrual disturbances, the mechanism of which is unknown. Women with CAH related to 21-hydroxylase deficiency were studied to evaluate the relationship between their menstrual history and their biochemical and genetic characteristics.

Methods.—The study included 21 women with classic CAH receiving follow-up at one hospital. Information on age at menarche and menstrual pattern was collected from each patient. Blood samples were obtained during the follicular phase of the menstrual cycle while the women were receiving their usual maintenance therapy. These samples were analyzed to determine serum luteinizing hormone, follicle-stimulating hormone, progesterone, 17-α-hydroxyprogesterone, testosterone, androstenedione, and plasma renin activity. Gas chromatography and mass spectrometry were performed to determine the women's urinary steroid profiles. In addition, leukocyte DNA was obtained for molecular genetic analysis of the 21-hydroxylase gene.

Findings.—Eighteen patients had spontaneous menarche. In this group, the effectiveness of adrenal suppression influenced the degree of menstrual disturbance and progesterone excess. The other 3 patients did not experience menarche while receiving standard medical therapy. This group had reduced endometrial thickening, nonsuppressible serum progesterone concentrations despite suppression of 17-α-hydroxyprogesterone, and progesterone metabolites in their urinary steroid profiles. The patients with and without elevated progesterone concentrations could not be distinguished by molecular genetic analysis.

Conclusion.—In women with classic CAH caused by 21-hydroxylase deficiency—regardless of the type of steroid therapy used—control of progesterone levels may occur independently of control of androgen levels. Some women with CAH will have nonsuppressible serum progesterone of adrenal origin, primary amenorrhea, and failure of endometrial thickening causing infertility. These patients have a characteristic urinary steroid profile that distinguishes them from other women with CAH and menstrual disturbances resulting from inadequate adrenal suppression.

▶ This is a concept that I have discussed on at least 1 other occasion in the YEAR BOOK.[1] Patients with CAH, particularly those who are seeking fertility, may have abnormalities in progesterone secretion. The magnitude of this alteration is not predictable and does not necessarily correlate with levels of 17-hydroxyprogesterone or the androgens. However, the rise in progesterone does explain menstrual irregularity, amenorrhea, and a reduction in fertility status. Therefore, it is extremely important, as first pointed out by Rosenfield from the Chicago group, that monitoring progesterone is vital for patients who are seeking fertility, and progesterone levels need to be normalized. The progesterone, in this instance, is clearly of adrenal origin, even though in patients with CAH an ovarian component can develop similar to patients who have polycystic ovary syndrome.

R.A. Lobo, M.D.

Reference

1. 1993 YEAR BOOK OF INFERTILITY, p 155.

Decreased Bone Formation and Increased Mineral Dissolution During Acute Fasting in Young Women
Grinspoon SK, Baum HBA, Kim V, Coggins C, Klibanski A (Harvard Med School, Boston)
J Clin Endocrinol Metab 80:3628–3633, 1995   1–18

Objective.—Although chronic undernutrition may compromise bone formation and lead to osteoporosis, the effects of short-term starvation on bone turnover remain uncertain. In this study, 14 healthy women 18–26 years of age, whose body weight averaged 105% of ideal weight, fasted totally for 4 days.

Methods.—The participants were randomized to either 2 mEq/kg daily of potassium bicarbonate to prevent acidosis or a control condition of 25 mEq of potassium chloride daily. Bone turnover was evaluated using 2 specific markers of bone formation—osteocalcin and type I procollagen carboxyl-terminal propeptide—and 2 markers of resorption—pyridinoline and deoxypyridinoline.

Observations.—The decline in serum bicarbonate was substantially less in patients given potassium bicarbonate. Venous pH decreased only in control subjects. Serum creatinine levels increased in both groups but remained well within the normal range. The subjects lost an average of 3.3 kg of body weight. Levels of insulin-like growth factor 1 decreased significantly in both groups. Urinary calcium increased and parathyroid hormone levels decreased only in control subjects. Bone formation decreased significantly in both groups after 4 days of fasting. Bone resorption decreased more in control subjects but did not change significantly in either group.

Conclusion.—Acute fasting depresses bone formation in healthy young women. Acidosis stimulates calcium release from bone and may, thereby, promote mineral dissolution and account for bony demineralization in chronic undernutrition.

▶ This study underlines the importance of nutrition for bone mass preservation. It is known that the status of bone density largely establishes the risk of fracture in women, and peak bone density occurs from the teen years to the late twenties. The amount of bone at this time is a critical risk factor for hip fracture later in life. Here we see a study in which 18- to 26-year-old women were subjected to short-term starvation. Even with short-term fasting, we see that bone formation is affected. As pointed out in Figure 3 in the original article using markers of bone formation, the short-term fast of 5 days inhibited bone formation. Thus, a chronic nutritional deprivation in these critical years of peak mass formation can be expected to have a damaging effect on the skeletal structure and increase the risk for fracture later in life. Of interest, acidosis was also studied here, and acidosis contributes to the release of calcium for bone, which is another aspect of this problem that needs to be remembered.

R.A. Lobo, M.D.

Body Fat Distribution and Steroid Hormone Concentrations in Obese Adolescent Girls Before and After Weight Reduction
Wabitsch M, Hauner H, Heinze E, Böckmann A, Benz R, Mayer H, Teller W (Univ of Ulm, Germany; Univ of Duesseldorf, Germany; Children's Hosp Hochried, Murnau, Germany)
J Clin Endocrinol Metab 80:3469–3475, 1995   1–19

Background.—Obese women produce increased amounts of ovarian and adrenal sex steroids, and there is increased peripheral conversion of androgens to estrogens. Women with abdominal or upper-body obesity are prone to have increased androgens, hirsutism, and abnormal menstrual function. They also are more likely than women with gluteal-femoral or lower-body obesity to have metabolic disorders, lipid abnormalities, and hypertension. Most studies have focused on adult women.

Objective.—Studies were done in 92 obese adolescent girls (average age, 15 years) in an attempt to relate body fat distribution to steroid hormone production before and after weight reduction.

Methods.—The participants received a mixed diet having an average energy content of 4,321 kJ per day for 6 weeks. In addition, they exercised under supervision for 1–2 hours each day. The body mass index (BMI), waist-to-hip circumference ratio (WHR), and subscapular-to-triceps skinfold ratio (STR) were monitored.

Results.—The average baseline BMI was 31 kg/m² and the average body fat was 39%. Serum androgens and insulin were elevated compared with normal-weight girls of similar age. The girls lost 8.3 kg of body weight

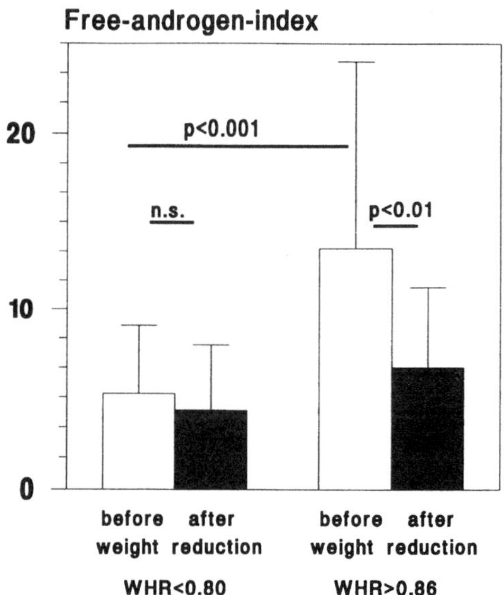

FIGURE 2.—Free androgen index before and after weight reduction in girls with abdominal obesity and those with gluteal-femoral obesity. (Courtesy of Wabitsch M, Hauner H, Heinze E, et al: Body fat distribution and steroid hormone concentrations in obese adolescent girls before and after weight reduction. *J Clin Endocrinol Metab* 80:3469–3475, Copyright 1995, The Endocrine Society.)

during the study, reducing the BMI to 28 kg/m² and the body fat to 36%. The WHR decreased significantly but the STR did not. Serum levels of estradiol and testosterone declined, whereas sex hormone–binding globulin levels increased significantly.

Correlations.—The WHR, but not the BMI or percentage of body fat, correlated positively with serum testosterone and inversely with the cortisol level at baseline. The girls with abdominal obesity had more marked changes in serum testosterone, cortisol, and the free androgen index during weight reduction than did those with gluteal-femoral obesity (Fig 2).

Conclusion.—Adolescent girls with abdominal obesity have a particularly adverse steroid hormone profile characterized by high androgenic activity. Elimination of excess body weight markedly reduces androgenic activity in these girls.

▶ This study was conducted in adolescent girls with an average age span of 14.5 to 16.8 years. It describes the positive relationship of the free androgen index to abdominal fat. This is aptly illustrated in Figure 2, showing that the girls who had central obesity and an increased WHR had a higher free androgen index. It was also this group of girls who had significant reductions with dieting, whereas the girls with gluteal obesity tended to have normal free androgen status and no change in the ratio with diet.

Abdominal obesity with an increased WHR is a significant factor for cardiovascular risk. Therefore, identification of this type of obesity—which may also signify increased androgen status—is an important identifying factor for evaluating the cardiovascular status of women.

Nevertheless, although there is a close association between free androgen status and WHR, it is not clear whether it is androgen, per se, that induces this body change or something about obesity that results in the increase in androgen status. Obesity alone can reduce sex hormone–binding globulin and increase insulin, and both factors result in higher free androgen. Perhaps it is obesity that first causes the androgen disturbance, which then leads to a change in body composition. It would be important to know what occurs with the use of oral contraceptives in adolescence. Even though androgen is often normalized, it is unclear whether the WHR is affected. These important variables will need to be dissected out in the years to come.

R.A. Lobo, M.D.

Disparate Effects of Weight Reduction by Diet on Serum Dehydroepi-androsterone-Sulfate Levels in Obese Men and Women
Jakubowicz DJ, Beer NA, Beer RM, Nestler JE (Fundación Cardiovascular Congreso National, Caracas, Venezuela; Med College of Virginia/Virginia Commonwealth Univ, Richmond)
J Clin Endocrinol Metab 80:3373–3376, 1995   1–20

Background.—Evidence suggests that the adrenal steroid dehydroepi-androsterone-sulfate (DHEA-sulfate) may have antiatherogenic and cardioprotective actions in men, but not in women. Insulin appears to reduce serum levels of DHEA-sulfate in men but not in women. This apparent sex-biased disparity in insulin action was studied in both men and women before and after dietary weight loss.

Methods.—Forty-seven obese, healthy subjects aged 28–62 years (29 women), who wished to lose weight by diet and who had a normal oral glucose tolerance test, were given a standardized 1,000–1,400 kcal diet for 2 months. At baseline and again at the end of the 2 months, fasting blood samples were drawn for determination of serum insulin, glucose, and DHEA-sulfate levels.

Results.—At baseline, age, body mass index (BMI), and serum insulin and glucose levels were similar in the men and women. However, baseline serum DHEA-sulfate levels were twofold higher in women (mean, 5.4 μm/L) than men (2.8 μm/L). After 2 months of dieting, the reduction in BMI was similar in the men (3.5 kg/m²) and women (3.2 kg/m²). Serum glucose fell slightly in both the men and the women, and both groups had similar decreases in serum insulin (men, 38%; women, 33%). However, although serum DHEA-sulfate levels did not change in the women, they increased by 125% in the men. After 2 months of dieting, the serum DHEA-sulfate levels were similar in the men (6.3 μm/L) and the women (5.2 μm/L).

Conclusion.—Dietary weight loss is associated with a marked rise in serum DHEA-sulfate levels in men, but not in women. These findings suggest that insulin reduces serum DHEA-sulfate levels in men only. Because a low serum DHEA-sulfate level is a risk factor for cardiovascular disease in men, these findings may be clinically relevant.

▶ The conclusion of this paper that the regulation of DHEA-sulfate is different in men than in women is certainly valid. Dehydroepiandrosterone-sulfate is a very interesting hormone that has implications for cardiovascular health as well as for immunology and for general health and longevity. A problem with this study is the fact that a large age span of women was studied; the women were both premenopausal and postmenopausal. This, however, may not have affected the results. It was interesting also that the DHEA-sulfate concentrations in the women were higher than those in men, which is not normally the case in premenopausal individuals.

The DHEA in women is produced by the ovaries. The levels of DHEA-sulfate which could be ovarian derived (via peripheral conversion of DHEA to DHEA-sulfate) could be substantial in some patients with polycystic ovary syndrome. Although a reciprocal relationship between insulin and DHEA-sulfate levels seems to be well validated in men, this is not the case in women. These studies lead us to the conclusion (and exemplify the fact) that we cannot extrapolate certain studies between men and women, particularly those that deal with cardiovascular disease.

R.A. Lobo, M.D.

Perimenopausal Changes in Serum Lipids and Lipoproteins: A 7-Year Longitudinal Study
Fukami K, Koike K, Hirota K, Yoshikawa H, Miyake A (Osaka Univ, Japan; Sumitomo Life Multiphasic Health Test System, Osaka, Japan)
Maturitas 22:193–197, 1995   1–21

Introduction.—Menopause appears to have a significant adverse effect on serum lipid and lipoprotein concentrations. However, the cause and extent of these changes are difficult to determine accurately. The changes in serum lipid and lipoprotein levels occurring around menopause were assessed in a 7-year longitudinal study.

Methods.—The study included 16 healthy, middle-aged women who underwent annual medical examinations in the 4 years before and 3 years after menopause. Age at menopause ranged from 47 to 56 years. At each examination, the women's total cholesterol, high-density lipoprotein (HDL) cholesterol, low-density lipoprotein cholesterol (LDL), and triglyceride levels were measured. Women who had hyperlipidemia before menopause were excluded.

Results.—Serum total cholesterol increased by an average of 25 mg/dL, or 14%, from the 4 years before to the first year after menopause. At the same time, LDL cholesterol increased by an average of 20 mg/dL, or 19%. Total cholesterol increased rapidly from 1 year before menopause until menopause, whereas the increase in serum LDL cholesterol occurred more slowly. Little or no change occurred in serum triglyceride or HDL cholesterol concentrations.

Conclusion.—Serum total and LDL cholesterol concentrations increase significantly around the time of menopause, and these changes are likely responsible for the increased risk of cardiovascular disease after menopause. This study is noteworthy for its relatively long follow-up and accurate information on menopausal status.

▶ Readers might note with interest why we are covering areas related to menopause in these reviews. Certainly it is of interest to us because of the ramifications of treating older women from a reproductive standpoint when estrogen replacement is used, and also because of the important health care consequences of rendering patients hypoestrogenic, such as with the use of gonadotropin-releasing hormone (GnRH) agonists. The latter point is relevant to this discussion, as there has been controversy regarding changes in lipids and lipoproteins around the time of menopause.

During the next 10 or 15 years after menopause, a woman's risk for the development of cardiovascular disease increases substantially. Among a multitude of mechanisms, the predominant theory for this increased risk has been the accelerated increase in cholesterol and LDL cholesterol. Controversy has arisen with the assumption that HDL cholesterol also decreases substantially after menopause. This is relevant to what we do when we treat premenopausal patients with GnRH agonist therapy, which renders women acutely hypoestrogenic.

As shown here and in confirmation of cross-sectional data from Framingham, at least for the first 3 years after menopause, HDL levels do not change substantially, whereas cholesterol and LDL concentrations increase dramatically. Thus, although oral estrogen substantially increases HDL concentrations, this effect may be viewed as a beneficial pharmacologic effect. Reductions of endogenous estrogen, like that which occurs at menopause, do not lead to a substantial reduction in HDL cholesterol.

R.A. Lobo, M.D.

The Effect of the Anti-Estrogen Tamoxifen on Cardiovascular Risk Factors in Normal Postmenopausal Women

Grey AB, Stapleton JP, Evans MC, Reid IR (Univ of Auckland, New Zealand)
J Clin Endocrinol Metab 80:3191–3195, 1995   1–22

Background.—Treatment with tamoxifen in women with breast cancer has been associated with a reduced risk of recurrent breast cancer, cardiovascular disease, and osteoporosis, but these effects have not been studied in healthy women. To assess the potential of tamoxifen therapy for reducing cardiovascular risk in normal women, the impact of 2 years of treatment was studied on major cardiovascular risk factors: serum lipids, fibrinogen, and body composition.

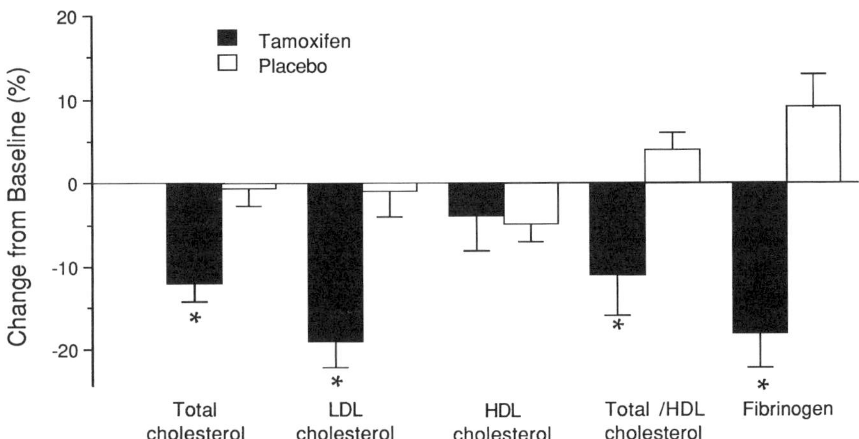

FIGURE 1.—Percentage change from baseline in serum lipids and fibrinogen after 2 years of tamoxifen or placebo therapy in normal postmenopausal women. The *horizontal bars* indicate standard error of the mean. *Asterisk* denotes $P < 0.001$ vs. placebo. *Abbreviations: LDL,* low-density lipoprotein; *HDL,* high-density lipoprotein. (Courtesy of Grey AB, Stapleton JP, Evans MC, et al: The effect of the anti-estrogen tamoxifen on cardiovascular risk factors in normal postmenopausal women. *J Clin Endocrinol Metab* 80:3191–3195, Copyright 1995, The Endocrine Society.)

Methods.—Fifty-seven healthy women at least 36 months postmenopausal were randomly assigned to receive either tamoxifen or placebo daily for 2 years. Forty-six completed the trial. At baseline, at 6 months, and at 2 years, blood specimens were obtained and analyzed for the serum lipid profile and fibrinogen concentration. Regional fat distribution was determined by calculating the ratio of android (waist) to gynoid (thigh) fat, as measured by dual-energy x-ray absorptiometry.

Results.—There were no significant differences between the groups in the studied variables at baseline. After treatment, the tamoxifen group had significantly lower levels of total cholesterol (12% fall), low-density lipoprotein (LDL) cholesterol (19%), ratio of total cholesterol to high-density lipoprotein (HDL) cholesterol (11%), and fibrinogen (18%) (Fig 1). The 2 groups had no significant differences in the levels of HDL cholesterol, HDL cholesterol subfractions, triglycerides, or glucose. The tamoxifen group also had a trend toward a higher apolipoprotein A1 level. Both groups had an increased ratio of android-to-gynoid fat, which was not altered by tamoxifen treatment.

Conclusion.—Tamoxifen treatment of normal postmenopausal women produces favorable changes in the levels of serum lipids and fibrinogen, which can substantially reduce the risk of cardiovascular disease.

▶ Because tamoxifen use is so widespread, it is important to know all of its metabolic ramifications. This paper only addresses the dose of 20 mg of tamoxifen for 2 years in postmenopausal women. It has been suggested that tamoxifen can have a cardioprotective effect as well as preventing bone resorption in postmenopausal women. The magnitude of this effect is unclear, although in the Scottish trial,[1] tamoxifen was suggested to have a relative risk of 0.7 or a 30% protective effect against heart disease. The mechanisms are unclear and, indeed, the mechanisms for cardioprotective effects of estrogen are multiple.

This study only really addresses the effects on lipoproteins and on fibrinogen. The reductions compared with those achieved by placebo were substantial in terms of total cholesterol, LDL cholesterol, and the total/HDL cholesterol ratio as shown in the figure. Indeed, the changes in total cholesterol and LDL cholesterol are mirror images of those findings with Premarin, 0.625 mg. However, HDL was not significantly altered, and this is distinctly different from the effects of oral estrogen. Similar to the effects of oral estrogen is the reduction in fibrinogen, which may be another independent risk factor for cardiovascular disease.

It is clear now that this antiestrogen tamoxifen has multiple different effects in different end organs and, indeed, the concept of an estrogen receptor antagonist has to be reevaluated because different agents are able to activate different parts of the receptor complex and, therefore, have different effects (sometimes agonistic and sometimes antiagonistic). Here the effects are primarily on the LDL receptor and less on hepatic lipase, which is one of the reasons HDL levels are increased with oral estrogen.

The reduction in fibrinogen is intriguing and thought to be beneficial. Grey et al. suggest that the magnitude of the reduction of fibrinogen may translate into a reduction in cardiovascular risk of 28%, which I think is a premature conclusion. Some of the other effects of estrogen on cardiovascular function involve non–receptor-mediated effects (such as vasodilation). It would be interesting to see whether tamoxifen influences these factors in any way.

R.A. Lobo, M.D.

Reference

1. McDonald CC: Fatal myocardial infarction in the Scottish Adjuvant Tamoxifen Trial. *BMJ* 303:435–437, 1991.

Dietary Intervention Study to Assess Estrogenicity of Dietary Soy Among Postmenopausal Women
Baird DD, Umbach DM, Lansdell L, Hughes CL, Setchell KDR, Weinberg CR, Haney AF, Wilcox AJ, McLachlan JA (Natl Inst of Environmental Health Sciences, Research Triangle Park, NC; Survey Research Assoc, Research Triangle Park, NC; Duke Univ, Durham, NC; et al)
J Clin Endocrinol Metab 80:1685–1690, 1995   1–23

Introduction.—Many fruits, vegetables, and grains have phytoestrogens, nonsteroidal plant compounds that produce estrogenic responses, and little is known about the biological effects of dietary phytoestrogen intake in human beings. Postmenopausal women were studied to evaluate the estrogenic effects of a soybean-supplemented diet.

Methods.—After a 2-week period to assess baseline measurements, 97 women were randomly assigned to a soy diet group or a control group. All women were younger than 65 years and were at least 2 years past menses.

During the next 4 weeks, the soy group substituted approximately one third of their daily caloric intake with soy foods (about 38 g of dry texturized vegetable protein or 114 g of dry whole soybeans and 25 g of soy splits; the controls ate as usual. The soy group had 165 mg/day of isoflavones, which is approximately equivalent to 0.3 mg/day of conjugated steroidal estrogen. Serum luteinizing hormone (LH), serum follicle-stimulating hormone (FSH), serum sex hormone–binding globulin (SHBG) and cytology of the vaginal epithelium were measured.

Results.—Nineteen percent of the soy group had increased vaginal superficial cells, indicative of estrogenicity, compared with 8% of the controls. No decreases were seen in FSH and LH, and there was no increase of SHBG. During the diet, there was little change in body weight or endogenous estradiol concentration. Estrogenic responses were similar among women with large increases in urinary isoflavone concentrations and in women with more modest increases.

Discussion.—Estrogenic effects were not seen with the 4-week soy-supplemented diet on the liver and pituitary in postmenopausal women, despite evidence of absorption of high quantities of estrogenic isoflavones. A small estrogenic effect was seen on vaginal cytology.

Meta-Analysis of the Effects of Soy Protein Intake on Serum Lipids

Anderson JW, Johnstone BM, Cook-Newell ME (Univ of Kentucky, Lexington)
N Engl J Med 333:276–282, 1995

1–24

Background.—The beneficial practice of eating plant products, especially soy protein, is well recognized in animals. Substituting plant protein for animal protein appears to reduce hypercholesterolemia and atherosclerosis in human beings as well. To determine the effect of eating soy products on total cholesterol, low-density lipoprotein (LDL) cholesterol, and triglycerides, a meta-analysis of all clinical studies that had compared intake of soy and animal protein was conducted.

Methods.—Twenty-nine articles from the medical literature representing 38 separate studies were chosen for analysis. All the studies selected had evaluated soy protein or soy products, had a crossover or parallel design, and had reported baseline values. Each study was analyzed in terms of initial serum lipid levels, the amount and type of soy product ingested, the age group studied, and the similarity of the soy-containing diet and the control diet. The change in lipid levels that occurred between ingestion of soy and animal protein was expressed as the mean difference. The effect of soy protein on lipid levels was determined. Predictive models were developed using hierarchical linear modeling. Regression analysis was used to interpret results.

Results.—In most of the studies, the amount of saturated and total fat were similar in control and soy diets. Isolated soy protein was used in 20 studies, textured soy protein in 15, and a combination of the 2 was used in 3 studies. Compared with patients ingesting control diets, all 3 measures—total cholesterol, LDL cholesterol, and triglycerides—were reduced in patients who ingested soy diets. Total cholesterol decreased by 9.3% and LDL cholesterol decreased by 12.9%. The net change for HDL cholesterol was an increase of 2.4%. Patients on soy diets who had moderate or severe hypercholesterolemia initially had the most significant reductions in total and LDL cholesterol concentrations. Although the amount of soy ingested was a significant factor, neither the type of soy used used nor the age of the subjects was a significant factor.

Discussion.—Based on the findings in the majority of the studies, ingestion of 31 to 47 g/day of soy protein, which is 2–3 servings of soy products, can significantly reduce serum and LDL cholesterol levels.

▶ These 2 papers are placed together because they tie together the metabolic effects of soy protein, an emerging area of interest because of the estrogenic effects that may impact on reproduction as well as having a role in the care of postmenopausal women. These studies are different in design, but the features are similar. In the first study (Abstract 1–23), a prospective trial was organized to determine the acute effects of a 4-week trial of soy protein on vaginal epithelial changes, as well as classic estrogenic effects on gonadotropins and SHBG. A previous study by Wilcox[1] had suggested in 1990 that there was an estrogenic effect of soy protein on the vaginal epithelium.

The study above was somewhat disappointing in that only a marginal estrogenic effect in the vaginal epithelium was encountered and there was no effect on gonadotropins or SHBG. The amount of soy was considered adequate and was validated by measurements of isoflavonoids in urine as a compliance measure. Nevertheless, an acute study might have required larger doses to show this, and, indeed, vaginal epithelial changes often take 3 months to occur rather than a short 4-week trial. In addition, the classic measures of estrogenicity such as LH/FSH and SHBG may be mediated through mechanisms other than by activation of the isoflavonoids, such as genistene.

Indeed, some of these estrogenic effects on the pituitary vs. the liver may involve mechanisms that are different from those of the classic estrogen receptor, and, even though the isoflavonoids may activate the estrogen receptor, there may be a greater propensity to activate different aspects of the receptor, given the different target organs involved. Therefore, one would conclude that there is some evidence that these doses do have mild estrogenicity. The assumption made in this paper that the effects should be equivalent to the effects of 0.3 mg of conjugated equine estrogens is really not valid. Such a conclusion would need to be based on a study that took into account the amount of soy protein ingested and the effects on multiple organ systems (liver, uterus, bone, etc.).

In the second study (Abstract 1–24), published in *The New England Journal of Medicine,* a meta-analysis was carried out, not on reproductive factors but on the effects of serum lipids. Of interest is the fact that this was not a parameter explored in the first study, although, again, usually 3 months of treatment is required to see stable changes in lipoprotein with any estrogenic substance. This meta-analysis used doses of soy that are comparable to the ones in the previous study. Indeed, there were significant changes in this meta-analysis on total cholesterol, LDL cholesterol, and triglycerides and a marginal increase in HDL cholesterol as well.

All of these trends are obviously healthy and suggest that a diet supplemented liberally with soy protein has beneficial effects on serum lipids. Although in a meta-analysis different regimens and different doses and types of patients are used in the various studies, I think the conclusion that 2–3 servings of supplement results in these effects is a valid conclusion. This information could be extrapolated to the first study, suggesting, perhaps, that this dose may have minimal estrogenic effects on the reproductive system.

R.A. Lobo, M.D.

Reference

1. Wilcox G, Wahlqvist ML, Burger HG, et al: Oestrogenic effects of plant foods in postmenopausal women. *BMJ* 301:905–906, 1990.

Can Progestin Be Limited to Every Third Month Only in Postmenopausal Women Taking Estrogen?
Hirvonen E, Salmi T, Puolakka J, Heikkinen J, Granfors E, Hulkko S, Mäkäräinen L, Nummi S, Pekonen F, Rautio A-M, Sundström H, Telimaa S, Wilen-Rosenqvist G, Virkkunen A, Wahlström T (Gynecologic Ctr, Helsinki; Turku Univ, Finland; Mikkeli Central Hosp, Finland; et al)
Maturitas 21:39–44, 1995   1–25

Background.—In women given hormone replacement therapy, progestin is used to counter the stimulatory effect of estrogen on the uterine endometrium and the consequent hyperplastic response. Regular bleeding generally takes place when progestin is added for 10–14 days each month, but progestins produce subjective side effects in some women.

Objective.—A prospective but nonrandomized trial was undertaken in 263 postmenopausal women to determine whether adding a progestin to estrogen replacement for 2 weeks every 3 months will prevent endometrial hyperplasia. All patients received 2 mg of estradiol valerate daily for 84 days. Medroxyprogesterone acetate, in a dose of 20 mg daily, was added on cycle days 71–84 and was followed by a 7-day drug-free interval.

Results.—The 227 women who completed a year of treatment represented 86% of those enrolled. All menopausal symptoms decreased significantly within 6 months. The average body weight gain was 0.4 kg after 1 year of treatment, and 0.8 kg after 2 years. Withdrawal bleeding took place on cycle day 87 on average (Fig 1). Bleeding lasted 6.3 days on average in the first cycle and 5.4 days after the first year of treatment. The frequency of heavy bleeding decreased from 23% at 3 months to 11.5% at 1 year. Seven women had unscheduled bleeding. Severe pain accompanying withdrawal bleeding became less frequent over time and was not seen in the second year of treatment. Initial endometrial samples showed a

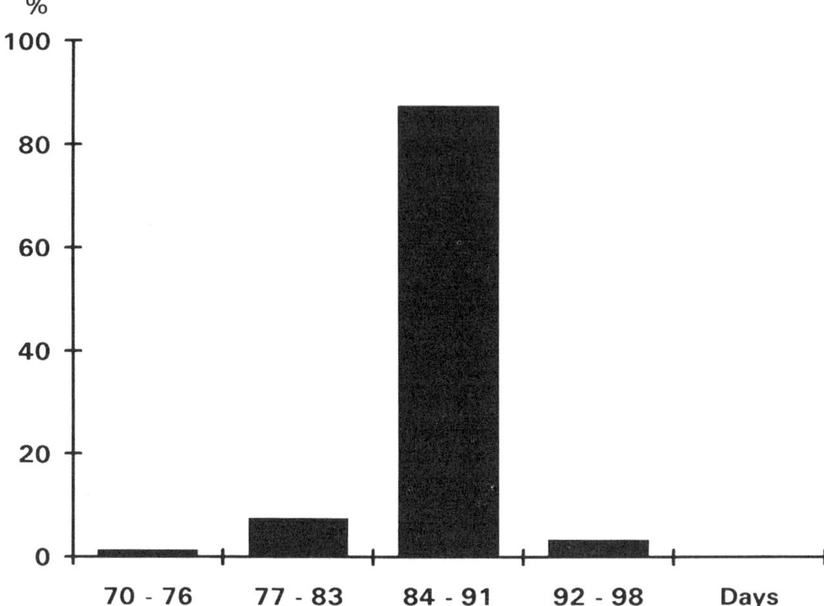

FIGURE 1.—Onset of bleeding during 3-month estrogen/progestogen treatment regimen (740 cycles). (Reprinted from *Maturitas,* Vol. 21, Hirvonen E, Salmi T, Puolakka J, et al: Can progestin be limited to every third month only in postmenopausal women taking estrogen? *Maturitas* pp 39–44, 1995, with kind permission from Elsevier Science Ireland Ltd., Bay 15K, Shannon Industrial State, Co. Clare, Ireland.)

progestogenic effect in 7% of women. Two women exhibited hyperplastic changes. Fourteen women (5%) withdrew at some point during the 2-year study because of side effects. Of 87 women who formerly had used a monthly combined regimen, 43% preferred the 3-month cycle and another 29% expressed no preference.

Implications.—Adding a progestin every 3 months to estrogen replacement therapy can prevent the development of endometrial hyperplasia. This regimen may be prescribed for women having normal or scanty bleeding, but it is not recommended for those who have been postmenopausal for less than 3 years.

▶ For all the reasons we give hormonal replacement, this study is 1 of several that have described the relative safety of using an intermittent regimen every 3 months to oppose the effects of estrogen on the endometrium. The amount and duration of progestin is going to be influenced by the dose and duration of the estrogen treatment. In this study, the 2 mg of estradiol valerate used caused moderate stimulation of the endometrium.

In studies by Bruce Ettinger and Howard Judd, medroxyprogesterone acetate at 10 mg for 14 days was able to prevent hyperplasia. This study used 20 mg of medroxyprogesterone acetate. The amount of progestin used also influences the amount of bleeding, and bleeding was fairly substantial in these women. Therefore, even though this reduces the frequency of bleeding, scheduled bleeding may be problematic for some patients, and it is not recommended that this form of therapy be used in patients within the first few years of menopause, as these younger women tend to have more bleeding, particularly if larger doses of estrogen are used.

R.A. Lobo, M.D.

Effect of Chronic Daily Oral Administration of 17β-Oestradiol and Norethisterone on the Isoforms of Serum Gonadotrophins in Post-Menopausal Women

Wilde L, Naessén T, Phillips DJ (University Hosp, Uppsala, Sweden)
Clin Endocrinol 42:59–64, 1995   1–26

Objective.—The increase in gonadotropin levels at menopause is accompanied by the appearance of more acidic—i.e., more negatively charged—isoforms of follicle-stimulating hormone (FSH) and luteinizing hormone (LH). These acidic isoforms can be offset by chronic treatment with 17-β-estradiol (E_2) implants. Many postmenopausal women receive oral hormone replacement therapy (HRT) containing an estrogen combined with a progestogen. The impact of this form of HRT on serum gonadotropin concentration and charge was evaluated.

Methods.—The study included sera from 20 postmenopausal women (mean age, 60 years). All of the women were taking continuous daily HRT consisting of 2 mg of E_2 and 1 mg of norethisterone acetate. Fluoroimmunoassays were performed to measure serum FSH, LH, and E_2. Electrophoresis in 0.1% agarose suspension was performed to assess the median charge and charge heterogeneity of the FSH and LH isoforms. The findings were compared with those of 20 postmenopausal women who were not taking HRT, and with published results of postmenopausal women treated with E_2 implants and normally menstruating women.

Results.—The women taking HRT had a serum E_2 level in the range of 198 to 610 pmol/L. These results were in the range expected during the midluteal phase of the menstrual cycle and were comparable to those reported in women with E_2 implants. The mean LH level in the women taking HRT was comparable to that seen during the luteal phase but significantly lower than the LH level in controls, in women with E_2 implants, and during the follicular phase of the menstrual cycle. The mean FSH level in the HRT group was comparable with that of the follicular phase and of women with E_2 implants but lower than in the non-HRT controls and higher than in the luteal phase of the menstrual cycle. For both FSH and LH, the median charge was less acidic in the women taking HRT than in the controls but more acidic than in women with E_2 implants and during different phases of the menstrual cycle. Compared with controls, the mean degree of charge heterogeneity of FSH was greater and that of LH was less in the HRT group. There was no significant difference in the mean sex hormone–binding globulin concentration among the women taking HRT, the non-HRT controls, and the women with E_2 implants.

Conclusion.—In postmenopausal women, chronic oral HRT with E_2 plus norethisterone produces a decrease in serum gonadotrophin levels. However, it does not completely prevent the formation of more acidic isoforms of FSH and LH. The charge is different for both FSH and LH between women with E_2 implants and those taking oral HRT. This could be related to the differing routes of administration of E_2 and/or to the effect of norethisterone.

▶ This paper was abstracted because of the concept of changes in charge of gonadotropins FSH and LH during the menopausal transition, and, indeed, data similar to these have been generated in patients with premature ovarian failure, so this is a deficiency in terms of sex steroid state as opposed to one that is induced as a function of age. So the more acidic forms of gonadotropins are associated with estrogen deficiency. One of the important points to be brought out from this and other work is the fact that hormonal replacement does not and should not interfere with measurements of the gonadotropins by routine immunoassay. Of interest in this report, is that perhaps by more sophisticated assays in which different charges of the gonadotropins can be ascertained, an early transition towards the menopause could be picked up. Because estrogen deficiency results in more acidic forms, the finding of a greater proportion of acidic forms in perimenopausal women might be helpful for determining the hormonal status of these patients, and a reduction in this pattern might be one way to monitor results of treatment. Clearly, there are differences with different forms of estrogen replacement, and what this is caused by is not entirely clear at the present time.

R.A. Lobo, M.D.

Effect of Oral Alendronate on Bone Mineral Density and the Incidence of Fractures in Postmenopausal Osteoporosis

Liberman UA, for the Alendronate Phase III Osteoporosis Treatment Study Group (Tel Aviv Univ, Petah-Tikva, Israel)
N Engl J Med 333:1437–1443, 1995   1–27

Background.—Alendronate has been shown to inhibit osteoclast-mediated bone resorption in animals and patients with osteoporosis at daily doses that do not affect bone mineralization. Two multicenter, randomized, double-blind, placebo-controlled dose-ranging studies evaluated the efficacy of continuous treatment with oral alendronate at 3 doses in postmenopausal women with osteoporosis.

Methods.—Postmenopausal women with osteoporosis between the ages of 45 and 80 years and living in 8 countries were randomly assigned to receive either placebo or daily oral alendronate at doses of 5 or 10 mg for 3 years or 20 mg for 2 years followed by 5 mg for 1 year. At baseline and

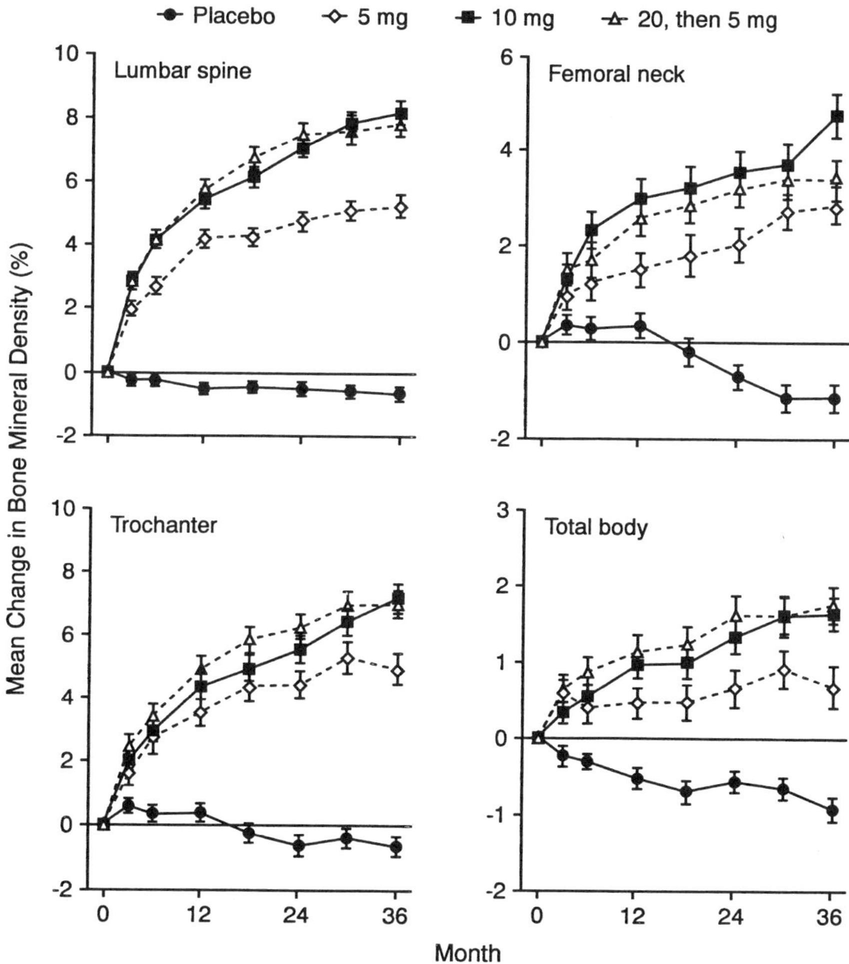

FIGURE 1.—Mean (± standard error) changes in bone mineral density from baseline values in women with postmenopausal osteoporosis receiving alendronate or placebo for 3 years. (Reprinted by permission of *The New England Journal of Medicine*, Liberman UA, for the Alendronate Phase III Osteoporosis Treatment Study Group: Effect of oral alendronate on bone mineral density and the incidence of fractures in postmenopausal osteoporosis. *N Engl J Med* 333:1437–1443, Copyright 1995, Massachusetts Medical Society.)

after 3 years, bone mineral density of the lumbar spine, femoral neck, trochanter, forearm, and total body was measured by dual-energy x-ray absorptiometry. Vertebral fractures and the progression of vertebral deformities were assessed with annual lateral spine films. Height was measured every 3 months.

Results.—The treatment groups had similar baseline characteristics and risk factors for fracture. The bone mineral density of the spine, femoral neck, trochanter, and total body increased significantly during all 3 years with all 3 doses of alendronate but decreased significantly in the placebo group (Fig 1). There were significantly greater increases in bone mineral density with the 10-mg dose of alendronate than with the 5-mg dose. The 10-mg dose was as effective as the 20-mg dose. New vertebral fractures occurred in 6.2% of the placebo group and 3.2% of the combined alendronate groups. The risk of new vertebral fractures was decreased with all doses of alendronate. There was an increase in the Spine Deformity Index of 33% in the alendronate groups and of 41% in the placebo group. At 3 years, the mean loss of height was 35% less in the alendronate group than in the placebo group—a difference of 0.7 mm annually. There was also a trend toward fewer nonvertebral fractures in the alendronate groups. There were no significant differences in adverse effects associated with placebo or alendronate treatment.

Conclusion.—Daily oral alendronate treatment for 3 years induced significant increases in bone mineral density and decreases in risk of fracture, vertebral deformities, and loss of height, suggesting increased bone strength in both the appendicular and the axial skeleton.

▶ This article is the result of a large international multicenter study using alendronate, which was recently approved in the United States for osteoporosis. It is important to note that alendronate has been approved for the treatment, rather than the prevention, of osteoporosis, and studies will emerge eventually as to whether it has additional efficacy in the latter regard. Alendronate, which inhibits osteoclast function, is different from etidronate because of its tremendous potency, and because only small doses are administered, mineralization is not interfered with. This was one of the drawbacks of etidronate, which required a sequential regimen of administration. Here, continuous doses can be administered and, as shown in the figure, there is clearly a dose-response relationship, with 10 and 20 mg clearly being more beneficial than 5 mg. However, even 5 mg is substantially different from placebo.

The importance of this work is that not only was bone mass shown to increase with the various doses, but that fracture rates were reduced by half in these osteoporotic women who were followed for 3 years. This is an important finding because criticism of other regimens for treating osteoporosis has been that even though bone density may be improved somewhat, the integrity of bone is different and fractures will still be sustained. Clearly, an agent that reduces fracture incidence will be of benefit to women. In the area of reproductive endocrinology other than the case of postmenopausal women, all women with estrogen deficiency—including those being treated long term with gonadotropin-releasing hormone analogues—will have to consider various prophylactic regimens for the maintenance of bone mass.

R.A. Lobo, M.D.

2 Epidemiology of Infertility

Infertility, Involuntary Infecundity, and the Seeking of Medical Advice in Industrialized Countries 1970–1992: A Review of Concepts, Measurements and Results
Schmidt L, Münster K (Univ of Copenhagen)
Hum Reprod 10:1407–1418, 1995   2–1

Objective.—Prevalence rates of infertility and involuntary infecundity, as well as care-seeking practices by infertile couples, were examined by reviewing 22 epidemiologic studies done in 8 countries, including the United States, in the years 1970–1992. In general, it proved difficult to compare the results of the various studies because researchers used different concepts, and there was considerable variation in how the study populations were delineated.

Infertility.—Reported rates of infertility in women of fertile age ranged from 3.6% to 14.3%, and lifetime prevalence rates ranged from 12.5% to 32.6%. In studies of women 25 to 45 years of age, primary infertility lasting longer than 1 year was identified in 13.3% to 16% of women and secondary infertility in approximately 17%. The lifetime prevalence of primary and/or secondary infertility is 24%. The extent to which infertility becomes more frequent with advancing age remains unclear. Lifetime prevalence rates are higher for women at the end of their fertile period than for the overall study population.

Involuntary Infecundity.—Other terms for this state include sterility, involuntary childlessness, and unresolved subfertility. Reported prevalence rates of primary involuntary infecundity range from 2.5% to 4.5% and of secondary infecundity, from 3.5% to 5.9%.

Care-Seeking.—From 32% to 95% of primarily infertile women in various populations have sought medical help. The figures for secondarily infertile women range from 22% to 79%. From 3.6% to 17% of the study populations themselves have sought medical advice for treatment of infertility.

▶ The studies analyzed in this report were mainly carried out in the United States, England, Scandinavia, and Finland, with 1 study from Australia. The results indicate that difficulty in achieving pregnancy at some time in a couple's life is fairly common, with a lifetime prevalence of 24%. Therefore, primary care physicians need to be educated as to how to perform a diagnostic infertility evaluation, as well as how to counsel infertile couples.

After a semen analysis is conducted and midluteal serum progesterone levels are analyzed, a hysterosalpingogram should be performed to determine whether there is tubal patency. Interpretation of the results of these 3 tests should allow the clinician to decide whether to treat the couple with controlled ovarian hyperstimulation and intrauterine insemination or refer them to an infertility specialist for more specific therapy, such as tubal reconstruction surgery or in vitro fertilization.

D.R. Mishell, Jr., M.D.

The Prognosis for Live Birth Among Untreated Infertile Couples
Collins JA, Burrows EA, Willan AR (McMaster Univ, Hamilton, Ont, Canada)
Fertil Steril 64:22–28, 1995
2–2

Objective.—To estimate the effects of infertility treatment for patients with a given set of clinical characteristics, it is first necessary to know the baseline prognosis for untreated patients. A prediction model incorporating key clinical data could be useful in producing more formal estimates. A cohort follow-up study was performed to assess the likelihood of live birth and the effects of prognostic factors for untreated couples with infertility.

Methods.—The study included 2,198 couples from 11 infertility clinics with an infertility history of longer than 1 year. They were followed for up to 7 years. The analysis included 18,364 untreated months of observation in 873 untreated couples and 9,761 untreated months of observation before the start of treatment. The likelihood of birth without treatment and the role of key prognostic factors were estimated by proportional hazards analysis. The resulting prediction score was then evaluated for reproducibility and reliability.

Results.—A total of 263 live birth conceptions occurred during 28,125 months of untreated observations. The 12-month cumulative rate of conceptions leading to live birth was 14% (Fig 1). The mean time to conception for untreated couples who had a live birth was 10 months. Couples with unexplained fertility had the highest live birth rate, 36-month cumulative live birth rate, and approximate fecundity. Pregnancy history, duration of infertility, the female partner's age, male defect, endometriosis, and tubal disease were the relevant prognostic factors for likelihood of live birth. When used in a prediction score, these factors would permit an accurate prediction in about 62% of cases.

Conclusion.—The estimates are sufficiently accurate to be used in the clinical management of infertility and in the planning of clinical trials. The likelihood that an infertile couple will have a live birth during untreated observation is affected by diagnostic and clinical covariates.

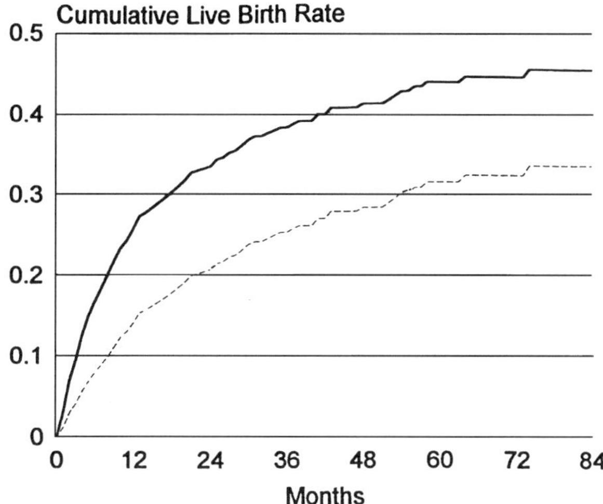

FIGURE 1.—Cumulative rate of conceptions leading to live birth. *Broken line* represents all couples (2,198), including pretreatment months for treated couples. The cumulative rate of live birth conception at 36 months was 25.2%. *Solid line* represents couples (873) who remained untreated throughout follow-up. The cumulative rate of live birth conception at 36 months was 38.2%. (From Collins JA, Burrows EA, Willan AR: The prognosis for live birth among untreated infertile couples. *Fertil Steril* 64:22–28, 1995. Reproduced with permission of the publisher, The American Society for Reproductive Medicine [The American Fertility Society].)

► Couples for whom no cause for their infertility can be found during the diagnostic evaluation are considered to have unexplained infertility. The results of this study indicate that without treatment about one third of these couples will have a live birth in 3 years. Abnormalities reducing the chance of a live birth in 3 years include anovulatory cycles, an abnormal semen analysis, tubal blockage, and endometriosis. However, the birth rates with these conditions range from 5% to 29%. In determining whether any treatment for infertility is superior to no treatment, clinical trials using placebo controls or historical controls, such as the ones in this report, need to be used.

Because it is difficult to perform randomized clinical trials involving a sufficient number of infertile couples, the pregnancy rates cited in this study can be used to serve as a comparison group when deciding whether a treatment for infertility is effective. These results can also be used when counseling infertile couples regarding their chance of conception without therapy.

D.R. Mishell, Jr., M.D.

Fertility in Men Exposed Prenatally to Diethylstilbestrol

Wilcox AJ, Baird DD, Weinberg CR, Hornsby PP, Herbst AL (Natl Inst of Environmental Health Sciences, Research Triangle Park, NC; Univ of Virginia, Charlottesville; Univ of Chicago)
N Engl J Med 332:1411–1416, 1995   2–3

Background.—Between the late 1940s and the early 1970s, diethylstilbestrol (DES) was frequently prescribed to prevent complications in pregnancy. However, the use of DES was banned when it was linked with the development of clear cell adenocarcinoma of the vagina and cervix in the daughters of the women treated with it during pregnancy. Prenatal exposure to DES is also known to cause infertility in women and has been suspected of causing infertility in men. The effects of prenatal DES exposure on male fertility were evaluated in a follow-up study of the sons of women who had participated in a randomized clinical trial of DES during pregnancy in the 1950s.

Methods.—Between 1950 and 1952, 1,646 pregnant women were randomly assigned to treatment with either DES or placebo. Of the 848 male infants born during the study, 548 were located in 1991 and 494 consented to be interviewed, including 253 DES-exposed and 241 unexposed men. In addition, 305 of their female partners who had been impregnated were interviewed. The interviewers were blinded to the exposure status.

Results.—There were no significant differences between the exposed and unexposed groups in height, weight, education, income, race or ethnicity, smoking status, or age at first marriage. The men who had been exposed to DES reported a significantly higher incidence of medically diagnosed genital malformations (15% vs. 5%), most commonly epididymal cysts and hypoplastic testes. Among the DES-exposed men, genital malformations were twice as common among those exposed to DES earlier than 11 weeks' gestation than among those exposed to DES later in the pregnancy (Table 2). However, the exposed and unexposed groups, re-

TABLE 2.—Reported Genital Abnormalities According to Diethylstilbestrol Exposure Status and Timing of Diethylstilbestrol Treatment

SITE OF ABNORMALITY*	EXPOSED (N = 253)		UNEXPOSED (N = 241)
	<11 WEEKS' GESTATION (N = 154)	≥11 WEEKS' GESTATION (N = 99)	
	percent		
Testicles	10	8	5
Epididymis	3	1	0
Other	6	2	1
Total with any genital abnormality	18	9	5

* Some men reported more than 1 abnormality.

(Reprinted by permission of *The New England Journal of Medicine,* Wilcox AJ, Baird DD, Weinberg CR, et al: Fertility in men exposed prenatally to diethylstilbestrol. *N Engl J Med* 332:1411–1416, Copyright 1995, Massachusetts Medical Society.)

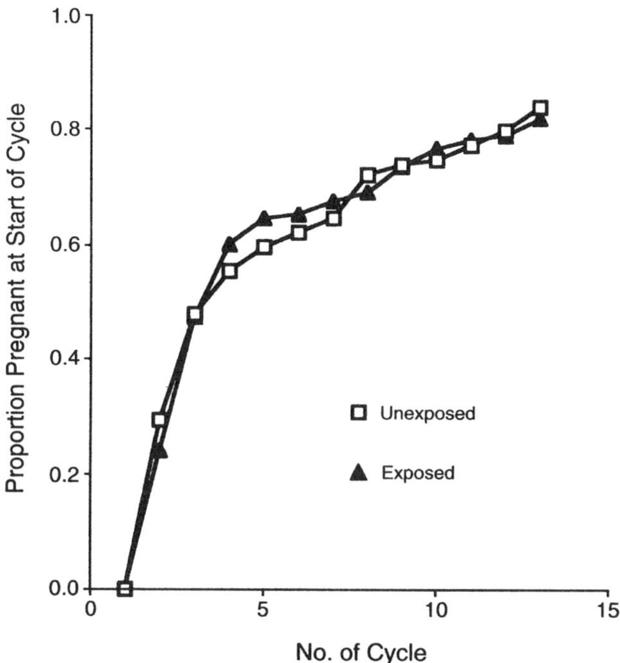

FIGURE 1.—Cumulative probability of conception per menstrual cycle for 119 couples in which the man was exposed prenatally to diethylstilbestrol and 104 couples in which the man was unexposed. (Reprinted by permission of *The New England Journal of Medicine,* Wilcox AJ, Baird DD, Weinberg CR, et al: Fertility in men exposed prenatally to diethylstilbestrol. *N Engl J Med* 332:1411–1416, Copyright 1995, Massachusetts Medical Society.)

gardless of the presence or absence of genital malformations, did not differ in measures of fertility, including fathering a child, age at the birth of their first child, total number of children, or medical diagnosis of infertility (Fig 1). In addition, more exposed than unexposed men reported accidental conception while using contraception. There was no difference in the length of time to conception in the 2 groups. Neither the timing of exposure to DES nor the presence of genital malformations reduced fertility.

Conclusion.—Prenatal exposure to DES significantly increased the risk of genital malformations in males, particularly when treatment began before 11 weeks' gestation. However, there was no evidence that prenatal exposure to DES impaired male fertility.

▶ Infertility induced by DES among the sons of women treated with the drug during pregnancy has been widely postulated. Exposed male rodents were noted to have an excess of genital malformations and infertility in adulthood. Until now, results of clinical studies have been equivocal. This well-designed study supports previous findings of increased genital malformations in exposed men but clearly shows that fertility is not compromised.

R.Z. Sokol, M.D., F.A.C.P.

Polycystic Kidney Disease and Infertility
van der Linden EFH, Bartelink AKM, Ike BW, van Leeuwaarden B (Eemland Hosp, Amersfoort, The Netherlands)
Fertil Steril 64:202–203, 1995   2–4

Introduction.—Patients with adult polycystic kidney disease (APKD) can have cysts in other organs in addition to the kidneys. A patient with cysts in the genital system, causing infertility, was described.

> *Case Report.*—Man, 32, was evaluated for infertility. He reported variable bilateral testicular pain and occasional pressure on the bladder. He had received a diagnosis of APKD. His physical examination revealed congestion of the epididymis, which was confirmed by ultrasonography. Laboratory examination of the ejaculate revealed low volume, total azoospermia, and extremely low levels of seminal fructose. Transrectal ultrasonography showing severely dilated seminal vesicles and supplementary CT showing cysts in the vesicles confirmed the presumptive diagnosis of obstructive azoospermia.

Discussion.—Cystic changes in the seminal vesicles resulting from APKD can cause obstructive azoospermia by compressing the ejaculatory duct. Transrectal ultrasonography can be used to detect and localize the obstruction. When the blockage is distal, it can be treated with transurethral resection. Cystic blockage in the genital system should be considered in infertile patients with APKD.

▶ Polycystic kidney disease is a relatively common inherited disease seen in patients between the ages of 20 and 40 years. Cysts in the kidney are associated with cysts in numerous other organs, including the testes, seminal vesicles, and epididymis. Azoospermia in a patient with APKD is a surgically correctable cause of male infertility.

R.Z. Sokol, M.D., F.A.C.P.

Is Congenital Bilateral Absence of Vas Deferens a Primary Form of Cystic Fibrosis? Analyses of the CFTR Gene in 67 Patients
Mercier B, Verlingue C, Lissens W, Silber SJ, Novelli G, Bonduelle M, Audrëzet MP, Férec C (Centre de Biogénétique, Brest, France; Univ Hosp, Brussels, Belgium; St Luke's Hosp, St Louis; et al)
Am J Hum Genet 56:272–277, 1995   2–5

Background.—An important cause of sterility in men is congenital bilateral absence of the vas deferens (CBAVD). The genetic mechanism of this condition is not known. However, some patients with CBAVD have been found to carry mutations in their cystic fibrosis transmembrane conductance regulator (CFTR) genes. The association of CBAVD and cystic fibrosis was investigated.

Methods and Findings.—The entire coding sequence of the CFTR gene was analyzed in 67 otherwise healthy men with CBAVD. Four novel missense mutations were identified—A800G, G149R, R258G, and E193K. Forty-two percent of the men carried one CFTR allele, and 24% were compound heterozygous for CFTR alleles. Thus, 76% of the subjects were identified as carrying 2 CFTR mutations. The family of 1 man was found to have CFTR haplotype segregation. This family included 2 brothers with identical CFTR loci but different phenotypes. One brother was fertile, and the other was not.

Conclusion.—Congenital bilateral absence of the vas deferens is a heterogenous, complex genetic disorder. One fifth to one fourth of CBAVD cases may actually represent very mild forms of cystic fibrosis. Thirty-four percent are apparently unassociated with the CF gene. The 43% incidence of cystic fibrosis mutations on just 1 allele of the rest of the patients with CBAVD may implicate a role for CFTR.

Mutations in the Cystic Fibrosis Gene in Patients With Congenital Absence of the Vas Deferens

Chillón M, Casals T, Mercier B, Bassas L, Lissens W, Silber S, Romey M-C, Ruiz-Romero J, Verlingue C, Claustres M, Nunes V, Férec C, Estivill X (L'Hospitalet de Llobregat, Barcelona; Univ Hosp, Brest, France; Inst of Urology, Nephrology, and Andrology, Barcelona; et al)

N Engl J Med 332:1475–1480, 1995   2–6

Background.—Mutations in the cystic fibrosis transmembrane conductance regulator (CFTR) genes have been documented in congenital bilateral absence of the vas deferens (CBAVD). The molecular basis of this form of male infertility is not well understood. Patients with cystic fibrosis have mutations in both copies of the CFTR gene, but most men with CBAVD have mutations in only 1 gene copy. Congenital bilateral absence of the vas deferens at the molecular level was studied.

Methods.—Cystic fibrosis transmembrane conductance regulator gene mutations in 102 patients with CBAVD were characterized. None of the men studied had clinical manifestations of cystic fibrosis. The 5T allele, a DNA variant, was also analyzed in a noncoding region of CFTR that decreases levels of the normal CFTR protein. For comparison, the parents of patients with cystic fibrosis, patients with non-CBAVD infertility, and healthy individuals were investigated.

Findings.—Mutations were found in both copies of the CFTR gene in 19 patients with CBAVD. None of these patients had the 5T allele. In 54 patients, a mutation was noted in 1 copy of CFTR. Sixty-three percent of the patients in this group had the 5T allele in the other CFTR gene. No

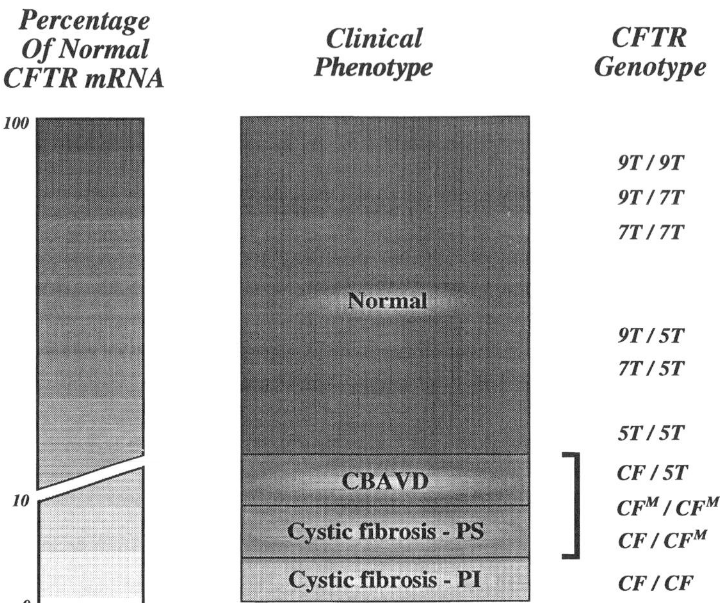

FIGURE 3.—Comparison of percentages of normal cystic fibrosis transmembrane conductance regulator (*CFTR*) messenger RNA (*mRNA*), clinical phenotypes, and CFTR genotypes. *Abbreviations:* *CBAVD*, congenital bilateral absence of the vas deferens; *PS*, pancreatic sufficiency; *PI*, pancreatic insufficiency; *CF*, a severe cystic fibrosis mutation; and *CF^M*, a moderate cystic fibrosis mutation. (Reprinted by permission of *The New England Journal of Medicine*, Chillón M, Casals T, Mercier B, et al: Mutations in the cystic fibrosis gene in patients with congenital absence of the vas deferens. *N Engl J Med* 332:1475–1480, Copyright 1995, Massachusetts Medical Society.)

CFTR mutations were discovered in 29 men, but 7 of these patients, or 24%, had the 5T allele. This allele occurred at a frequency of about 5% in the general population.

Conclusion.—Mutations in the CFTR gene occur in most men with CBAVD. The most common cause of this condition is the combination of the 5T allele in 1 copy of the CFTR gene and a cystic fibrosis mutation in the other. The clinical manifestations of the 5T allele mutation range widely. The 5T allele mutation is found in patients with CBAVD, in those with moderate forms of cystic fibrosis, and in fertile men (Fig 3).

▶ The association of bilateral vasal agenesis and cystic fibrosis was first reported by Kaufman and colleagues in 1986. Since then, we have learned that approximately 55% of men with congenital agenesis of the vas are carriers of the cystic fibrosis gene. Abstracts 2–5 and 2–6 expand our understanding of the molecular basis and inheritance pattern of congenital absence of the vas.

R.Z. Sokol, M.D., F.A.C.P.

Have Sperm Counts Been Reduced 50 Percent in 50 Years? A Statistical Model Revisited

Olsen GW, Ross CE, Bodner KM, Lipshultz LI, Ramlow JM (Dow Chemical Company, Midland, Mich; Shell Oil Company, Houston; Baylor College of Medicine, Houston)

Fertil Steril 63:887–893, 1995

2–7

Background.—The allegation that human sperm counts have decreased by about 50% worldwide since the beginning of World War II is attracting much attention. This allegation comes mainly from 1 paper published by a Danish research group in 1992. This group—Carlsen et al.—reviewed 61 studies on semen quality among fertile men published between 1938 and 1991 and, using a linear regression model, predicted that mean seminal volume had declined from 3.4 to 2.75 mL and that mean sperm counts had dropped from 113 to 66 $\times$ 10^6/mL between 1940 and 1990. Given the public health concerns that have been raised by this paper, a reassessment of the data analyzed by Carlsen et al. seems warranted.

Methods.—A visual examination of the Carlsen et al. data suggested that several alternative statistical models would be of value. These included a quadratic curve and 2 nonlinear models: a spline fit and a stairstep model.

Findings.—The original linear regression analysis was reproduced exactly. However, the quadratic model provided a better fit to the data. Because there were few data points before 1970, the statistical models used were inconsistent in representing the transition from high to low sperm counts over time. None of the 4 models used had an exceptional fit, even when data were abundant. The best-fitting stairstep model still did not account for 50% of the total between-studies variation.

Conclusion.—Inferring a 50% reduction in mean sperm counts in the past 50 years from the published linear regression model is not appropriate. There are several reasons for this. Most important is that a variety of other mathematical models better describe the data and suggest very different hypotheses. The available data on sperm counts are only robust during the past 20 years of the Carlsen et al. analysis, and all models but the linear one suggest that sperm counts have remained constant or slightly increased in the past 20 years.

Decline in Semen Quality Among Fertile Men in Paris During the Past 20 Years

Auger J, Kunstmann JM, Czyglik F, Jouannet P (Université Paris Sud)

N Engl J Med 332:281–285, 1995

2–8

Objective.—The suggestion of a decline in the quality of semen in normal men during the past 30 years prompted this retrospective study of semen quality in 1,351 healthy fertile men.

Methods.—Semen quality data collected from 1,351 fertile men from 1973 to 1992 at 1 sperm bank in Paris were analyzed. The data included volume of seminal fluid, sperm concentration, and percentages of motile and morphologically normal spermatozoa. The data from each calendar year were analyzed as a function of the age of the patient, the year of the donation, the year of birth, and the duration of sexual abstinence before semen collection.

Results.—The mean seminal fluid volume remained the same throughout the study (3.8 mL). However, during the same period, significant decreases were noted in mean sperm concentration (2.1%; from 89 × 10^6/mL to 60 × 10^6), motile spermatozoa (0.6%), and normal spermatozoa (0.5%). When the data were adjusted for age and duration of sexual abstinence and analyzed by multiple regression, 2.6%, 0.3%, and 0.7% of the yearly declines in sperm concentration, motility, and normal morphology, respectively, were found to be associated with each successive calendar year of birth. The sperm concentration decreased by 3.7% in a group of 382 men who were matched for age and duration of sexual abstinence. The decline in percentage of normal spermatozoa per year in this subgroup (0.7%) was also more pronounced than in the entire study population.

Conclusion.—Unexplainable declines in concentration of sperm and in the percentages of motile and normal spermatozoa with each successive year of birth were documented in 1,351 men. There was no concomitant decline in seminal volume. Increased age of the donor and the duration of sexual abstinence before semen collection correlated with more pronounced declines in sperm concentration, motility, and normal morphology.

▶ Are sperm concentrations really declining? Here are two different studies (Abstracts 2–7 and 2–8) that reach opposite conclusions. The more cynical investigators among us would suggest that the documented decline is a reflection of technician expectations. During the years spanned by these studies, the "normal" range for sperm concentration has declined from greater than 60 million sperm/c³ to greater than 20 million sperm/c³. Thus, the individual performing the semen analysis 20 years ago would be more inclined to err on the high side than that person would today. In support of this hypothesis is a table in the first article showing that before 1963, only 2 of the 10 studies demonstrated average sperm counts of less than 100 million/c³. Finally, the issue of clinical relevance must be addressed. The decline noted in the second paper is minimal. Epidemiologic data do not support the existence of a corresponding decline in fertility rates among men of reproductive age. Of course, there may be a delay between the documentation of a decline in sperm concentration and the manifestation of a decline in sperm concentration and the manifestation of a decline in fertility rates.

R.Z. Sokol, M.D., F.A.C.P.

Chromosomal Analysis of Sperm From Men With Idiopathic Infertility Using Sperm Karyotyping and Fluorescence In Situ Hybridization
Moosani N, Cox DM, Pattinson HA, Rademaker AW, Carter MD, Martin RH (Univ of Calgary, Alberta, Canada; Alberta Children's Hosp, Calgary, Canada; Calgary Gen Hosp, Alberta, Canada; et al)
Fertil Steril 64:811–817, 1995   2–9

Background.—Apart from constitutional chromosomal abnormalities, infertility may possibly be related to chromosomal instability. The frequency of chromosomal abnormalities in the sperm of infertile men was investigated.

Methods.—Sperm chromosomal complements from 5 somatically normal, infertile men were analyzed. Assays were done using the human sperm–hamster oocyte fusion system and the disomy frequencies for chromosomes 1 and 12. Sex chromosomes were determined using fluorescence in situ hybridization. Sperm were fused with hamster oocytes, resulting in sperm chromosomes, or sperm nuclei were prepared for fluorescence in situ hybridization. The main outcome measures were structural and numerical abnormalities determined by sperm karyotypes and disomy frequency assessed by fluorescence in situ hybridization analysis.

Findings.—The subjects had increased frequencies of numerical abnormalities and total abnormalities, determined by sperm karyotyping. There was also a significant increase in the frequency of disomy for chromosome 1 and XY disomy on analysis of sperm nuclei by fluorescence in situ hybridization.

Conclusion.—This analysis using sperm karyotyping and fluorescence in situ hybridization indicates that sperm from infertile men may have an increased frequency of chromosomal abnormalities. The X-Y pairing, as well as the pairing of the autosomes, may be affected, resulting in spermatogenic disruption.

▶ With the advent of intracytoplasmic sperm injection (ICSI), it is more important than ever that we understand the genetic inheritance patterns of male factor infertility. A number of studies have established that there is an increase in the frequency of constitutional chromosomal abnormalities in the infertile population relative to the general population. Even men with a somatically normal karyotype may have a chromosomal abnormality limited exclusively to the germ cells. Therefore, there is a theoretical risk that microinjected spermatozoa may result in a chromosomally abnormal conceptus. Additional studies such as this one must be conducted to ensure adequate prenatal genetic counseling prior to ICSI. As noted by Silber and colleagues in Abstract 2–10, if we rely solely on ICSI as the therapy for male infertility, we can expect a higher incidence of severe male factor infertility in future generations.

R.Z. Sokol, M.D., F.A.C.P.

The Use of Epididymal and Testicular Spermatozoa for Intracytoplasmic Sperm Injection: The Genetic Implications for Male Infertility

Silber SJ, Nagy Z, Liu J, Tournaye H, Lissens W, Ferec C, Liebaers I, Devroey P, Van Steirteghem AC (St Luke's Hosp, St Louis; Dutch-Speaking Brussels Free Univ, Belgium; Centre de Biogenetique, Brest, France)
Hum Reprod 10:2031–2043, 1995   2–10

Background.—Intracytoplasmic sperm injection (ICSI) may provide a means of improving fertilization and pregnancy rates in patients with congenital absence of the vas deferens (CAV), failed vasoepididymostomy, and inoperable obstructions. The results of using testicular and epididymal spermatozoa with ICSI in patients with severe infertility were reviewed.

Patients and Findings.—Microsurgical epididymal sperm aspiration (MESA) was performed in 72 patients with CAV and irreparable obstructive azoospermia. Normal embryos obtained by ICSI were used for transfer and fertilization in 90% of patients. Consistently good results were obtained using epididymal sperm with ICSI compared with conventional in vitro fertilization (Table 1). An overall fertilization rate of 46% was achieved. Normal cleavage was noted in 68%. The pregnancy rate per transfer was 58%. The delivery rate per transfer was 37%, and the delivery rate per cycle was 33%. In instances in which epididymal spermatozoa were not available, testicular sperm extraction (TESA) was used for sperm retrieval. Although the transfer rate was lower with TESA (84% vs. 96%) and the spermatozoa could not be frozen and saved for future cycles, the difference in achieved pregnancy rates when using epididymal or testicular spermatozoa was minimal (Table 4). The cause of the obstruction—CAV or failed vasoepididymostomy—did not have an effect on outcome. The age of the woman appeared to be the only significant factor influencing treatment success (Table 6).

Conclusion.—The use of testicular and epididymal spermatozoa with ICSI provides consistently good results. Therefore, ICSI should be consid-

---

TABLE 1.—Comparison of Microsurgical Epididymal Sperm Aspiration–Intracytoplasmic Sperm Injection With Conventional Microsurgical Epididymal Sperm Aspiration In Vitro Fertilization in a Similar Patient Population

Method	Cycles	Mature eggs	2PN	Fertilization rate (%)	Transfers (%)	Pregnancy rate (% delivered)
IVF–MESA	67	1427	98	7	13/67 (19)	3/67 (4.5)
ICSI–MESA*	33	431	201	47	31/33 (94)	12/33 (36.3)

* This does not include results with frozen epididymal sperm cycles and testicular sperm cycles.

Abbreviations: 2PN, 2 pronuclei; *IVF,* in vitro fertilization; *MESA,* microsurgical epididymal sperm aspiration; *ICSI,* intracytoplasmic sperm injection.

(Courtesy of Silber SJ, Nagy Z, Liu J, et al: The use of epididymal and testicular spermatozoa for intracytoplasmic sperm injection: The genetic implications for male infertility. *Hum Reprod* 10:2031–2043, 1995, by permission of Oxford University Press.)

TABLE 4.—Pregnancy and Delivery Rates After Intracytoplasmic Sperm Injection With Epididymal and Testicular Biopsy Spermatozoa

Source of spermatozoa	No. patient cycles	No. transfers (%)	No. clinical pregnancies per transfer (%)	No. delivered per transfer (%)	No. delivered per cycle (%)
Fresh epididymal (MESA)	33	31 (94)	20 (65)	12 (39)	36
Frozen epididymal	7	7 (100)	4 (57)	2 (28)	28
Testicular biopsy (TESE)	32	27 (84)	14 (52)	10 (37)	31
Totals	72	65 (90)	38 (58)	24 (37)	33

Abbreviations: MESA, microsurgical epididymal sperm aspiration; *TESE*, testicular sperm extraction.
(Courtesy of Silber SJ, Nagy Z, Liu J, et al: The use of epididymal and testicular spermatozoa for intracytoplasmic sperm injection: The genetic implications for male infertility. *Hum Reprod* 10:2031–2043, 1995, by permission of Oxford University Press.)

TABLE 6.—Fertilization and Pregnancy Rate After Intracytoplasmic Sperm Injection With Epididymal and Testicular Spermatozoa in Relation to Age of Female Partner

Age of female partner	No. of patients	No. of eggs (MII)	2PN (%)	No. of cleaved embryos (%)	No. of embryos transferred per patient	No. pregnancies (%)	No. delivered (%)
<30	20	293	138 (47)	91/138 (66)	54 (2.7)	15 (75%)	12 (60)
30–38	35	479	220 (46)	160/220 (73)	104 (3.0)	19 (54%)	11 (31)
>38	17	190	85 (45)	51/85 (60)	51 (3.0)	4 (24%)	1 (6)
Totals	72	962	443 (46)	302/443 (68)	209 (2.9)	38 (53%)	24 (33)

Note: Delivery rate for wives < 38 years of age was 23 of 55 (42%).
Abbreviation: 2PN, 2 pronuclei.
(Courtesy of Silber SJ, Nagy Z, Liu J, et al: The use of epididymal and testicular spermatozoa for intracytoplasmic sperm injection: The genetic implications for male infertility. *Hum Reprod* 10:2031–2043, 1995, by permission of Oxford University Press.)

ered essential for all MESA patients. Even in instances of nonobstructive azoospermia, including Sertoli cell only, or maturation arrest, there typically are some small foci of spermatogenesis. Thus, patients with azoospermia caused by lack of spermatogenesis or a block in meiosis will generally have a few spermatozoa available in the testis that will be sufficient for ICSI. Some forms of severe male factor infertility are genetically transmitted. Therefore, sons of infertile couples may also need ICSI should they desire to start their own families.

▶ This article includes an excellent review of the inheritance patterns of cystic fibrosis and CAV. Cystic fibrosis is one of the most common autosomal recessive genetic disorders in human beings. Whereas virtually all patients with cystic fibrosis also have CAV, only 60% of CAV males are found to be carriers of a cystic fibrosis mutation upon routine screening. The inheritance of CAV on the cystic fibrosis gene seems to follow simple mendelian rules. Genetic counseling is essential before performing ICSI, and preimplantation embryo diagnosis should be considered if both the man and his partner are carriers of the cystic fibrosis gene.

R.Z. Sokol, M.D., F.A.C.P.

Gonadal Hormones and Semen Quality in Male Runners: A Volume Threshold Effect of Endurance Training

De Souza MJ, Arce JC, Pescatello LS, Scherzer HS, Luciano AA (Univ of Connecticut, Farmington; New Britain Gen Hosp, Conn)
Int J Sports Med 15:383–391, 1994   2–11

Background.—Intense endurance training has been associated with a spectrum of menstrual abnormalities in female athletes. In male athletes, endurance training has not been related to a specific "volume-threshold" of training. In fact, data showing a distinct, consistent effect of intense endurance training on male reproductive function are very limited.

Methods.—Eleven high mileage runners (HRs), 9 moderate mileage runners (MRs), and 10 sedentary controls (SCs) of similar age were assessed to determine the effects of volume of endurance training on reproductive function in male runners. Levels of reproductive, adrenal, and thyroid hormones were measured during a 1-hour period of serial blood sampling. Urinary excretion of 24-hour luteinizing hormone (LH) was determined on 2 separate days. Semen examinations and assessment of sperm penetration of standard cervical mucus were performed on 2–5 occasions.

Findings.—Levels of total testosterone and free testosterone were significantly lower in HRs than in MRs and SCs. The 3 groups were comparable in urinary LH, serum LH, follicle-stimulating hormone, and prolactin. There were no other hormonal differences. Compared with SCs, total motile sperm count and density were reduced in HRs. Compared with MRs and SCs, decreased sperm motility and an increased population of immature sperm and round cells were noted in HRs. Sperm penetration of bovine cervical mucus was also lower in HRs than in SCs. Training volume was significantly associated with sperm motility, density, and number of round cells. Number of round cells and total testosterone were significantly correlated.

Conclusion.—There appear to be well-defined differences in reproductive function between HRs and MRs. These include reduced gonadal steroids and disturbed semen quality that are not seen in runners participating in more moderate volumes of training. A volume-threshold training effect appears to be coincident with high volumes of endurance running.

▶ These investigators hypothesized that the greater the volume of training, defined as kilometers per week and hours per week, the greater the disruption of the hypothalamic-pituitary axis. They found that men who ran a minimum of 104 km/wk had subclinical alterations in semen parameters and a subclinical decline in serum testosterone. Men who ran 40–56 km/wk did not. Interestingly, 3 of 9 men among the HRs had a history of infertility. No change in circulating gonadotropins was found, but serial sampling to analyze changes in LH pulsatility was not performed. Because hypercortisolism has been shown both to adversely influence the gonadal axis and to occur in intense athletes, plasma adrenocorticotropic hormone and 24 hour urinary free cortisol were measured. No evidence of hypercortisolism was found. An interesting study would be one reevaluating the high-endurance athletes after a hiatus from exercise to see whether all parameters normalize. This article is highly recommended because of its excellent review of the literature.

R.Z. Sokol, M.D., F.A.C.P.

Prospective Study of Hormonal and Semen Profiles in Marathon Runners

Jensen CE, Wiswedel K, McLoughlin J, van der Spuy Z (Univ of Cape Town, South Africa)
Fertil Steril 64:1189–1196, 1995   2–12

Background.—The long-term effects of endurance training on reproductive function in men have not yet been studied prospectively. Endocrine and semen parameters were investigated in a group of male marathon runners over a 1-year period.

Methods.—Twenty-four healthy men aged 25–64 years were included in the study. The results of hormonal and semen analyses were correlated with the intensity of these runners' training.

Findings.—Training intensity significantly increased in the first 5 months of the study. A significant increase in serum prolactin levels and a decline in progesterone levels accompanied this increase in training intensity. There were no significant changes in plasma levels of total testosterone, luteinizing hormone, follicle-stimulating hormone, or estradiol. There was a significant decline in semen volume as well as sperm motility and morphology during training. However, sperm counts were not significantly affected.

Conclusion.—Endurance training can modify hormonal profiles and semen quantitatively and qualitatively in male marathon runners. The low percentage of morphologically normal sperm documented in the current study is of clinical concern as it may affect fertility rates. It is not clear whether the hormonal and semen parameter changes, as defined in this study, will cause a decrease in fertility potential. Further research is needed.

▶ In this study, marathon runners were followed before and after a period of intense training. Although again some significant changes were noted in sperm motility and morphology, no values fell below the normal ranges. Based on the results of the studies outlined in Abstracts 2–11 and 2–12, one can counsel the marathon runner that although some subclinical changes may occur during the most intense period of training, there is no evidence that fertility is compromised.

R.Z. Sokol, M.D., F.A.C.P.

Occupationally Related Magnetic Field Exposure and Male Subfertility
Lundsberg LS, Bracken MB, Belanger K (Yale Univ, New Haven, Conn)
Fertil Steril 63:384–391, 1995   2–13

Background.—Little research has been done on the reproductive hazards of occupationally related electromagnetic field exposure. Possible relationships between occupationally related magnetic field exposure and male subfertility—as determined by sperm morphology, motility, and concentration—were investigated.

Methods.—The male partners of couples seeking diagnosis and treatment at an infertility clinic were included in the analysis. Data on the first semen analysis and interview information were complete for all men. Case groups consisted of 177 men with abnormal motility, 135 with abnormal morphology, and 172 with abnormal concentration findings. Three hundred four men with normal findings on all 3 parameters made up the control group.

Findings.—Men with high job exposure to magnetic fields had an odds ratio of 0.6 for abnormal morphology, 1.1 for abnormal motility, and 1.0 for abnormal concentrations. Medium levels of magnetic field exposure were unrelated to abnormalities in any of these parameters. Risk estimates were not changed substantially after adjustment for selected risk factors in a multivariate analysis.

Conclusion.—Occupational exposure to magnetic fields is unassociated with male subfertility as defined by morphology, motility, and concentration. Thus, these data do not support theories that magnetic fields have a deleterious effect on male reproductive health.

▶ Electromagnetic fields are the result of electrical power generation. With the advent of the computer age, patients frequently express concern that repeated exposure to the magnetic field of a computer monitor may be harmful to spermatogenesis and fertility. These data indicate that the answer is "no."

R.Z. Sokol, M.D., F.A.C.P.

Breast and Ovarian Cancer Incidence After Infertility and In Vitro Fertilisation
Venn A, Watson L, Lumley J, Giles G, King C, Healy D (La Trobe Univ, Carlton, Australia; Natl Perinatal Epidemiology Unit, Oxford, England; Anti-Cancer Council of Victoria, Carlton, Australia; et al)
Lancet 346:995–1000, 1995

2–14

Background.—Some recent studies have suggested that exposure to fertility drugs may be correlated with an increased risk of ovarian cancer. Studies of cancer in women experiencing infertility have been hampered by low statistical power and the inability to distinguish between the effects of fertility drug exposure and the effects of the underlying ovulation disorder. Studying cancer incidence in women having undergone in vitro fertilization (IVF) allows this distinction because most patients exposed to ovarian stimulation for IVF do not have abnormal ovulatory patterns. The incidence of cancer in a cohort of women referred for IVF was analyzed in an effort to determine whether cancer risk is increased by exposure to fertility drugs.

Methods.—The records of 10,358 women referred for IVF during a 14-year period were evaluated. Ovarian stimulation (to produce multiple folliculogenesis) was performed in 5,564 women; the remaining 4,794 women were either untreated or underwent natural cycle treatment without fertility drug exposure. The duration of follow-up ranged from 1 to 15 years. Record linkage with data from population-based cancer registries was used to identify women with cancer.

Results.—Invasive ovarian cancer developed in 6 women; invasive breast cancer developed in 34. The expected numbers of cases of cancer, as determined by application of age-standardized general population rates, were compared with the statistics from the cohort, resulting in a 0.89 standardized incidence ratio (SIR) for breast cancer in the exposed group and a 0.98 SIR for breast cancer in the unexposed group. Women exposed to fertility drugs had a 1.70 SIR for ovarian cancer; unexposed women had an SIR of 1.62. The incidence of cancers among women exposed to fertility drugs was also evaluated as to number of IVF cycles. The risk of cancer did not appear to increase in association with greater exposure to stimulated treatment cycles. The rate of all cancers among the cohort did not differ significantly from that of the general population. After adjustment for age and infertility type, treated women had a relative risk of breast cancer of 1.11 relative to untreated women and a relative risk of ovarian cancer of 1.45 relative to untreated women. Risks of ovarian cancer and body-of-uterus cancer were increased in women with unexplained infertility relative to those with known causes of infertility, independent of IVF exposure. The combined group of treated and untreated women had an increased risk of cancer of the body of the uterus.

Conclusion.—The incidence of breast cancer in women treated with fertility drugs for IVF was not significantly greater than either that of women referred for IVF but not treated or that of the general population. The incidence of body-of-uterus cancer appeared higher in the cohort, but this could be an artifact of the increased gynecologic surveillance of women experiencing infertility. Little evidence existed to establish a link between fertility-drug use and incidence of ovarian cancer. However, this study was limited by the rarity of ovarian cancer and the relatively short follow-up. Lack of reliable information regarding parity is also a limitation because nulliparity, which is likely to be more prevalent among women in the cohort than among the general population, is a risk factor for several cancers.

▶ The risk of ovarian cancer in women is inversely associated with parity. The risk is also reduced by the use of oral contraceptives, with the extent of the reduction in risk directly related to the duration of oral contraceptive use. Therefore, it has been hypothesized that the risk of ovarian cancer is directly related to the number of times a woman ovulates in her lifetime. There has been a suggestion that administration of ovulation-inducing agents to anovulatory women may increase their risk of ovarian cancer, but there are no definitive studies to support this assumption. Infertile women undergoing IVF usually ovulate regularly and are nulliparous.

The results of this study indicate that with only a few years of follow-up, there is little evidence that administration of agents that induce multiple ovulations increases the risk of either ovarian cancer or breast cancer. Obviously, further studies with a longer follow-up (until the age when ovarian cancer becomes more common) are needed to determine whether the use of agents that induce multiple ovulations in ovulatory women affects these risks for any type of cancer.

D.R. Mishell, Jr., M.D.

3 Diagnostic Evaluation of the Female Partner

Infertility Evaluation in Fertile Women: A Model for Assessing the Efficacy of Infertility Testing
Guzick DS, Grefenstette I, Baffone K, Berga SL, Krasnow JS, Stovall DW, Naus GJ (Univ of Pittsburgh, Pa)
Hum Reprod 9:2306–2310, 1994

3–1

Background.—The standard infertility workup consists of semen analysis, hysterosalpingography, a postcoital test, an endometrial biopsy, and laparoscopy. These tests, although clinically well grounded, have not been proven to consistently distinguish infertile from fertile couples.

Objective.—Thirty-two matched pairs of fertile and infertile couples underwent the standard infertility tests and, in addition, were tested for sperm antibodies and had cervical culture for *Mycoplasma hominis* and *Ureaplasma urealyticum*. The average duration of infertility was approximately 4 years. Fertile women, matched with the infertility group for age and race, had been delivered of a child within the past 2 years and were scheduled for laparoscopic tubal ligation.

Results.—Twenty-two of the 32 fertile couples (69%) had at least 1 abnormal test. All types of infertility factors other than endometriosis were identified. In many cases, the abnormalities related to male, tubal, and luteal-phase deficiency factors would have been considered moderate in severity. Endometriosis and tubal damage, but not other abnormalities, were significantly more prevalent in the infertile couples

Implications.—Two thirds of fertile couples in this study proved to have at least one infertility factor, and many of these factors were as prevalent as in the matched infertile couples. Some infertility tests—such as semen analysis and endometrial biopsy—may best be investigated in large samples.

▶ When abnormal results occur in many of the diagnostic tests clinicians use to evaluate infertile couples, it has not been shown that the abnormality is a cause of the infertility. Therapy for luteal-phase insufficiency, antisperm antibodies, mild abnormalities in the semen analysis that do not persist, mild degrees of hyperprolactinemia in ovulatory women, and mild or minimal endometriosis have not been shown in randomized trials to be more effective than no therapy in the treatment of infertile couples. Therefore, there is no need to perform these tests to determine whether results are abnormal as the tests are costly and do not aid in the treatment of the infertile couples. As shown in this study, many of these abnormalities are also present in the majority of couples with proven fertility.

D.R. Mishell, Jr., M.D.

Chlamydia trachomatis Antibody Titers and Hysterosalpingography in Predicting Tubal Disease in Infertility Patients

Meikle SF, Calonge BN, Zhang X, Hamman RF, Marine WM, Betz G (Univ of Colorado, Denver; Colorado Permanente Med Group, Denver)
Fertil Steril 62:305–312, 1994

3–2

Background.—Infertility from tubal disease affects 10% to 20% of couples in North America. The number of diagnostic laparoscopies done on women without tubal adhesive disease may be reduced by testing for tubal disease with *Chlamydia trachomatis* antibody titers and hysterosalpingography (HSG), singly or together.

Methods.—Seven hundred three patients with infertility who had *C. trachomatis* antibody titers done between 1988 and 1992 were included in the study. The final study group included 218 patients with antibody titers, HSG, and laparoscopy.

Findings.—Hysterosalpingography had a sensitivity and negative predictive value of 78% and 85%, respectively. For *C. trachomatis* titers, the sensitivity and negative predictive value were 78% and 82%, respectively. There was no significant difference. False negative rates were the same for the 2 tests, but false positive rates were lowest for HSG and series testing (Table 2).

Conclusion.—To minimize false positive tests and unnecessary laparoscopies, HSG can be done alone or combined with the *C. trachomatis* antibody titer as series tests. This strategy is associated with a significantly

TABLE 2.—Diagnostic Test Results

HSG/chlamydia titer results	Tubal Disease on Laparoscopy		Total
	+	−	
+HSG/+Titer	53	7	60
+ HSG/−Titer	15	14	39
−HSG/+Titer	15	40	55
−HSG/−Titer	4	70	74
Total	87	131	218

Abbreviation: HSG, hysterosalpingography
(From Meikle SF, Calonge BN, Zhang X, et al: Chlamydia trachomatis antibody titers and hysterosalpingography in predicting tubal disease in infertility patients. *Fertil Steril* 62:305–312, 1994. Reproduced with permission of the publisher, the American Society for Reproductive Medicine [The American Fertility Society].)

lower false positive rate. In this series, when both tests were negative, tubal disease was identified on laparoscopy in only 5% of subjects.

▶ As shown in Table 2, of 74 patients with normal HSG results and a negative titer of antibodies to *C. trachomatis,* only 4 had evidence of tubal disease at the time of diagnostic laparoscopy for infertility. A laparoscopy is a costly invasive procedure. Hysterosalpingography and measurement of antibodies to *C. trachomatis* are much less costly.

In view of the fact that if these 2 tests are negative only 5% of women will have tubal disease, it does not appear to be cost-effective to perform a diagnostic laparoscopy on all women with infertility who have normal HSG results and a negative antibody titer for *C. trachomatis.* If the semen analysis of the male partner reveals a sufficient number of mobile sperm to fertilize an egg and the woman is ovulatory, several cycles of controlled ovarian hyperstimulation followed by intrauterine insemination should be tried before proceeding with a diagnostic laparoscopy.

D.R. Mishell, Jr., M.D.

Infertile Couples With a Normal Hysterosalpingogram: Reproductive Outcome and Its Relationship to Clinical and Laparoscopic Findings
Cundiff G, Carr BR, Marshburn PB (Univ of Texas, Dallas)
J Reprod Med 40:19–24, 1995   3–3

Background.—Hysterosalpingography (HSG) is useful for examination of the intraluminal environment of the fallopian tube and endometrial cavity. If abnormalities are detected at HSG, this examination is followed with more invasive and costly laparoscopy or hysteroscopy. However, if the HSG findings are normal, it is not clear what course to follow. A retrospective review of infertile couples with normal HSG results was performed to assess subsequent fertility and laparoscopic findings.

Subjects.—A retrospective analysis was performed of 132 couples with normal HSG results, who were evaluated at the University of Texas Southwestern Medical Center between 1986 and 1991. Inclusion criteria were normal HSG results during infertility evaluation and at least 6 months of follow-up. Hysterosalpingograms were obtained using water-soluble contrast medium. Of the 132 patients, 33 underwent subsequent diagnostic laparoscopy. At presentation, the couples had an average age of 29 years, with at least 3 years of infertility. They were monitored for an average of 17 months.

Findings.—During the 3 months after the HSG, there was a fourfold higher rate of pregnancy than during any other 3-month period. Among the patients who received laparoscopy, 56% had pelvic pathology. There was an increased proportion of abnormal findings with an increasing time interval between HSG and laparoscopy. Abnormal uterine bleeding was correlated with abnormalities at laparoscopy. Prior use of oral contraceptives was negatively correlated with pelvic pathology.

Conclusion.—When infertile couples have normal results of HSG, laparoscopy should not be performed for at least 3 months, because HSG with water-soluble contrast medium appears to have a beneficial effect on fertility during that period. Women who have not conceived within 1 year of HSG should have laparoscopy, as there is a high incidence of pelvic pathology in this group, which can affect treatment.

▶ Of the 33 women who had normal HSG results, 14 had normal laparoscopic results, 11 had some type of pelvic adhesions, and 2 had some degree of endometriosis. It is probable that most of the women with adhesions would have a positive *Chlamydia* antibody titer and most of the women with endometriosis would have had a history of dysmenorrhea, pelvic pain, or an elevated serum CA 125. It is unlikely that women with a negative *Chlamydia* antibody titer and no symptoms or signs of endometriosis would have sufficient pelvic pathology to cause them to be infertile. Therefore, in such instances, the cost-effectiveness of diagnostic laparoscopy should be questioned.

D.R. Mishell, Jr., M.D.

In-Vitro Cervical Mucus–Sperm Penetration Tests and Outcome of Infertility Treatments in Couples With Repeatedly Negative Post-Coital Tests
Farhi J, Valentine A, Bahadur G, Shenfield F, Steele SJ, Jacobs HS
(Middlesex Hosp, London)
Hum Reprod 10:85–90, 1995   3–4

Objective.—Negative postcoital test (PCT) results may be associated with a wide range of clinical problems including anovulation, structural abnormalities of the cervix, problems in deposition, and abnormal semen. The results of the in vitro cervical mucus–sperm penetration test (CMSPT) and cross-hostility testing were examined in 178 infertile couples having repeatedly negative PCT results. The average duration of infertility was 3.3 years.

Methods.—All couples received 3 cycles of intrauterine insemination (IUI) alone and 3 further cycles of IUI combined with ovulation induction using human menopausal gonadotropins or follicle-stimulating hormone. The CMSPT was timed to coincide with the urinary luteinizing hormone surge. A cross-hostility test was done in each case using fresh donor semen.

Results.—In cases of male factor infertility, the number of sperm and the percentage of motile spermatozoa were significantly lower in husband samples than in donor samples. Failure of the husbands' spermatozoa to penetrate cervical mucus did not, however, indicate deficient fertilizing potential in vivo. The performance of donor sperm in the cervical mucus correlated with the pregnancy rate. The overall pregnancy rate after 6 cycles of IUI was 28%. Pregnancy was possible by IUI alone when the husband's spermatozoa failed to penetrate cervical mucus. The cross-hostility test clearly distinguished the abnormal factor.

Implications.—Before advising assisted reproduction on the grounds of failed sperm penetration in male factor infertility, it would be best to attempt IUI. Women with polycystic ovaries and repeatedly negative PCTs should be suspected of having low-quality cervical mucus. In these cases, IUI should be accompanied by ovulation induction.

▶ The finding of several PCTs in which sperm do not penetrate the cervical mucus is most likely a cause of infertility. However, because the treatment of this problem is the same as treatment of unexplained infertility, controlled ovarian hyperstimulation and IUI, it is no longer necessary to perform the emotionally bothersome diagnostic PCT as part of the diagnostic infertility evaluation. Even though the sperm cannot penetrate the cervical mucus, they usually have the capacity to fertilize the ovum in vivo as shown in this study by the 28% pregnancy rate after 6 cycles of intrauterine insemination.

D.R. Mishell, Jr., M.D.

4 Diagnostic Evaluation of the Male Partner

Hyaluronidase Activity in Human Semen: Correlation With Fertilization In Vitro
Abdul-Aziz M, MacLusky NJ, Bhavnani BR, Casper RF (Univ of Toronto)
Fertil Steril 64:1147–1153, 1995   4–1

Background.—Traditional semen analysis supplies information about sperm count, motility, and morphologic characteristics, but it cannot be used alone to predict the success of in vitro fertilization (IVF). An acrosomal enzyme, hyaluronidase, is important during fertilization. The relationships between hyaluronidase activity and traditional semen analysis results, and between hyaluronidase activity and fertility rates in vitro were investigated prospectively.

Methods.—A total of 408 semen samples were collected from men involved in an IVF program, men attending fertility clinics, and healthy sperm donors. Sperm count and motility were assessed using the Cellsoft computer-assisted semen analysis system. Morphologic features were assessed using World Health Organization standards for semen analysis. A modification of the method described by Singer et al., which involves measuring areas of substrate hydrolysis in agar dishes, was used to measure hyaluronidase activity.

Results.—The hyaluronidase activity was similar in fresh and frozen semen specimens. Significant correlations were found between hyaluronidase activity and the sperm concentration, percentage of mobile sperm, and percentage of sperm with normal morphologic features. In the 160 IVF samples studied, the correlation between the fertilization rate and the hyaluronidase activity (ring size) was high. Whatever the sperm count, motility, or morphologic profile in the 14 samples tested, a ring size of $\leq$ 3 mm was associated with a zero fertility rate. The median fertility rate in the 55 samples with a ring size of 3.1–5.5 mm was 57%, in the 78 samples with a ring size of 5.6–8 mm was 70%, and in the 23 samples with a ring size of 8.1–11 mm was 87%.

Conclusions.—The measurement of semen hyaluronidase activity may be a useful means to assess sperm function in human beings. If the semen hyaluronidase activity is very low, intracytoplasmic sperm injection without a prior attempt at IVF should be considered.

▶ Except for the classic parameters of sperm concentrations, motility, and morphologic characteristics, which are measured in the semen analyses, there are no other tests that can reliably quantitate the degree to which sperm can effect fertilization of the ovum. Measurement of semen hyaluronidase activity is not a difficult technical procedure. The results of this study indicate that it may be useful to determine the amount of hyaluronidase activity in the semen sample to help predict the ability of the sperm to fertilize the ovum.

D.R. Mishell, Jr., M.D.

Sperm Morphology and In Vitro Fertilization Outcome: A Direct Comparison of World Health Organization and Strict Criteria Methodologies
Morgentaler A, Powers RD, Fung MY, Alper MM, Harris DH (Harvard Med School, Boston; Boston IVF, Brookline, Mass)
Fertil Steril 64:1177–1182, 1995   4–2

Background.—Kruger et al. have described a set of strict criteria for normal sperm morphology that are highly correlated with in vitro fertilization (IVF) outcome. In contrast, studies using World Health Organization (WHO) criteria have shown mixed results. Strict criteria were directly compared with WHO criteria in a prospective study.

Methods.—Data from of 132 of 141 consecutive couples undergoing IVF were adequate for analysis. Morphology assessment of semen using strict criteria was done by technicians specifically trained in this technique. Later, the same slides were assessed in a different laboratory by a blinded technician trained only in the WHO morphology method. The WHO morphology technique primarily differs from the strict criteria in that it classifies borderline sperm head forms as normal.

Results.—When WHO criteria with a threshold of $\geq$ 40% were used, 71% of men had normal sperm morphology. When strict criteria with a threshold $\geq$ 4% were used, 58% of men had normal sperm morphology. One or more eggs were fertilized in 90 of the 132 couples. The WHO morphology scores $\geq$ 65% were associated with a fertilization rate of 90%. The fertilization rate for men with WHO scores < 40% was only 32%. The fertilization rate for men with strict criteria scores < 4% was 64%. More than 2 fertilized eggs were present in only 1 case in which the WHO criteria score was < 40%. In contrast, up to 5 fertilized eggs were found with the lowest strict criteria scores. The WHO criteria scores were associated with a significantly higher sensitivity (87% vs. 61%) and negative predictive value (68% vs. 36%) for IVF than strict criteria scores.

Conclusions.—The WHO criteria for assessing sperm morphology are more predictive of IVF outcomes than strict criteria. Because WHO criteria results are a good predictor of IVF outcomes, further studies of the WHO sperm morphology assessment method and male fertility are warranted.

▶ The results of this study indicate that the WHO criteria used to assess sperm morphology yield an adequate correlation with the degree to which these sperm can fertilize an ovum in an in vitro system. If the semen analyses showed more than 40% normal sperm head forms, fertilization occurred in more than 80% of the IVF cycles. However, if there were less than 40% normal sperm head forms, the fertilization rate was only 32%. Thus, the established criteria of 40% normal morphology appears to be a reasonable place to separate normal from abnormal sperm head morphology.

D.R. Mishell, Jr., M.D.

Selenium Supplementation Enhances the Element Concentration in Blood and Seminal Fluid But Does Not Change the Spermatozoal Quality Characteristics in Subfertile Men
Iwanier K, Zachara BA (Municipal Hosp, Grudziądz, Poland; Univ School of Med Sciences, Bydgoszcz, Poland)
J Androl 16:441–447, 1995   4–3

Background.—The sperm selenium (Se) level in infertile men has been found to be lower than that in fertile men. Low sperm motility has been associated with reduced sperm Se concentration. More recently, Se supplementation in subfertile men was shown to increase sperm motility to a degree not achieved by any of the other antioxidant micronutrients given. In that research, however, the effect of Se supplementation on seminal fluid Se levels, glutathione peroxidase (GSH-Px) activity, sperm count, and sperm morphologic characteristics was not measured. The effects of supplementation with 2 forms of Se on Se levels and GSH-Px activity in seminal fluid and on spermatozoal quality characteristics in subfertile men were investigated.

Methods.—Thirty-three men received 200 μg Se/day for 12 weeks. Sixteen men, comprising group 1, were given yeast-rich Se, and 17 men, comprising group 2, were given sodium selenite. Blood samples and sperm were obtained at the beginning of the study and 2, 4, 8, and 12 weeks after Se supplementation.

Findings.—Levels of Se in whole blood and plasma were significantly increased during the course of treatment. This effect was more pronounced in the group given yeast-Se. Both groups also had an increase in Se concentration in seminal fluid, but the effect of yeast-Se was substantially greater than that of selenite. In both groups, Se levels in plasma were significantly associated with seminal fluid. In the yeast-Se group, GSH-Px activity in seminal fluid rose significantly, reaching a plateau after 2 weeks. In the selenite group, the activity did not change during the course of treatment. Selenium levels were weakly correlated with GSH-Px activities in seminal fluid. The relationship between these values was significant only in the yeast-Se group. No response in sperm count, motility, or morphologic characteristics was observed in either group.

Conclusions.—Supplementation of subfertile men with yeast-rich Se had a more marked effect on Se levels and GSH-Px activities in blood components and seminal fluid than did selenite. However, supplementation with Se did not improve sperm count, motility, or morphologic characteristics.

▶ Because GSH-peroxidase is an Se-containing antioxidant enzyme, Se supplementation has been suggested as a therapy for idiopathic male infertility. Although Se supplementation resulted in an increase in Se seminal plasma concentration, no improvement was noted in sperm count or motility. Improvement in fertility potential as reflected in changes in sperm function test results was not studied.

R.Z. Sokol, M.D., F.A.C.P.

Excretion of Alpha-Tocopherol Into Human Seminal Plasma After Oral Administration
Moilanen J, Hovatta O (Family Federation of Finland, Infertility Clinic, Helsinki)
Andrologia 27:133–136, 1995   4–4

Introduction.—Alpha-tocopherol (α-tocopherol), a lipid-soluble antioxidant, protects spermatozoa against damage from free radicals in vitro. It is possible to increase the α-tocopherol level in seminal plasma by 1 month of oral supplementation.

Study Plan.—Fifteen unselected males, 9 of them outpatients at an infertility clinic and 6 with no history of infertility, were given d-α-tocopherol in a dose of 600, 800, or 1,200 mg daily for 3 weeks in the form of 200-mg capsules.

Results.—Plasma levels of α-tocopherol increased significantly after 1 week of treatment, most markedly in those given 800 mg daily. Plasma vitamin E levels increased significantly more in patients given this dose than in those given 600 mg daily. Seminal plasma levels of α-tocopherol increased significantly, from 0.54 to 0.75 µmol/L, after 3 weeks of treatment. After this time the changes in blood and seminal plasma levels correlated to a significant degree. No significant improvement was noted in the movement characteristics of spermatozoa.

Conclusion.—Oral administration of d-α-tocopherol increases the level in seminal plasma, but not to the extent that it protects spermatozoa in vitro against peroxidative damage.

Magnolol Protects Human Sperm Motility Against Lipid Peroxidation: A Sperm Head Fixation Method

Lin MH, Chao HT, Hong CY (Inst of Traditional Medicine, Natl Yang-Ming Univ, Taipei, Taiwan, Republic of China; Veterans Gen Hosp, Taipei, Taiwan, Republic of China)
Arch Androl 34:151–156, 1995

4–5

Background.—Free radical damage by toxic oxygen metabolites has been implicated in impaired sperm function. Magnolol is a component of the bark of a Chinese medical herb that reputedly possesses antibacterial activity, has a muscle relaxant effect, inhibits central nervous function, and counters platelet aggregation. Magnolol is nearly one thousand times more potent than vitamin E in suppressing lipid peroxidation in rat heart mitochondria.

Objective and Methods.—The effects of magnolol on human spermatozoa, particularly on motility and lipid peroxidation, were studied using samples of human semen obtained from healthy subjects by masturbation. Tail beat frequency was estimated using a sperm-head fixation method. Lipid peroxidation was induced by $FeSO_4$.

Findings.—Tail beat frequency was significantly depressed when sperm were exposed to $FeSO_4$, and this effect was reversed by as little as 10^{-9} mol of magnolol. The formation of malondialdehyde induced by $FeSO_4$ was significantly inhibited by magnolol in concentrations that reversed approximately 40% of the suppressive effect on tail beat frequency.

Conclusion.—Magnolol appears to maintain sperm motility by inhibiting iron-induced lipid peroxidation.

▶ Reactive oxygen species (ROS) are oxidizing agents categorized as free radicals. Free radicals contain one or more impaired electrons. The ROS of importance in fertility include the superoxide anion, hydrogen peroxide, peroxyl radicals, and nitric oxide. A delicate balance exists between the production of ROS and the ability of antioxidants (superoxide dismutase, catalase, glutathione-peroxidase, and glutathione-reductase) to dispose of ROS. A shift in the balance in either direction has been associated with altered sperm function. Mammalian spermatozoa, because they are rich in polyunsaturated fatty acids, are suspectile to ROS. Lipid peroxidation alters the sperm membrane, possibly leading to deleterious effects on sperm capacitation and the acrosome reaction.

Investigations into the protective effects of antioxidants on peroxidative damage of spermatozoa yield variable results. A number of compounds have been studied including vitamin E, magnolol, and selenium. Vitamin E (α-tocopherol) is a lipid-soluble antioxidant naturally present in cell membranes. It interferes with the free radical reaction by forming a relatively stable tocopheroxyl radical. The seminal plasma levels required for protection against peroxidative damage in vitro cannot be achieved by oral vitamin E supplementation. Magnolol, an active component isolated from the bark of a Chinese medicine herb, inhibits lipid peroxidation of spermatozoa in vitro. Its usefulness in a clinical setting has not been studied.

R.Z. Sokol, M.D., F.A.C.P.

Predicting the Fertilizing Potential of Human Sperm Suspensions In Vitro: Importance of Sperm Morphology and Leukocyte Contamination
Sukcharoen N, Keith J, Irvine DS, Aitken RJ (Univ of Edinburgh, Scotland)
Fertil Steril 63:1293–1300, 1995   4–6

Introduction.—Failed fertilization could result from any of the many different aspects of sperm physiology. In couples undergoing in vitro fertilization (IVF), some sperm function tests do appear to provide information that is correlated with the in vitro fertilizing potential of the spermatozoa. Relationships between various criteria of semen quality and the fertilization of human ova in vitro were studied.

Methods.—The analysis included 41 infertile couples undergoing IVF-ET. The spermatozoa's ability to achieve fertilization in vitro was compared with various criteria of semen quality. These included the conventional semen profile, computer-aided assessment of sperm movement, ionophore-induced acrosome reaction, acridine orange staining, sperm morphology, and chemiluminescent signals induced by phorbol ester and N-formyl-methionyl-leucyl-phenylalanine (FMLP).

Results.—Fertilization rates were significantly correlated with several sperm attributes. These included aspects of sperm function, as assessed by acrosome reaction; movement, as assessed by percentage motile, hyperactivation, and amplitude of lateral sperm head displacement; morphology, as assessed by normal morphologic characteristics, midpiece defects, and multiple anomalies index; nuclear normality, as assessed by acridine orange staining; and reaction oxygen species generation, as assessed by chemiluminescence induced by phorbol ester and FMLP (Fig 1). Stepwise multiple regression analysis permitted accurate prediction of fertilization rates using a multiple regression equation. Of the 6 variables included in this equation, sperm morphology and FMLP-induced chemiluminescence had the best predictive ability.

Conclusions.—The criteria identified in this study can accurately predict the in vitro fertilization potential of human sperm suspensions. Sperm morphology and degree of leukocyte contamination appear to be particularly important in this regard. Future studies aimed at optimizing IVF-ET procedures should include a systematic evaluation of the best techniques for counteracting the disruptive effects of leukocytes.

▶ As discussed in the previous 2 abstracts (Abstracts 4–4 and 4–5), excessive generation of reactive oxygen species in semen, mainly by neutrophils, but with some contribution by abnormal spermatozoa, may lead to infertility. In this study, an attempt was made to determine in a prospective manner whether selected sperm function tests are predictive of success in an IVF

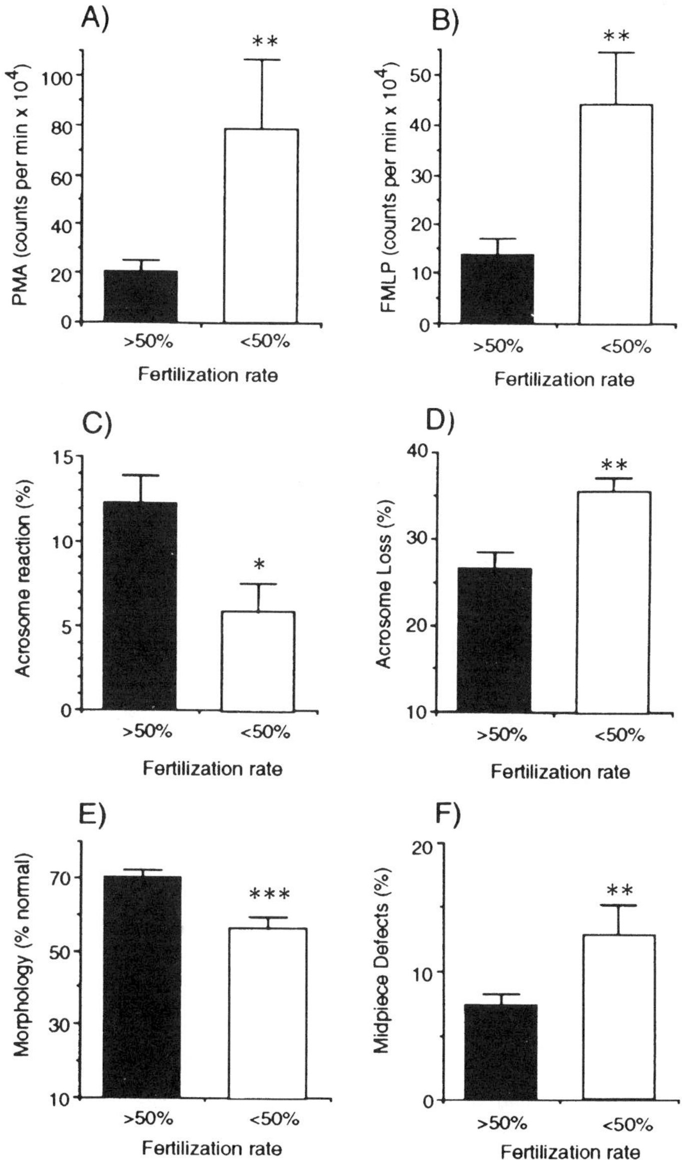

FIGURE 1.—Quality of the sperm suspensions in relation to the fertilizing potential of the spermatozoa in vitro. Samples fertilizing < 50% of ova were characterized by significantly higher levels of (**A**) phorbol ester- and (**B**) *N*-formyl-methionyl-leucyl-phenylalanine (*FMLP*)-induced luminol-dependent chemiluminescence, (**C**) significantly lower levels of A23187-induced acrosome reaction, (**D**) significantly higher levels of complete acrosome loss in response to ionophore, (**E**) a significantly lower proportion of morphologically normal spermatozoa, and (**F**) a significantly higher incidence of midpiece defects. Data are presented as means ± SEM. (From Sukcharoen N, Keith J, Irvine DS, et al: Predicting the fertilizing potential of human sperm suspensions in vitro: Importance of sperm morphology and leukocyte contamination. *Fertil Steril* 63:1293–1300, 1995. Reproduced with permission of the publisher, the American Society for Reproductive Medicine [The American Fertility Society].)

setting. The percentage of normal forms based on World Health Organization criteria and the presence of reactive oxygen species in seminal plasma were positively (morphologic) and negatively (oxygen radicals) correlated with IVF outcome.

R.Z. Sokol, M.D., F.A.C.P.

Sperm Morphology Using Strict Criteria After Percoll Density Separation: Influence on Cleavage and Pregnancy Rates After In-Vitro Fertilization
Yue Z, Meng FJ, Jørgensen N, Ziebe S, Andersen AN (Herlev Univ Hosp, Copenhagen; Rigshospitalet, Copenhagen)
Hum Reprod 10:1781–1785, 1995   4–7

Background.—Both the swim-up procedure and separation on discontinuous Percoll gradients increase the percentage of morphologically normal spermatozoa, but the latter has the greatest recovery. Studies of the clinical importance of the Percoll technique have yielded conflicting results. Percoll separation mainly selects motile sperm cells. Sperm morphology is normally assessed on a fixed smear from the original sperm sample, which includes motile as well as immotile and presumably dead sperm cells. The use of morphology evaluation using strict criteria on the sperm sample after Percoll separation was investigated.

Methods.—A consecutive, unselected series of 213 oocyte aspirations in 159 women were assessed. One hundred seventy-seven aspirations were from patients with tubal infertility, and 36 from patients with unexplained infertility. The analysis included 197 aspirations in which the semen sample used for insemination had a normal sperm concentration. Of 1,413 oocytes aspirated, 863 were fertilized and cleaved. A total of 492 preembryos were transferred in 193 cycles, resulting in a 42% pregnancy rate per transfer.

Findings.—Percoll separation significantly increased the percentage of sperm cells with normal morphologic characteristics from 7.7% to 11.3%. In a sperm morphology analysis, Percoll separation was found to reduce the number of sperm samples in the group with a poor prognosis pattern from 31% to 13% and increased the number of samples considered normal from 16% to 33%. After Percoll separation, the group with the poor prognosis pattern had a 46% cleavage rate, which was significantly lower than in the groups with normal and good prognosis patterns. However, compared with the normal group, the group with poor prognosis had a significantly greater pregnancy rate. The groups with poor prognosis and good prognosis patterns had significantly greater rates of ongoing pregnancies, deliveries, and implantation than the normal group.

Conclusions.—A reduced cleavage rate and a significant but marginally decreased number of embryos transferred were predicted by less than 4% normal spermatozoa. However, rates of pregnancy and delivery were at least as good as in couples with normal morphology scores.

▶ This study by Yue and associates confirms the association between a low percentage of morphologically normal spermatozoa as defined by the strict criteria and a low cleavage rate. However the predictability of pregnancy rates is not conclusive. Indeed, the group with < 4% normal forms and the group with 4% to 14% normal forms resulted in pregnancy rates of 52% and 32%, respectively, which were greater than the group with > 14% normal forms (13% pregnancy rate). These morphology assessments were done, however, on sperm harvested after Percoll gradient separation, a technique that selects for specific sperm populations. Percoll gradients also help to remove neutrophils, which as discussed in the previous abstract (Abstract 4–6) decrease the amount of oxygen radicals available to inhibit fertilization. This might explain the results of this experiment. Pre- and post-Percoll white blood cell content would have been useful information.

R.Z. Sokol, M.D., F.A.C.P.

A Quality Control System for the Optimized Sperm Penetration Assay
Johnson A, Bassham B, Lipshultz LI, Lamb DJ (Baylor College of Medicine, Houston)
Fertil Steril 64:832–837, 1995   4–8

Background.—The sperm penetration assay (SPA) is used to assess the functional events necessary for sperm capacitation and egg penetration. Although some researchers have found an excellent association between SPA results and in vitro fertilization outcomes, others have reported a poor correlation and high false negative rates. Technical and/or biological problems may produce assay variability. A quality control system for the

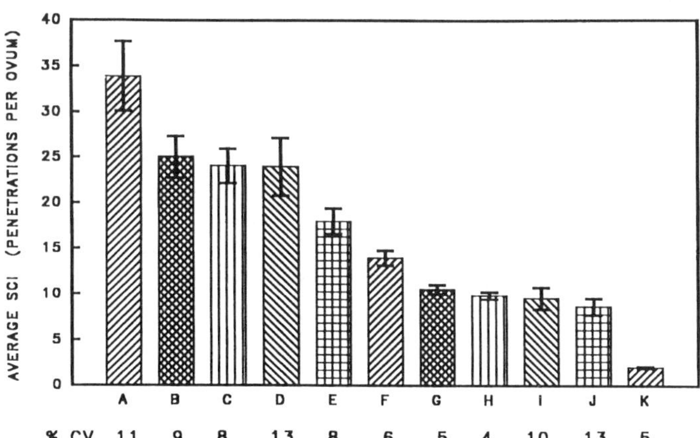

FIGURE 2.—Intra-assay variability in the optimized SPA. Semen from 11 donors was divided into 3 equal portions for assay in triplicate in the optimized SPA. Results are expressed as the average sperm capacitation index (mean ± 1 SD). The coefficients of variation (CV) were A, 11%; B, 9%; C, 8%; D, 13%; E, 8%; F, 6%; G, 5%; H, 4%; I, 10%; J, 13%; and K, 5%. (From Johnson A, Bassham B, Lipshultz LI, et al: A quality control system for the optimized sperm penetration assay. *Fertil Steril* 64:832–837, 1995. Reproduced with permission of the publisher, the American Society for Reproductive Medicine [The American Fertility Society].)

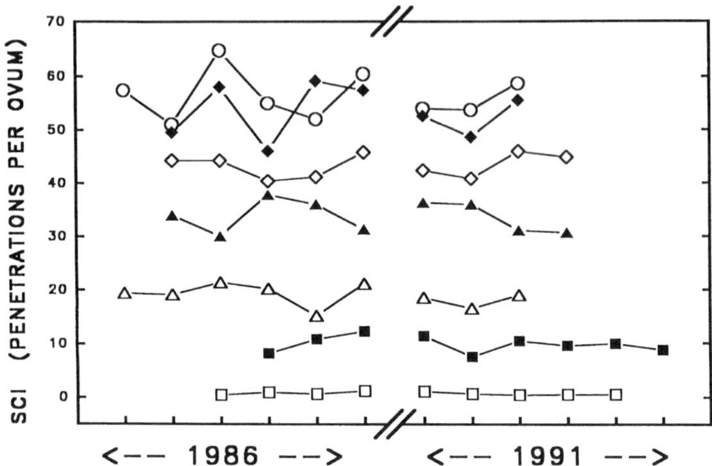

FIGURE 3.—Analysis of 7 cryopreserved semen specimens in the optimized sperm penetration assay (*SPA*): assay stability over a 5-year period. Semen from 7 individuals was frozen in aliquots and then used as a control in the optimized SPA in 1986 and again in 1991. Results are expressed as the sperm capacitation index obtained in each assay. The figure shows the assay results over a 1-month period for each specimen because many of the straws from different controls were tested in different assays. (From Johnson A, Bassham B, Lipshultz LI, et al: A quality control system for the optimized sperm penetration assay. *Fertil Steril* 64:832–837, 1995. Reproduced with permission of the publisher, the American Society for Reproductive Medicine [The American Fertility Society].)

optimal SPA was developed and used to monitor interassay variability and stability over time.

Methods.—Four semen donors underwent consecutive testing for 7–139 weeks with the SPA. Mean semen analyses and SPA scores were assessed to monitor natural biological variation. Intra-assay variation was determined by dividing 11 semen samples into 3 aliquots and assessing each one separately. Single ejaculates were obtained from 7 men, aliquoted, and frozen to serve as control samples. These aliquots were tested on different days in 1986 and 1991 to determine assay stability over time.

Findings.—Coefficients of variation in consecutive weekly semen analyses and SPAs ranged from 20% to more than 40%. These variations were much wider than intra-assay variations. The frozen specimens assessed in several SPAs also exhibited a low coefficient of variation. When aliquots were tested 5 years later, the values were the same, demonstrating remarkable stability of the SPA over time. The lower limit of the normal fertile range was unchanged over 2 years (Figs 2 and 3).

Conclusions.—Fresh semen samples are not adequate positive controls in the SPA. The use of frozen semen controls overcomes this problem. Using frozen specimens for quality control, the optimized SPA developed by the authors is very reproducible and meets the strict criteria needed for clinical laboratory certification.

▶ This study is important for a number of reasons. The SPA, first introduced in the 1970s, has a checkered history. Whereas some investigators consider it to be a reliable indicator of fertility potential, others do not. The lack of reliability is most likely attributable to the lack of assay standardization, which leads to assay variability. This variability is secondary to inconsistencies in the processing of the sperm and ova. Using an optimized SPA developed in their laboratory, Lamb and co-workers introduce quality control procedures that will enhance the reliability and sensitivity of the assay. Specific technical details for optimizing the SPA are included in the paper.

The use of frozen semen standards to assess quality control is an excellent approach. Laboratories will be able to exchange cryobanked semen for parallel testing, providing a method for both assay quality control and proficiency testing. With the advent of intracytoplasmic sperm injection (ICSI), the SPA may become an important tool for determining whether standard in vitro fertilization or ICSI should be used.

R.Z. Sokol, M.D., F.A.C.P.

Analysis of TEST (TES and Tris) Yolk Buffer Effects on Human Sperm
Jacobs BR, Caulfield J, Boldt J (Albany Med College, NY)
Fertil Steril 63:1064–1070, 1995   4–9

Background.—The sensitivity of the sperm penetration assay (SPA) may be increased through the use of alternative sperm preparation methods. In these procedures, semen samples are incubated at a low temperature in TEST yolk buffer (TYB). However, the biological basis for improvement in sperm penetration capacity after TYB treatment is not well understood. The biological effects of TYB treatment on sperm function were assessed.

Methods and Findings.—Sperm penetration levels in the SPA and acrosomal loss were assessed in donor sperm using a fluorescent lectin staining method. The rate of acrosomal loss was higher in sperm incubated in TYB for 42–46 hours at 4°C than in sperm capacitated in Biggers-Whitten-Whittingham (BWW) media for 20–22 hours, but the difference was nonsignificant. When insemination concentrations were normalized to identical acrosome-reacted sperm levels, specimens treated in TYB had much greater penetration levels than BWW specimens. Penetration levels were identical in samples incubated in BWW and in TYB for 42–46 hours at 4°C before heat shock. Penetration levels were significantly greater in samples washed with 37°C BWW than in those washed with 4°C BWW.

Conclusions.—Although TYB increases acrosome reactions, this treatment alone does not explain the substantial rise in penetration levels occurring in SPA. Treatment with TYB is not needed to enhance penetration. The heat shock step of TYB appears to be the most important aspect for enhancing sperm fusion ability in the SPA.

▶ This study confirms the findings of the previous study (Abstract 4–8) that the thermal shock step is a prerequisite for the optimized SPA assay.

R.Z. Sokol, M.D., F.A.C.P.

Is One Testicular Specimen Sufficient for Quantitative Evaluation of Spermatogenesis?

Gottschalk-Sabag S, Weiss DB, Folb-Zacharow N, Zukerman Z (Shaare Zedek Med Ctr, Jerusalem; Sackler School of Medicine, Tel Aviv, Israel)
Fertil Steril 64:399–402, 1995   4–10

Purpose.—Fine-needle aspiration (FNA) has been preferred over biopsy for analysis of the spermatogenic process in infertile men with azoospermia or oligospermia. The advantages of FNA include simplicity, reliability, tolerability, and lack of complications. The adequacy of using a single testicular FNA for quantitative evaluation of spermatogenesis was assessed.

Methods.—The study included FNA specimens from 1 testis of 13 men with azoospermia or severe oligospermia. Specimens were taken from the upper, middle, and lower pole of each testis. Five hundred Sertoli cells and cells at each stages of spermatogenesis were identified, counted, and classified by cell type in each aspirate. For each cell type in each aspirate, a quantitative cell type index was calculated, and this information was used to calculate mean cell type indexes for each cell type in the 3 aspirates of each patient. Comparisons were then made between the variations of a given sample and its mean.

Results.—Wide deviations from the mean were noted between each aspirate and the mean of the 3 aspirates for that patient. Cell type indexes by spermatogenic stage ranged from 0.8% to 200% for spermatogonia, 1.4% to 94.3% for spermatocytes, 2.9% to 200% for spermatids, and 0.7% to 128% for spermatozoa. Most of the patients had a cell type index score in at least 1 aspirate that was significantly different from the other 2 aspirates.

Conclusions.—Quantitative evaluation of spermatogenesis in infertile men appears to require more than one testicular FNA specimen. Taking FNAs from several sites of the testes is recommended when such quantitative analyses are performed. With the FNA technique, these multiple specimens can be taken without harming the patient.

▶ Fine-needle aspiration of the testis is a relatively noninvasive, reliable method for obtaining testicular tissue for cytologic evaluation. However, a simple specimen may not be representative of spermatogenesis throughout the testis. These results indicate that aspirations of multiple sites are required to accurately quantitate spermatogenesis. It is not clear, however, that multiple aspirates are needed to determine whether a specimen has spermatogenic elements present.

R.Z. Sokol, M.D., F.A.C.P.

The Use of a Seminal Vesicle Specific Protein (MHS-5 Antigen) for Diagnosis of Agenesis of Vas Deferens and Seminal Vesicles in Azoospermic Men

Barak M, Calderon I, Abramovici H, Gruener N, Yavez H, Paz G, Homonnai ZT (Carmel Med Ctr, Haifa, Israel; Tel Aviv Univ, Israel)

J Androl 15:603–607, 1994　　　　　　　　　　　　　　　　　　4–11

Background.—Azoospermia is detected in 8% of infertile males. Agenesis of both the vas deferens (VD) and the seminal vesicles (SV) is the reason for infertility in 10% of these azoospermic men. About 70% of the human ejaculate is composed of products of the SV. A monoclonal antibody, MHS-5, has recently been developed that recognizes a protein that is specific to SV secretions, the seminal vesicle-specific protein (SVSP). The use of MHS-5 was evaluated as a diagnostic marker of SV secretion in azoospermic men.

Methods.—The study group consisted of 7 patients with previously diagnosed azoospermia resulting from VD and SV agenesis. The control group consisted of 8 normozoospermic volunteers and 3 azoospermic patients with primary testicular failure. All 18 semen samples were coded and examined in a blinded fashion.

Results.—The antigen recognized by the MHS-5 monoclonal antibody SVSP was detected in the seminal plasma of all normozoospermic participants and in the 3 patients with azoospermia attributable to testicular failure. This antigen was not detected in the seminal plasma from any patients with azoospermia resulting from SV and VD agenesis. The prostate-specific antigen (PSA) was detected in the seminal plasma from all study participants.

Conclusions.—The MHS-5 monoclonal antibody that specifically binds the seminal vesicle-specific protein, SVSP, can be used as an accurate, reliable, and sensitive method for the diagnosis of SV and VD agenesis in azoospermic infertile men.

▶ The measurement of SVSP in the azoospermic patient will aid in the clinical diagnosis of the man with agenesis of the vas and seminal vesicles.

R.Z. Sokol, M.D., F.A.C.P.

TEST-Yolk Media and Sperm Quality

Jeyendran RS, Gunawardana VK, Barisic D, Wentz AC (Andrology Lab Services Inc, Chicago; Northwestern Univ, Chicago; Univ of Peradeniya, Sri Lanka)

Hum Reprod Update 1:73–79, 1995　　　　　　　　　　　　　　　4–12

Background.—Media prepared with egg yolk and the buffers TES and TRIS, or TEST-yolk, positively affect the survivability, fertilizing ability, and storage potential of human spermatozoa. Egg yolk lipoproteins are the important compounds, having a synergistic effect because of the TES-TRIS buffer component. The uses of TEST-yolk media were discussed.

Uses of TEST-Yolk Media.—Many of the uses of TEST-yolk buffer have clinical significance in the diagnosis and treatment of male infertility. Its use in the sperm penetration assay (SPA) is well documented. One research team showed that TEST-yolk treatment of spermatozoa from fertile donors with normal semen parameters increased zona binding, possibly because of increased numbers of capacitated but nonacrosome-reacted spermatozoa after TEST-yolk treatment. Also, preincubation with TEST-yolk enhances human oocyte penetration in vitro. In 1980, the efficacy of TEST-yolk as a low-temperature storage medium for spermatozoa for donor artificial insemination was established. This use of TEST-yolk improved the availability of donor semen over time. TEST-yolk has also been used as a cryoprotectant. There appear to be few disadvantages associated with the use of TEST-yolk, though controlled studies are needed to assess the therapeutic effects in the treatment of male infertility.

Conclusions.—Over the past decade, TEST-yolk medium has been found to be superior to conventional media for sperm function tests assessing fertilizing potential, for short-term spermatozoa storage, and for cryopreservation. Controlled studies are needed to assess its therapeutic effects in clinical applications. Further research is also needed to investigate the value of TEST-yolk medium in the hemizona assay and immunobead test and as a storage medium for oocytes. A research priority is that of TEST-yolk's therapeutic influence on sperm function.

▶ This is a comprehensive review article on the use of TEST-yolk medium in sperm function testing and the therapeutic efficacy in intrauterine insemination and in vitro fertilization.

R.Z. Sokol, M.D., F.A.C.P.

Pregnancy Following Discontinuation of a Calcium Channel Blocker in the Male Partner
Hershlag A, Cooper GW, Benoff S (Cornell Univ Med College, Manhasset, NY)
Hum Reprod 10:599–606, 1995   4–13

Background.—Studies have found an association between the fertilization potential of human sperm and mannose lectin translocation within the plasma membrane to the equatorial/postacrosomal segment of the head plus spontaneous acrosome exocytosis. There is evidence that men treated with calcium ion channel blockers have spermatozoa that express little head-directed mannose ligand receptors and do not demonstrate spontaneous acrosome loss. In vitro studies have shown that several lipophilic agents change the physical characteristics of the plasma membrane, thereby causing infertility. The effects on fertility parameters of the cessation of calcium ion channel blockers were studied.

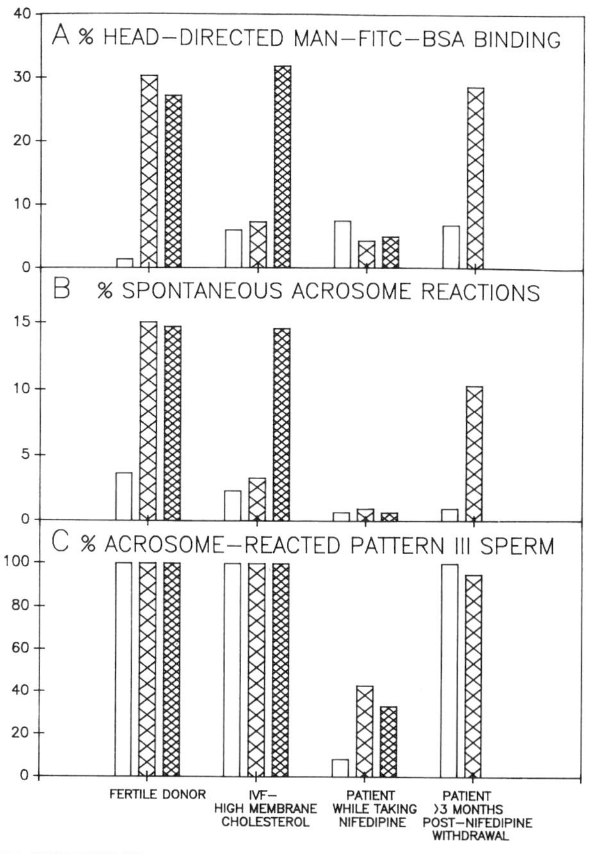

FIGURE 1.—Comparison of mannose receptor expression and acrosome status in motile sperm populations from a donor of known fertility (*fertile donor*), an in vitro fertilization (*IVF*) failure resulting from high membrane cholesterol content (*IVF-high membrane cholesterol*) and the husband in this case study (*patient*) while maintained on a calcium antagonist (nifedipine) and 3 months after nifedipine withdrawal. **A,** percentage of spermatozoa exhibiting head-directed (patterns II and III) man–fluorescein isothiocyanate (*FITC*)-neoglycoprotein binding; **B,** percentage of spermatozoa exhibiting spontaneous loss of acrosome content; and **C,** relationship between the percentage of spermatozoa exhibiting pattern III man-FITC-neoglycoprotein binding and acrosome status, as determined by double labeling with tetramethylrhadamine isothiocyanate–labeled *Pisam savitum* agglutinin. *Abbreviation: RT,* room temperature. (Courtesy of Hershlag A, Cooper GW, Benoff S: Pregnancy following discontinuation of a calcium channel blocker in the male partner. *Hum Reprod* 10:599–606, 1995, by permission of Oxford University Press.)

Methods.—Semen specimens were obtained from 3 men: 1 donor with known fertility, 1 with a high membrane cholesterol content, and 1 who had been treated with a maintenance regimen of nifedipine after a myocardial infarction. The specimens were analyzed in 3 preparations: fresh swim-up preparations, after incubation for 16–20 hours at 37°C, or after incubation for 3 days at room temperature. The frequency of D-mannose binding sites and acrosome status were assessed by microscopic inspection after fluorescein labeling.

Results.—The semen analysis of the patient receiving nifedipine showed that 68% had morphologically normal forms. The spermatozoa from the fertile donor and the donor with high membrane cholesterol both demonstrated time dependent increases in head-directed mannose-binding sites and spontaneous acrosome loss. Both parameters were significantly reduced in the patient receiving nifedipine. However, 3 months after discontinuing nifedipine therapy, he had a normal mannose lectin response to capacitation and spontaneous loss of acrosome content, with a return to the normal phenotype (Fig 1). Conception occurred after the wife was treated with just 2 cycles of Pergonal and intrauterine insemination.

Conclusions.—Although patients treated with calcium ion channel blockers have predominantly morphologically normal sperm in normal concentrations, they may be unable to fertilize. However, these findings indicate that the surface expression of D-mannose–specific lectin in the plasma membrane at the sperm head and acrosome reaction are valid molecular markers for human sperm fertilizing potential. After the discontinuation of calcium ion channel blockers, these markers returned to normal and conception occurred.

▶ This well-documented case report indicates that ingestion of calcium ion channel blockers may adversely affect spermatozoa so that they are unable to fertilize human ova. However, there is no effect of the calcium channel blockers on the parameters usually measured in the semen analysis. The changes affect mannose-lectin expression and the acrosome reaction. If the male member of an infertile couple is taking calcium channel blockers and has a normal semen analysis but conception does not occur with usual therapy, temporary discontinuation of the medication, if medically appropriate, should be advised.

D.R. Mishell, Jr., M.D.

5 Pathophysiology of Male Infertility

Insulin-Like Growth Factor I (IGF-I) and IGF Binding Proteins in Seminal Plasma Before and After Vasectomy in Normal Men
Ovesen P, Flyvbjerg A, Ørskov H (Aarhus Kommunehospital, Denmark)
Fertil Steril 63:913–918, 1995   5–1

Background.—Insulin-like growth factor I (IGF-I) apparently functions as an autocrine and/or paracrine factor in the testis. Previous studies have documented the presence of IGF-I, insulin-like growth factor binding protein (IGFBP)-2, IGFBP-3, and IGFBP-4 in human seminal plasma. Whether these substances originate from the testes or accessory sex glands, however, is not known. The content of IGF-I and IGFBPs in semen was examined in healthy men before and after vasectomy.

Methods.—Fifteen men aged 34–44 years were enrolled in the study. All were in good general health and had fathered at least 2 children. Seminal plasma and serum levels of IGF-I and IGFBP-1 and IGFBP-3 were assessed by commercially available assay. Samples were also subjected to Western ligand blotting.

Findings.—Mean seminal plasma IGF-I levels were 18 µg/L before and 12.5 µg/L after vasectomy, a significant difference. When the total ejaculate content of IGF-I was determined, the figures were decreased by half after vasectomy. Mean seminal IGFBP-3 levels were 844.9 µg/L before and 816.5 µg/L after vasectomy. Determination of the total ejaculate IGFBP-3 content showed a 36% decrease after vasectomy.

Conclusions.—A substantial amount of seminal plasma IGF-I and IG-FBP-3 may originate in the testis. Although the physiologic importance of IGF-I and IGFBPs in male reproduction is still unclear, the presence of these substances in the testes supports the functional role of gonadal function regulation.

▶ Growth hormone may be involved in the regulation of spermatogenesis. Support for this hypothesis is found in studies reporting that patients with spermatogenic maturation arrest have low growth hormone levels. Growth hormone may aid in stimulating spermatogenesis in patients with hypogonadotropic hypogonadism.

R.Z. Sokol, M.D., F.A.C.P.

The Paternal Inheritance of the Centrosome, the Cell's Microtubule-Organizing Center, in Humans, and the Implications for Infertility
Simerly C, Wu G-J, Zoran S, Ord T, Rawlins R, Jones J, Navara C, Gerrity M, Rinehart J, Binor Z, Asch R, Schatten G (Univ of Wisconsin, Madison; Univ of Irvine Med Ctr, Orange, Calif; Rush Univ, Chicago; et al)
Nature Med 1:47–52, 1995   5–2

Background.—Fertilization in human beings is achieved when parental chromosomes intermix at first mitosis. This requires centrosome restoration and microtubule-mediated motility. The role of microtubules in inseminated human oocytes was studied during the union of the pronuclei and first cell cycle.

Methods and Findings.—Microtubules and DNA were imaged during fertilization in inseminated human oocytes. Microtubules were detected only in the metaphase-arrested second meiotic spindle. Within 6 hours of insemination, the sperm aster was observed extending from the male pronucleus and incorporated sperm tail. The sperm aster enlarges as the male pronucleus decondenses, and by 16.5 hours, the pronuclei are adjacent in the bipolar, eccentric array. Spindle bipolarity occurs by prophase in the first mitosis.

In oocytes from infertile couples, development was arrested after sperm penetration. Nearly half of the oocytes studied were penetrated. Fertilization was arrested at several stages, including sperm incorporation, microtubule nucleation, incomplete sperm aster elongation, sperm aster detachment from male pronucleus, "silent" polyspermy, androgenesis, metaphase, and defective female pronuclear reconstitution.

Conclusions.—Imaging of inseminated human oocytes demonstrated that the sperm introduces the centrosome, which then nucleates the new microtubule assembly to form a sperm aster. This step is essential for successful fertilization. Complete fertilization fails in some infertile patients because of defects in uniting the sperm and egg nuclei. This failure to properly effect the cytoplasmic motions uniting the nuclei leads to infertility.

▶ Microtubules, cytoskeletal elements, are essential for the separation of chromosomes during mitosis and meiosis. They are also required for the migration of the sperm and egg nuclei during fertilization. The centrosome determines microtubule orientation and polarity. The sperm aster is a radial microtubule array, which is thought to be essential for the union of the male and female pronuclei. This research demonstrates that the sperm introduces the centrosome. Based on their findings, these investigators suggest that some intracytoplasmic sperm injection (ICSI) failures may be attributable to defective microtubule functioning and centrosome reconstitution. They speculate that exogenous centrosome introduction may form the basis of a therapy for potentially related ICSI failures.

R.Z. Sokol, M.D., F.A.C.P.

On the Epididymis and Its Role in the Development of the Fertile Ejaculate

Turner TT (Univ of Virginia, Charlottesville)
J Androl 16:292–298, 1995

5–3

Role of the Epididymis in Sperm Maturation.—Mammalian sperm are known to mature within the epididymis. In studies of a number of species, maturation is most evident in the segment between the distal caput epididymidis and the proximal cauda and is essentially complete when reaching the latter structure. After vasoepididymostomy, the possibility of a fertile ejaculate increases with the length of available epididymis for sperm to transit. Some sperm exposed to only a short part of the epididymis—or to no epididymis at all—nevertheless remain capable of fertilizing an egg in vivo.

Is the Epididymis Necessary?—Although in general the human epididymis, like that of other species, is required for a normally fertile ejaculate, some spermatozoa become fertile after only a brief exposure to the epididymal environment or to the vas deferens. After efferentiovasostomy, the minority of sperm cells that are disposed to mature early may be adequately stimulated in the vas deferens and so reach functional maturity. Sperm that are aspirated for use in in vitro fertilization need not have the full motility and survival abilities found in cells that attempt natural fertilization.

Epididymal Functions.—The epididymis transports sperm from the testis to the vas deferens. Regulation of fluid movement in the epididymal lumen may be an important aspect of sperm transport. Sperm are concentrated by fluid reabsorption resulting from antiluminal electrolyte transport. In addition to sperm maturation, more than half of all epididymal sperm are stored in the cauda epididymis in most species. Fertile sperm may be stored for longer than 2 weeks.

▶ This excellent review of the role of the epididymis in sperm maturation and fertility potential helps to clarify why sperm aspiration and subsequent assisted reproductive technology leads to fertilization.

R.Z. Sokol, M.D., F.A.C.P.

Acrosome Reaction Inducibility Predicts Fertilization Success at In-Vitro Fertilization

Calvo L, Dennison-Lagos L, Banks SM, Dorfmann A, Thorsell LP, Bustillo M, Schulman JD, Sherins RJ (Genetics & IVF Inst, Fairfax, Va)
Hum Reprod 9:1880–1886, 1994

5–4

Background.—Specialized sperm function testing appears to predict in vitro fertilization (IVF) success better than traditional semen parameters. Specialized testing takes into account the series of intricate steps required for fertilization, beginning with sperm capacitation, followed by binding to the zona pellucida and acrosome discharge, binding to the oolemma, and finally penetrating the ooplasm. The predictive value of the acrosome reaction (AR) for successful fertilization was investigated using a cohort of 232 infertile patients participating in IVF.

Methods and Findings.—Overall, the median percentage of eggs fertilized was 25%. One to 29 oocytes were available for insemination. As the percentage of spermatozoa able to undergo AR increased, the median percentage of eggs fertilized at IVF increased. Spermatozoa with a failed AR fertilized only 12% of eggs, compared with 50% of eggs fertilized by spermatozoa with AR values exceeding 9%. The specificity of the assay was 0.75, the sensitivity was 0.55, and the odds ratio was 2.9. Thus AR-positive patients were 2.9 times more likely to have successful fertilization than patients with a failed AR. Receiver operator characteristic (ROC) curves developed for AR, sperm concentration, and percentage of normal forms in semen were potentially useful for predicting the success of fertilization. Acrosome reaction and morphologic characteristics seemed superior to sperm concentration by ROC analysis. On the basis of traditional semen characteristics, including morphology, patients were divided into 4 well-defined subgroups. The median percentage of eggs fertilized declined as traditional mean characteristics deteriorated, from a median of 46% for patients with excellent sperm concentration, motility, and morphology to 29% for those with suboptimal semen quality to 0% for those whose semen was severely impaired. In each subgroup, the median percentage of eggs fertilized was threefold to fourfold greater for patients with a positive AR than for those with a failed AR. This suggests that AR has a greater effect on fertilization rate than traditional semen parameters, including morphology.

Conclusions.—Some men with good semen characteristics have an unexpectedly poor AR and a markedly decreased fertilization rate, whereas those with poor traditional semen characteristics unexpectedly retain AR and perform relatively well at IVF. Morphologic characteristics, by contrast, appeared to have little effect on fertilization success. As acrosome reaction has a much greater predictive value for IVF success than traditional parameters, including morphology, AR assessment is a clinically useful diagnostic tool for determining a patient's likelihood for successful fertilization at IVF.

Characterization and Frequency Distribution of Sperm Acrosome Reaction Among Normal and Infertile Men
Calvo L, Dennison-Lagos L, Banks SM, Sherins RJ (Genetics & IVF Inst, Fairfax, Va)
Hum Reprod 9:1875–1879, 1994   5–5

Objective.—In assessing male fertility, sperm function is fundamental to determining fertilizing capacity. Because the acrosome reaction (AR) is a prerequisite to fertilization, this study compared the AR reaction in spermatozoa from fertile males with that of infertile males to determine sperm fertilizing ability.

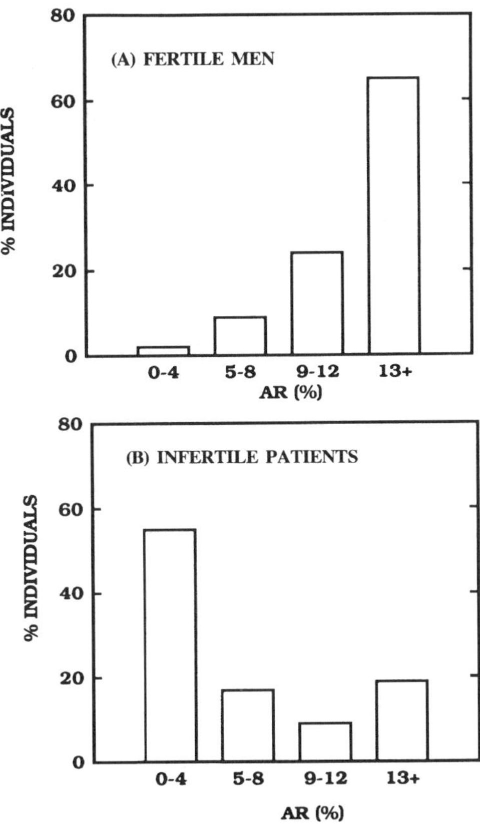

FIGURE 1.—Frequency distribution of acrosome reaction (*AR*) values for 58 fertile men (**A**) and 232 infertile patients (**B**). (Courtesy of Calvo L, Dennison-Lagos L, Banks SM, et al: Characterization and frequency distribution of sperm acrosome reaction among normal and infertile men. *Hum Reprod* 9:1875–1879, 1994, by permission of Oxford University Press.)

Methods.—Semen characteristics were determined for 58 healthy fertile volunteers and 232 male partners of infertile couples seeking in vitro fertilization (IVF).

Results.—The mean AR was 17% for fertile males and 3% for infertile males. Acrosome reaction inducibility was > 9% in 83% of fertile males and 3% in infertile males. Only 2% of fertile males had an AR < 5%, whereas 60% of infertile males had an AR < 5% (Fig 1). Individual variability was 4 AR units. Low AR levels were significantly correlated with poor semen quality. Acrosome reaction inducibility was significantly correlated with morphology, progression, and motility in infertile patients. Of the patients with satisfactory concentration, motility, and morphology, there were 20% with a low AR, and of the patients with low quality semen, there were 29% with a satisfactory AR. Acrosome reaction apparently provides fertility information in addition to that obtained from measurement of traditional semen parameters. Frequency distributions provide some insight. A quadrant analysis of AR and morphologic characteristics showed that although fertile men were equally distributed in the 4 quadrants, infertile men fell into the < 10% morphologically normal forms and < 20% AR quadrant.

Conclusion.—The AR provides information about male fertilization capacity in addition to that derived from conventional semen analysis.

▶ Ejaculated sperm must undergo capacitation and AR to fertilize ova. During the AR, the outer membrane of the acrosome breaks down, releasing the hydrolytic enzymes needed for sperm penetration into the oocyte. The AR is assessed by incubating spermatozoa under capacitating conditions and quantifying binding of FHC-labeled lectin. Used in combination with other sperm function tests, the AR may aid in the prediction of success in IVF.

R.Z. Sokol, M.D., F.A.C.P.

Nuclear Decondensation of Sperm Head and Failure at In-Vitro Fertilization: An Ultrastructural Study

Chitale AR, Rathaur RG (Jaslok Hosp and Research Centre, Bombay, India)
Hum Reprod 10:594–598, 1995   5–6

Objective.—Unexplained male infertility leads to low fertilization rates even when in vitro fertilization (IVF) is used. Although conventional semen analysis determines count, motility, and morphologic characteristics, light microscopy is not powerful enough to assess structural integrity of spermatozoa. The results of an electron microscopy study of spermatozoa in failed vs. successful cases of fertilization to determine baseline abnormalities were evaluated.

Methods.—Patients were divided into 3 groups: group A contained 25 normal, healthy, fertile men aged 25–35 years; group B contained 13 men who had successful IVF; and group C contained 13 men who had unsuccessful IVF. For each patient, an average of 330 sperm heads and 660 sperm tails were studied under the electron microscope.

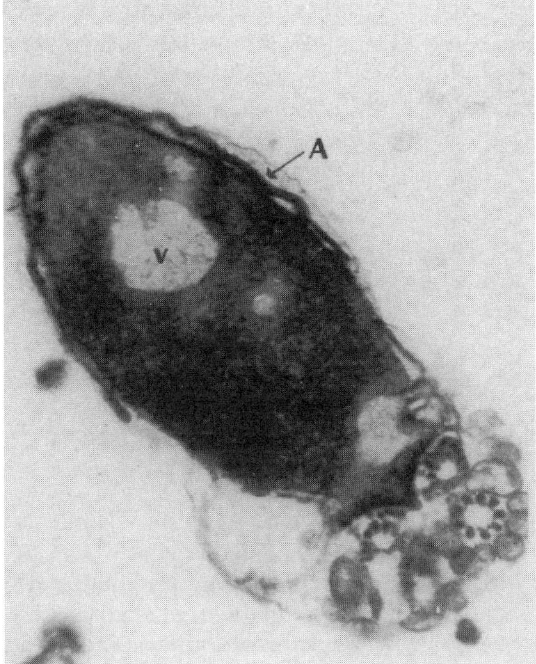

FIGURE 1.—Nuclear chromatin defect (mild decondensation) with intranuclear vacuole (*V*) and intact acrosome (*A*). Original magnification, ×12,000. (Courtesy of Chitale AR, Rathaur RG: Nuclear decondensation of sperm head and failure at in-vitro fertilization: An ultrastructural study. *Hum Reprod* 10:594–598, 1995, by permission of Oxford University Press.)

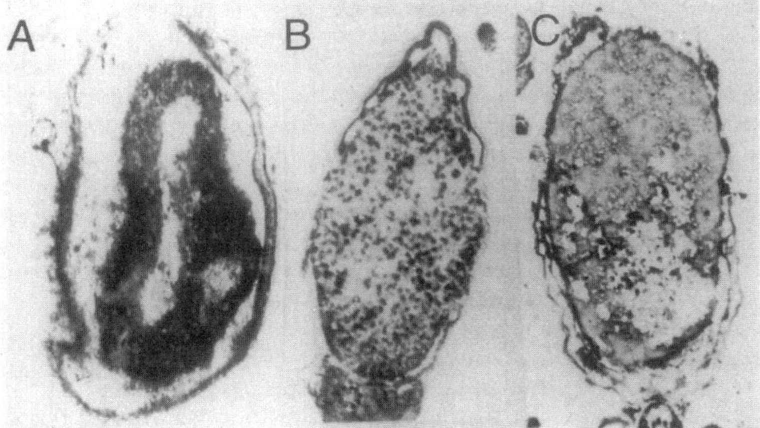

FIGURE 3.—Decondensed nuclear chromatin in sperm heads. **A**, acrosome separated from head; **B**, half acrosome; **C**, hypoplastic acrosome. Original magnification, ×12,000. (Courtesy of Chitale AR, Rathaur RG: Nuclear decondensation of sperm head and failure at in-vitro fertilization: An ultrastructural study. *Hum Reprod* 10:594–598, 1995, by permission of Oxford University Press.)

Results.—Mean sperm motility and concentration were normal for groups B and C. In group C, there were significantly more severe head (79%), acrosome (50.3%), and tail abnormalities (49%) than in group B and a significantly greater proportion of nuclear decondensation (Figs 1 and 3).

Conclusion.—Electron microscopy is useful for determining the cause of unexplained male infertility. Structural integrity of spermatozoa appear to be more important than motility and sperm count in assessing fertility.

▶ This article includes excellent photomicrographs of ultrastructural abnormalities in the various anatomical components of spermatozoa.

R.Z. Sokol, M.D., F.A.C.P.

Some Cases of Human Male Infertility Are Explained by Abnormal In Vitro Human Sperm Activation

Brown DB, Hayes EJ, Uchida T, Nagamani M (Univ of Texas, Galveston)
Fertil Steril 64:612–622, 1995   5–7

Background.—Sixteen percent of all couples seeking treatment for infertility receive diagnoses of unexplained infertility. The men in such couples produce sperm that appear normal in standard semen analyses, which include assessment of sperm density, progressive motility, sperm morphologic characteristics, and semen volume. However, these techniques have a limited ability for evaluating male fertility. Of the variety of other tests developed to assess male fertility, the sperm penetration assay is the only one that directly assays sperm activation events occurring after the sperm nucleus enters the egg. The value of the human sperm activation assay in this population was investigated.

Methods.—Sperm were obtained from 59 men with idiopathic infertility and 59 age-matched fertile men. Specimens were assayed in the human sperm activation assay, and the findings were compared. A portion of the sperm from the infertile men was also used in assisted reproductive technology (ART).

Findings.—Twenty-two percent of the infertile men produced sperm that responded abnormally in the assay, compared to only 1.7% of fertile men. A significantly higher percentage of abnormal responders in the infertile group showed unexplained infertility than in the fertile group. No sperm samples responding abnormally in the human sperm activation assay resulted in pregnancies when used in ART (Fig 1).

Conclusions.—The human sperm activation assay is a useful tool for assessing a subgroup of infertile men who would otherwise have unexplained infertility. This assay should be included in the evaluation of a couple's fertility before expensive ART is attempted.

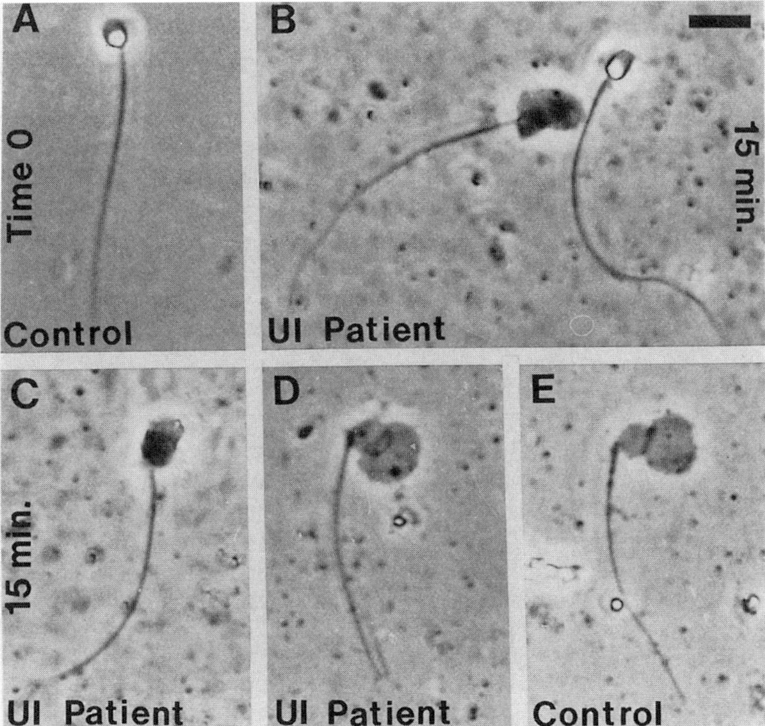

FIGURE 1.—Phase-contrast photographs of nuclei having normal and abnormal decondensation in the human sperm activation assay, taken using a 40× objective. *Bar,* 10 μm. **A,** time zero. Permeabilized sperm from a fertile male with no extract treatment. **B–D,** permeabilized sperm from a male with unexplained infertility incubated 15 minutes in egg extract. In (**B**) is shown an example of sperm that did not decondense, near a partially decondensed sperm. Another partially decondensed sperm is shown in (**C**). A fully decondensed sperm is shown in (**D**). The idiopathic infertile male whose sperm are shown in (**B–D**) had a decondensation score that was 57% of the control. **E,** a fully decondensed sperm from a fertile male incubated 15 minutes in egg extract. *Abbreviation: UI,* unexplained infertility. (From Brown DB, Hayes EJ, Uchida T, et al: Some cases of human male infertility are explained by abnormal in vitro human sperm activation. *Fertil Steril* 64:612–622, 1995. Reproduced with permission of the publisher, the American Society for Reproductive Medicine [The American Fertility Society].)

▶ Sperm activation is defined as a sequence of events, which include chromatic decondensation, formation of a pronucleus, DNA synthesis, chromatic recondensation, and breakdown of the pronucleus in preparation for the mitotic division that produces a two-cell embryo.[1] Electron microscopy allows a more accurate assessment of decondensation of nuclear chromatin (see Abstract 5–6) than light microscopy. The human sperm activation assay uses *Xenopus laevis* frog egg extract from unfertilized eggs arrested at the second meiotic metaphase. Prepared spermatozoa are mixed with the frog egg extract. The percent decondensation and DNA synthesis of the patient's sperm are compared with those of normal control sperm. This assay may be particularly useful in identifying couples who will benefit from intracytoplasmic sperm injection (ICSI) because ICSI bypasses all sperm function defects except sperm activation.

R.Z. Sokol, M.D., F.A.C.P.

Reference

1. Long FJ, Kunkle M: Transformations of sperm nuclei upon insemination. *Curr Top Dev Biol* 12:149–184, 1978.

Fertility Index Analysis in Cryptorchidism

McAleer IM, Packer MG, Kaplan GW, Scherz HC, Krous HF, Billman GF (Univ of California, San Diego)
J Urol 153:1255–1258, 1995

5–8

Introduction.—There is debate concerning the optimal timing for surgery to correct cryptorchidism, especially in terms of the impact on fertility potential. The fertility index, defined as the number of spermatogonia per tubule on cut sections of testis, has been used to predict future fertility potential. This index was used to examine the possibility of a critical time for orchiopexy in patients with undescended testis.

Methods.—The study included 226 boys with cryptorchidism who underwent orchiopexy or orchiectomy at the age of 6 months to 16 years, median age 2.5 years. A total of 355 open testis biopsy specimens were obtained at the time of surgery, and the preserved tissues were examined by light microscopy for measurement of the fertility index. There were 184 patients with unilateral cryptorchidism—87 of whom also underwent biopsy of the contralateral testis—and 42 patients with bilateral cryptorchidism. Fertility index measurements were compared with previously reported data on normal testes, and between undescended and descended testes of boys with unilateral cryptorchidism.

Results.—Patients aged 1 year or younger showed no significant differences in the fertility indexes of the undescended vs. descended testes. All other age groups did have significant differences in fertility index measurements between testes. Patients with unilateral cryptorchidism in all age groups had significantly subnormal fertility index measurements. The same was true for all patients with bilateral cryptorchidism except those aged 13–18 months. Fertility index measurements in the descended testes of boys with unilateral cryptorchidism were similar to the normal values.

Conclusions.—Fertility potential may be significantly reduced in undescended testes compared to normal testes, according to fertility index measurements. This is so regardless of the age at which the undescended testis is discovered. In some age groups, fertility potential may also be decreased in the contralateral testes of boys with unilateral cryptorchidism. Fertility potential might be preserved by performing orchiopexy during the first year of life.

Paternity After Cryptorchidism: Lack of Correlation With Age at Orchidopexy
Lee PA, O'Leary LA, Songer NJ, Bellinger MF, LaPorte RE (Univ of Pittsburgh, Pa)
Br J Urol 75:704–707, 1995   5–9

Background.—The effects of cryptorchidism—or the age at which it is corrected—on fertility are unknown. There is no solid evidence linking unilateral cryptorchidism to reduced ability to father children. Men with a history of unilateral or bilateral cryptorchidism were studied to determine the effects of their condition, and of age at orchiopexy, to paternity.

Methods.—A questionnaire was sent to 363 men who underwent orchiopexy at 1 children's hospital from 1955 to 1969, and to a group of 336 age-matched control men who underwent unrelated minor surgery during the same period. Data on age at orchiopexy and testicular size and position were collected from the medical records.

Results.—The cryptorchid group included 313 men with a history of unilateral cryptorchidism and 50 with a history of bilateral cryptorchidism. Three fourths of the men in the unilateral cryptorchid and control groups who had been married had fathered children. In contrast, only 53% of married men in the bilateral cryptorchid group had fathered children. Compared to the other 2 groups, the men with bilateral cryptorchidism had relatively fewer conceptions during the first year of regular intercourse with no contraception, but more conceptions after the first year. On separate examination of the men with unilateral and bilateral cryptorchidism, age at orchiopexy was unrelated to paternity or the duration of unprotected intercourse before conception.

Conclusions.—Although men with a history of bilateral cryptorchidism appear to have compromised paternity, those with a history of unilateral cryptorchidism do not. The age at which orchiopexy is performed has no influence on paternity. The reasons for decreased paternity in men with bilateral cryptorchidism are unknown.

Clinical and Anatomopathological Study of 2000 Cryptorchid Testes
Gracia J, González N, Gómez ME, Plaza L, Sánchez J, Alba J (Miguel Servet Children's Hosp, Zaragoza, Spain)
Br J Urol 75:697–701, 1995   5–10

Background.—The morphologic lesions in cryptorchid testes may result from damage induced by the extrascrotal position or may represent a congenital lesion. Whether age at the time of surgery and location of the testes helped determine the anatomicopathologic lesions was investigated.

Methods.—A total of 2,000 testes in 1,342 children, aged from newborn to 14 years (mean, 5.9 years), were studied. The tubular fertility index (TFI) and the tubular diameter (TD) were correlated with age at intervention and location of the testes.

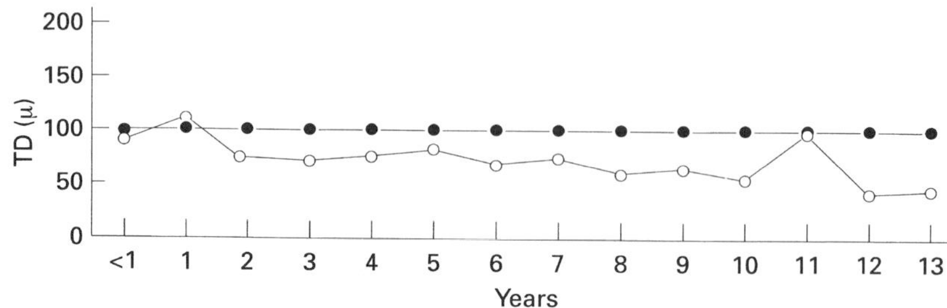

FIGURE 2.—Tubular diameter at age of surgery. *Open circles,* cryptorchid (% of the control values); *filled circles,* control values. (Courtesy of Gracia J, González N, Gómez ME, et al: Clinical and anatomopathological study of 2000 cryptorchid testes. *Br J Urol* 75:697–701, 1995.)

Findings.—The most "normal" measured values were found in children younger than 2 years. The TFI was low in 24%, very low in 55%, and normal (> 60%) in 21%. The TFI did not differ significantly between children younger than 2 years and those older than 7 years, suggesting that the TFI did not deteriorate progressively with age. Only 8% of the TD were very low, 51% were low and 41% were normal. The TD differed significantly between children younger than 2 years and those older than 7 years, but with a higher mean in the oldest age group. Parametric and nonparametric tests did not show a correlation between the TFI or TD and the time of surgery or testicular location (Figs 2 and 3).

Conclusion.—On the basis of these findings, no particular age can be recommended at which surgery should be performed for cryptorchid testes in relation to the anatomicopathologic damage.

▶ These articles (Abstracts 5–8 through 5–10) attempt to determine whether early orchiopexy prevents the compromise of the fertility potential of the cryptorchid testis and whether the fertility of the contralateral testis is also compromised. Previous histologic studies demonstrated a correlation between degenerative tubular changes and age of surgical correction. Clinical studies reported varying rates of paternity after unilateral or bilateral orchiopexy. McAleer and co-workers (Abstract 5–8) and Gracia and co-

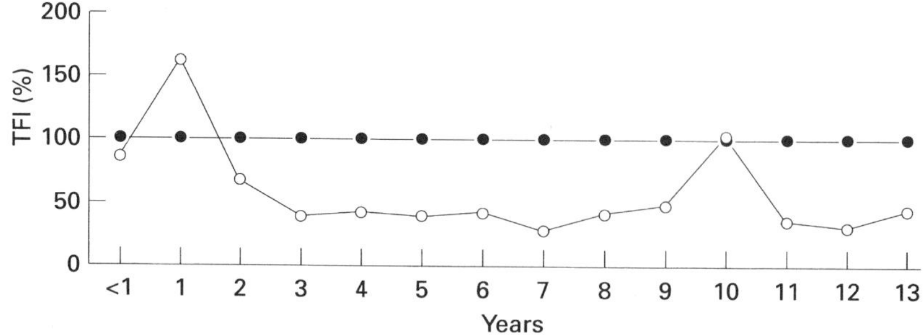

FIGURE 3.—Tubular fertility index (*TFI*) depending on the age at surgery. *Open circles,* cryptorchid (%) of the control values; *filled circles,* control values. (Courtesy of Gracia J, González N, Gómez ME, et al: Clinical and anatomopathological study of 2000 cryptorchid testes. *Br J Urol* 75:697–701, 1995.)

workers (Abstract 5–10), in an attempt to quantify fertility potential histologically, evaluated testicular biopsy specimens using the fertility index (FI). This assessment of the number of spermatogonia per tubule on cut sections correlates with fertility potential defined as the ability to conceive. The McAleer group compared FI among biopsy specimens from unilateral and bilateral cryptorchid testis and normally descended testicles. The observed FI in the cryptorchid testis was significantly less than the index in the normally descended testicles in children older than 1 year. In a similar study, Gracia et al. studied testicular biopsies collected from 1,432 children with crytorchidism. The children ranged in age from newborn to 14 years. They noted a preservation of the FI in children younger than 2 years. Both studies suggest that orchiopexy should be performed before the second year of life. The finding of a normal FI in the descended testicle as compared with the undescended testicle in the same child may explain the finding of Lee et al. (Abstract 5–9) that paternity is not compromised after unilateral cryptorchidism. The descended testicle seems to compensate for the abnormal testicle.

R.Z. Sokol, M.D., F.A.C.P.

Effects of Smoking on Testicular Function, Semen Quality and Sperm Fertilizing Capacity

Sofikitis N, Miyagawa I, Dimitriadis D, Zavos P, Sikka S, Hellstrom W (Tottori Univ, Yonaqo, Japan; Japanese-Greek Fertility Inst, Athens, Greece; Univ of Kentucky, Lexington; et al)
J Urol 154:1030–1034, 1995

5–11

Introduction.—Many men of reproductive age still smoke, and there is considerable evidence that smoking has adverse effects on the concentration and motility of spermatozoa. Its effect on human Leydig cell function remains uncertain, although animal studies suggest that function may be compromised.

Objective and Methods.—A number of assays known to correlate with sperm-fertilizing potential and the outcome of in vitro fertilization were performed in 49 men 21–38 years of age who had smoked more than a pack of cigarettes per day for longer than 3 years, and 28 of similar age who had never smoked. The acrosin assay, zona-free hamster oocyte sperm penetration assay, and hypoosmotic swelling test were carried out, and Sertoli cell secretion was evaluated. Semen samples were collected by intercourse a month before hernia repair, and a testicular biopsy specimen was obtained at the time of surgery. Semen and blood were collected again 6 months postoperatively.

Findings.—Smokers had lower percentages of morphologically normal spermatozoa, poorer morphometric parameters, and less motile sperm than did nonsmokers. Sperm function tests demonstrated significantly poorer function in the smokers (Table 2). In addition, they had signifi-

TABLE 2.—Effect of Smoking on the Outcome of Sperm Function Tests

Group	Smoking	Serum Cotinine Level (ng/ml)	Hypoosmotic Swelling Test (%)	Zona-Free Hamster Oocyte Sperm Penetration Assay (%)	Acrosin Activity (μIU/10^6 sperm cells)
1:*	Yes	—	48 ± 12	36 ± 15	12 ± 5
1A†	Yes	Less than 100	61 ± 6	53 ± 7	17 ± 3
1B	Yes	100 to less than 400	49 ± 7	38 ± 7	12 ± 3
1C	Yes	400 or more	36 ± 7	18 ± 6	7 ± 3
2	No	—	73 ± 10	65 ± 9	31 ± 8
3‡	Yes	—	55 ± 8	44 ± 7	13 ± 4
	No	—	69 ± 6	63 ± 6	21 ± 4

Note: Values are expressed as means ± 1 SD.

* Results of all sperm function tests were significantly higher in group 2 than in group 1 ($P < 0.05$).

† Results of all sperm function tests were significantly higher in group 1A than in group 1B, and in group 1B than in group 1C.

‡ Within group 3 all sperm function tests were significantly higher ($P < 0.05$) after the participants stopped smoking.

(Courtesy of Sofikitis N, Miyagawa I, Dimitriadis D, et al: Effects of smoking on testicular function, semen quality, and sperm fertilizing capacity. *J Urol* 154:1030–1034, 1995, Williams & Wilkins.)

cantly lower testosterone levels in the left testicular vein than nonsmoking men, and lower in vitro androgen-binding protein secretion rates.

Conclusions.—Sperm-fertilizing potential is reduced in men who smoke, possibly because of alterations in the sperm cytoskeleton during either spermatogenesis or sperm maturation in the epididymis. The primary defect may be deficient secretory function of the Leydig and Sertoli cells.

▶ These investigators approached the question of whether smoking alters fertility potential in a new way. In addition to the standard semen analysis, they evaluated the effects of smoking on assays known to correlate with the outcome of in vitro fertilization and monitored changes in the assays after cessation of smoking. In addition, they studied possible detrimental effects of smoking on Leydig cell secretory function by measuring testosterone levels in the left testicular vein, and possible adverse effects of smoking on the Sertoli cell secretory function as reflected in changes in the testicular androgen-binding protein secretion rate. Their hypothesis of diminished fertilizing capacity in smokers is supported at the chromosomal level. A significantly higher ratio of single-stranded–to–double-stranded DNA spermatozoa was found in smokers. Single-stranded DNA spermatozoa have lower fertilizing capacity than do double-stranded DNA spermatozoa.

R.Z. Sokol, M.D., F.A.C.P.

A Study in Patients With Erectile Dysfunction Comparing Different Formulations of Prostaglandin E1

Vanderschueren D, Heyrman RM, Keogh EJ, Casey RW, Weiske W-H, Ogrinc FG, De Koning Gans HJ, on behalf of the Alprostadil Study Group (Catholic Univ of Leuven, Belgium; Sir Charles Gardner Hosp, Nedlands, Australia; C.A.R.E. Centre, Mississauga, Ont, Canada; et al)

J Urol 154:1744–1747, 1995

5–12

Background.—Erectile dysfunction is effectively treated by injecting prostaglandin E_1 (PGE_1) into the corpora cavernosa of the penis. Current treatment employs a 25-fold dilution of a sterile solution containing 500 µg of PGE_1 in 1 mL of dehydrated alcohol. Penile pain during injection or erection is a frequent side effect that may be related to either inappropriate dilution or the presence of alcohol. Priapism is not a common occurrence, but it may be a result of the current formulation.

Objective.—Two new formulations of PGE_1 now are available. A multicenter double-blind, placebo-controlled, crossover trial was planned to determine the pharmacodynamic equivalence of the conventional pediatric sterile solution, a sterile powder form of PGE_1, and a nonalcoholic sterile solution. The freeze-dried sterile powder contains 20 µg/mL of PGE_1.

Methods.—Two hundred ten men 29–70 years of age received either single injections of each of 3 placebo formulations, or injections of 2.5, 5, 10, or 20 µg of PGE_1 from each of the 3 active formulations. The patients had been unable to achieve adequate erections for at least 4 months but were known to respond stably to intracavernous PGE_1. Most often erectile dysfunction was psychogenic and/or vasculogenic in origin.

Results.—All active preparations in all dosages were comparably effective in producing rigid erections, defined as 70% rigidity persisting for at least 10 minutes by RigiScan. The patients themselves expressed no preference for a particular preparation or dosage. No patient had priapism or blood pressure changes. Penile pain was most prevalent (17%) when the nonalcoholic sterile solution was used, but 11% of placebo recipients also reported pain.

Conclusion.—The 3 PGE_1 preparations tested in this study were pharmacodynamically equivalent and comparably safe.

▶ Newer formulations of PGE_1 offer an advantage in that they are "ready to use" and thus avoid preparation errors. All compounds seem to produce minimal side effects.

R.Z. Sokol, M.D., F.A.C.P.

The Interaction *In Vitro* of Human Spermatozoa With Epithelial Cells From the Human Uterine (Fallopian) Tube

Pacey AA, Hill CJ, Scudamore IW, Warren MA, Barratt CLR, Cooke ID
(Jessop Hosp for Women, Sheffield, England)
Hum Reprod 10:360–366, 1995

5–13

Background.—The fallopian tube environment plays an important role in fertility. In animals, the fallopian tube has been demonstrated to regulate and maintain sperm function. The role of the human fallopian tube has not been as well defined. The interaction between human spermatozoa and epithelial cells from the human fallopian tube was examined.

Methods.—Fallopian tubes were obtained from 20 fertile premenopausal women during routine hysterectomy. The fallopian tubes were dissected and the epithelium was isolated. Either epithelial tissue or dispersed epithelial cells were maintained in culture overnight. Motile spermatozoa were obtained from the semen of donors of proven fertility. Interaction experiments were performed within 24 hours of obtaining hysterectomy tissue. The interaction of spermatozoa and epithelial cells was investigated by live video observation, light microscopy, and electron microscopy.

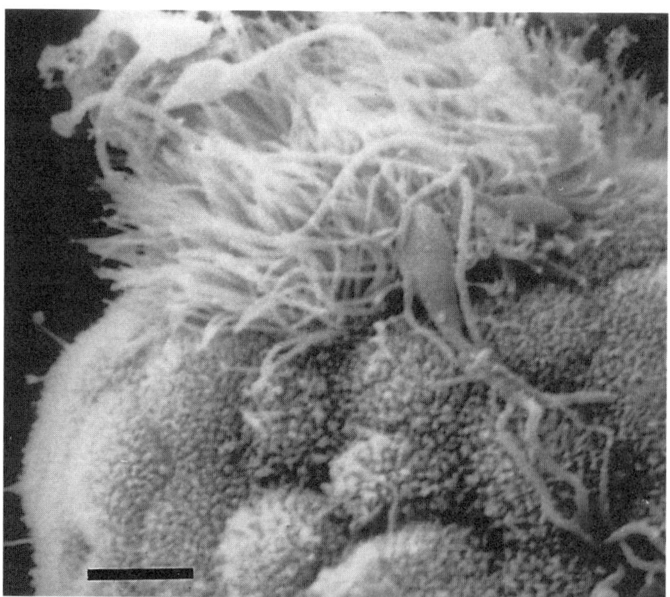

FIGURE 2.—Scanning electron micrograph showing spermatozoa attached to a ciliated area of uterine (fallopian) tube epithelium. The epithelial cells had been allowed to adhere overnight to the base of a tissue culture plate before the start of incubation and had been dissociated from tissue explants by incubation in collagenase. The preparation was fixed 1 hour after the addition of spermatozoa. Scale bar = 4 μm. (Courtesy of Pacey AA, Hill CJ, Scudamore IW, et al: The interaction in vitro of human spermatozoa with epithelial cells from the human uterine (fallopian) tube. *Hum Reprod* 10:360–366, 1995, by permission of Oxford University Press.)

Results.—Epithelial cells were identified by their morphologic characteristics and beating cilia. The thickness of the epithelial explants interfered with illumination, so observation was easier with dispersed epithelial cells. When sperm preparations were incubated with epithelial cells, there was no evidence of taxis. Random contact did lead to an interaction between spermatozoa and epithelial cells that suggested binding. Only a small amount of the total sperm was bound at any given time. The contact was through the sperm head and the sperm flagella continued to beat. The bound spermatozoa could not be easily dissociated. Their connection was maintained through fixation with glutaraldehyde, which permitted examination by electron microscopy (Fig 2). Transmission electron microscopy demonstrated that the 2 membranes were so close that it was not always possible to distinguish between the plasma membrane of the bound spermatozoa and the plasma membrane of the epithelial cell to which it was bound. All bound spermatozoa had intact acrosomal vessicles.

Conclusions.—The observations presented in this report suggest that interactions between spermatozoa and epithelial cells may be common during the time the sperm are in the fallopian tube. These observations are similar to those that have been made in animals. Although the function of this interaction is not known, it may play a role in normal human fertility. It is possible that defects in this interaction may be responsible for some cases of infertility of unknown cause.

▶ How sperm travel through the female reproductive system is unclear. Spermatozoa appear to move by a combination of self-propulsion and retrograde myometrial and myosalpingeal contraction. A combination of mechanisms, including innate sperm motility, cilial propulsion, fluid flow, and tubal contractility, aid in sperm transport. Sperm capacitation, a prerequisite for the acrosome reaction, occurs in the oviduct. The exact nature of the interaction of sperm with the epithelial cells of the fallopian tube in the human being is not well understood. These investigators describe a human epithelial cell culture system that will aid in the study of sperm tube physiology.

R.Z. Sokol, M.D., F.A.C.P.

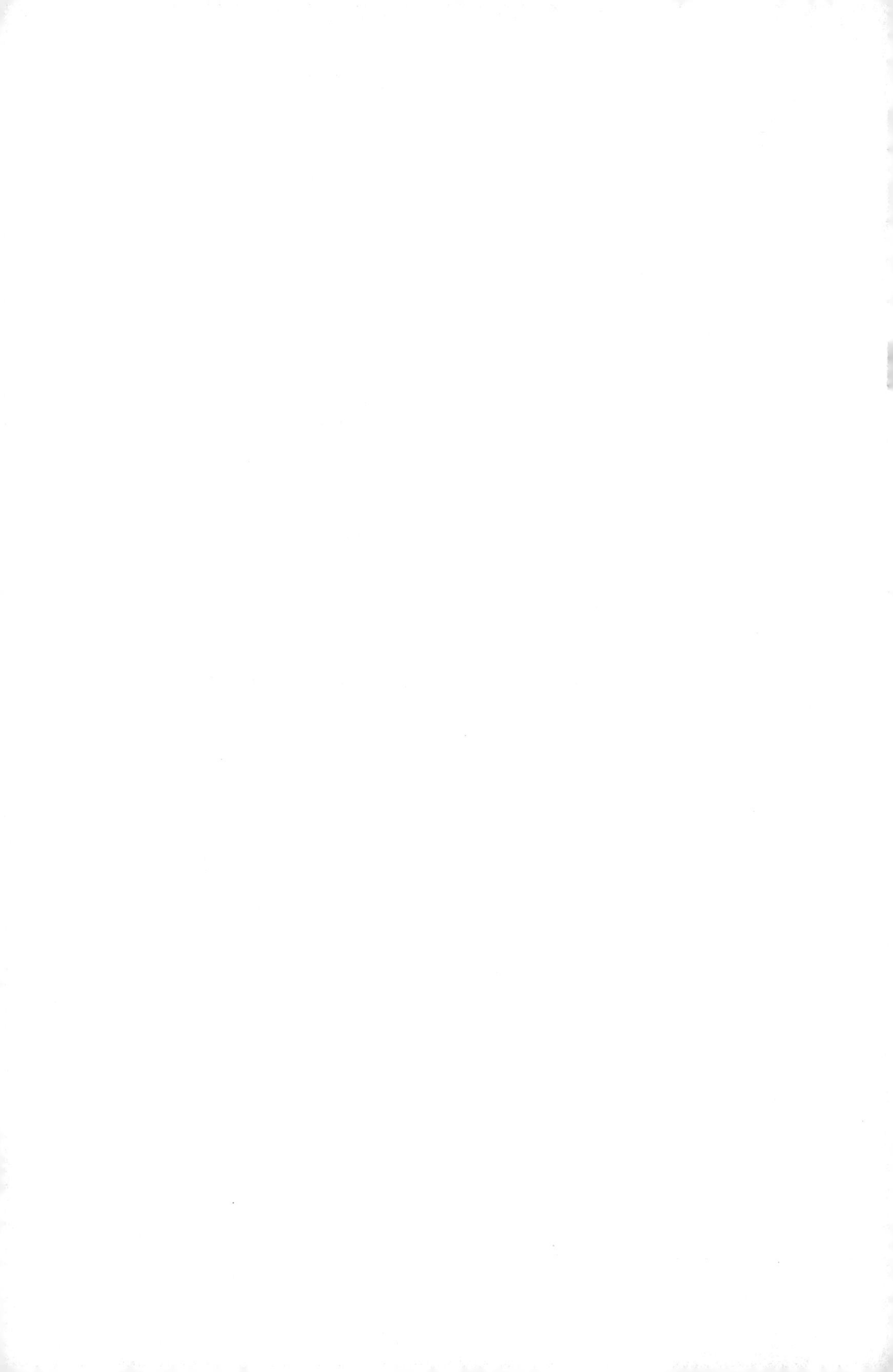

Moving?

I'd like to receive my *Year Book of Infertility & Reproductive Endocrinology* without interruption. Please note the following change of address, effective:

Name: ________________________________

New Address: ________________________________

____

City: ________________ State: ________ Zip: ________

Old Address: ________________________________

____

City: ________________ State: ________ Zip: ________

Reservation Card

Yes, I would like my own copy of *Year Book of Infertility & Reproductive Endocrinology*. Please begin my subscription with the current edition according to the terms described below.* I understand that I will have 30 days to examine each annual edition. If satisfied, I will pay just $69.95 plus sales tax, postage and handling (price subject to change without notice).

Name: ________________________________

Address: ________________________________

City: ________________ State: ________ Zip: ________

Method of Payment
O Visa   O Mastercard   O AmEx   O Bill me   O Check (in US dollars, payable to Mosby, Inc.)

Card number: ________________________ Exp date: ________________

Signature: ________________________________

LS-0909

*Your Year Book Service Guarantee:

When you subscribe to the *Year Book*, we'll send you an advance notice of future volumes about two months before they publish. This automatic notice system is designed to take up as little of your time as possible. If you do not want the *Year Book*, the advance notice makes it quick and easy for you to let us know your decision, and you will always have at least 20 days to decide. If we don't hear from you, we'll send you the new volume as soon as it's available. And, of course, the *Year Book* is yours to examine free of charge for 30 days (postage, handling and applicable sales tax are added to each shipment.).

BUSINESS REPLY MAIL
FIRST CLASS MAIL   PERMIT No. 762   CHICAGO, IL

POSTAGE WILL BE PAID BY ADDRESSEE

Chris Hughes
Mosby-Year Book, Inc.
200 N. LaSalle Street
Suite 2600
Chicago, IL 60601-9981

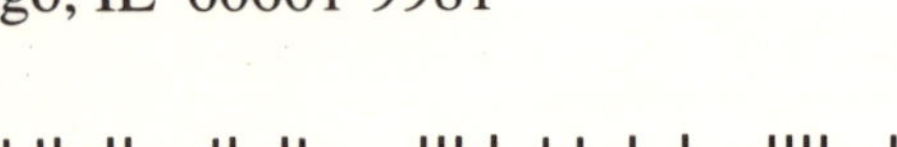

BUSINESS REPLY MAIL
FIRST CLASS MAIL   PERMIT No. 762   CHICAGO, IL

POSTAGE WILL BE PAID BY ADDRESSEE

Chris Hughes
Mosby-Year Book, Inc.
200 N. LaSalle Street
Suite 2600
Chicago, IL 60601-9981

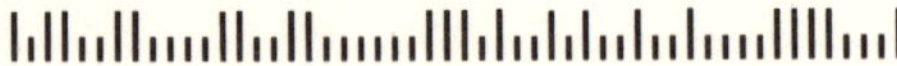

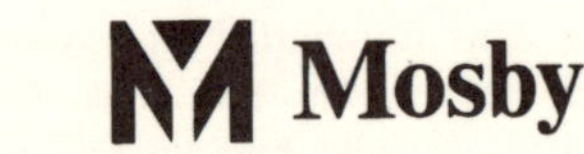

Dedicated to publishing excellence

6 Treatment of Male Infertility

The Result of Intracytoplasmic Sperm Injection Is Not Related to Any of the Three Basic Sperm Parameters
Nagy ZP, Liu J, Joris H, Verheyen G, Tournaye H, Camus M, Derde M-P, Devroey P, Van Steirteghem AC (Free Univ, Brussels, Belgium)
Hum Reprod 10:1123–1129, 1995   6–1

Objective.—Intracytoplasmic sperm injection (ICSI) reportedly is an effective approach to andrologic infertility, but how the results relate to sperm characteristics remains uncertain. For this reason the results of 683 ICSI cycles were analyzed in relation to total sperm count, motility, and sperm morphology.

Methods.—Intracytoplasmic sperm injection was done using freshly ejaculated semen when fertilization had been inadequate in standard in vitro fertilization cycles or when the ejaculate contained fewer than 500,000 progressively motile spermatozoa. The ovaries were stimulated with buserelin combined with human menopausal gonadotropin and human chorionic gonadotropin. Progesterone was administered intravaginally to support the luteal phase.

Findings.—The total pregnancy rate per transfer was 40.9%, and the ongoing pregnancy rate was 28.5%. Neither the type nor severity of sperm impairment significantly influenced the outcome of ICSI. High rates of fertilization and pregnancy were achieved in the most marked cases of male factor infertility when the initial semen sample exhibited cryptozoospermia, total asthenozoospermia, or total teratozoospermia. The only condition that compromised the results of ICSI was the injection of an immotile spermatozoon into the oocyte.

Conclusion.—Intracytoplasmic sperm injection is successful in even the most extreme cases of male factor infertility, providing that at least one living spermatozoon is present for each oocyte.

Intracytoplasmic Sperm Injection: A Major Advance in the Management of Severe Male Subfertility
Harari O, Speirs AL, Bourne H, Johnston WIH, McDonald M, Baker HWG, Richings N (Royal Women's Hosp, Carlton, Australia; Univ of Melbourne, Parkville, Victoria, Australia)
Fertil Steril 64:360–368, 1995   6–2

Background.—Male infertility has proven more difficult to treat than other types of infertility. A new technique involving injection of a single sperm into the egg cytoplasm, intracytoplasmic sperm injection, holds promise in the treatment of male infertility. The results of treatment of male infertility by intracytoplasmic sperm injection during 119 treatment cycles between July and December 1993 at a tertiary infertility sevice were assessed.

Subjects.—There were 31 patients with severe oligospermia, 21 with oligoasthenoteratospermia, 22 with asthenoteratospermia, 19 with genital tract obstructions, and 21 patients with a low fertilization rate in vitro who participated in this study.

Results.—Of 1,185 oocytes treated by intracytoplasmic sperm injection in this series, normal fertilization and cleavage occurred in 717 of the 1,073 that survived the procedure. This is a normal fertilization rate of 67%. Abnormal fertilization occurred in 11% and 10% of the oocytes did not survive the procedure. The implantation rate was 7.4%. In this group there were 36 clinical pregnancies, of which 24 were delivered or ongoing. Patients with genital tract obstruction had a higher fertilization rate than patients with sperm defects.

Conclusions.—These results confirm intracytoplasmic sperm injection as a valuable technique for the treatment of patients with various types of severe male infertility.

The Effect of Sperm Parameters on the Outcome of Intracytoplasmic Sperm Injection
Mansour RT, Amin YM, Aboulghar MA, Ramzi AM, Serour GI (Egyptian IVF-ET Ctr, Cairo, Egypt; Cairo Univ, Egypt; Al Azhar Univ, Cairo, Egypt)
Fertil Steril 64:982–986, 1995   6–3

Objective.—Most centers now use intracytoplasmic sperm injection (ICSI) as the preferred means of in vitro fertilization (IVF) in cases of male factor infertility. The influence of sperm parameters on the chances of fertilization and conception after ICSI was studied in a series of 130 cycles treated for male factor infertility of varying severity. Infertility had been present for 8½ years on average.

Results.—A total of 1,071 oocytes at the metaphase II stage were injected and 96% of them were intact afterward. Normal fertilization took place in 58% of oocytes. Of 130 ovum pick-up cycles, all but 2 reached the embryo transfer stage. The average number of embryos transferred was

3.5. There were 46 clinical pregnancies, for a success rate of 35%. Twelve of them were multiple pregnancies. Ten pregnancies ended in abortion. The fertilization and pregnancy rates were not significantly influenced by previous failure of conventional IVF; subfertile semen; or a sperm count less than 10^6/L. Teratospermia greater than 95% also was not a factor in the outcome. Fertilization was achieved in all 6 patients with 100% midpiece abnormalities, and 4 of them conceived.

Conclusion.—Sperm quality does not influence the outcome of ICSI as long as properly shaped, motile sperm are injected.

▶ The results of these studies (Abstracts 6–1 through 6–3) indicate that the results of ICSI are unrelated to the degree of morphologic abnormalities, quantity of motile sperm, or sperm concentration in the semen samples. As long as a single normally shaped motile spermatozoon is available for injection into the oocyte, fertilization can be achieved. This technique is a major advance in the treatment of infertility resulting from abnormalities in the semen. A few years ago, male factor infertility had one of the worst prognoses for pregnancy. With the use of ICSI, the prognosis for fertility when this problem exists is excellent.

D.R. Mishell, Jr., M.D.

Intracytoplasmic Sperm Injection: Achievement of High Pregnancy Rates in Couples With Severe Male Factor Infertility Is Dependent Primarily Upon Female and Not Male Factors
Oehninger S, Maloney M, Veeck L, Toner J, Lanzendorf S, Muasher S (Jones Inst for Reproductive Medicine, Eastern Virginia Med School, Norfolk, Va)
Fertil Steril 64:977–981, 1995   6–4

Objective.—Factors influencing the outcome of intracytoplasmic sperm injection (ICSI) were examined in a prospective series of 92 consecutive couples with severe male factor infertility who underwent a total of 102 cycles of in vitro fertilization (IVF) augmented with ICSI. In 50 cases at least one previous attempt at fertilizing mature preovulatory oocytes had failed. In the other 42 cases, sperm parameters were unsuitable for conventional IVF.

Findings.—The diploid fertilization rate for 1,163 preovulatory oocytes was 61%, and the cleavage rate was 99%. Normal fertilization was achieved in 97% of treatment cycles. An average of 4 embryos were transferred per cycle. The clinical implantation rate was 12%, and the clinical pregnancy rate per transfer was 32%. Twenty-six ongoing pregnancies were achieved in 97 transfers. They included 8 twin and 4 triplet gestations. No basic sperm parameters significantly influenced fertilization or pregnancy rates after ICSI (Table 1). Women who became pregnant had an average age of 34 years, compared with 36 years for those who did not conceive. Age was significantly related to both the basal serum follicle-stimulating hormone level and the outcome of pregnancy (Table 2).

TABLE 1.—Normal Fertilization and Pregnancy Outcome in Patients Undergoing Intracytoplasmic Sperm Injection According to Sperm Quality and/or Quantity

Sperm	Cycles	No. of fertilized per no. of inseminated oocytes	No. of pregnancies per no. of patients
Concentration ($\times 10^6$/mL)			
<1	9	67/115 (58.3)	4/9 (44.4)
1 to 4.9	26	180/305 (59.0)	9/26 (34.6)
5 to 9.9	7	54/82 (65.9)	3/7 (42.9)
10 to 49.9	36	273/438 (62.3)	10/36 (27.8)
≥50	24	134/223 (60.1)	5/24 (20.8)
Progressive motility (%)			
<5	10	70/127 (55.1)	4/10 (40.0)
5 to 19.9	25	204/327 (62.9)	5/25 (20.0)
≥20	67	434/709 (61.2)	22/67 (32.8)
Morphology (% normal forms)†			
<1	10	65/109 (59.6)	4/10 (40.0)
1 to 3.9	40	270/445 (60.7)	11/40 (27.5)
≥4	48	341/538 (63.4)	15/48 (31.3)

Note: Values in parentheses are percentages.
* Not available on 4 patients because of inadequate samples.
(Courtesy of Oehninger S, Maloney M, Veeck L, et al: Intracytoplasmic sperm injection: Achievement of high pregnancy rates in couples with severe male factor infertility is dependent primarily upon female and not male factors. *Fertil Steril* 64:977–981, 1995. Reproduced with permission of the publisher, the American Society for Reproductive Medicine [The American Fertility Society].)

Conclusions.—Female factors are the chief determinant of the outcome after IVF with ICSI. Intracytoplasmic sperm injection is a promising approach to couples with male infertility resistant to conventional IVF.

TABLE 2.—Intracytoplasmic Sperm Injection Results According to Female Age

Age	No. of cycles	No. of transfers	Fertilization rate	No. of embryos transferred	Clinical pregnancy rate per transfer†	Clinical implantation rate‡	Ongoing pregnancy rate per transfer§
≤ 34	49	45	349/571 (61.1)	165/45 (3.7)	22/45 (48.9)	35/165 (21.2)	17/45 (37.7)
35 to 39	36	35	262/424 (61.8)	152/35 (4.3)	8/35 (22.9)	11/152 (7.2)	8/35 (22.8)
≥40	17	17	97/168 (57.7)	73/17 (4.3)	1/17 (5.9)	1/73 (1.4)	1/17 (5.9)
	102	97	708/1,163 (60.9)	390/97 (4.0)	31/97 (31.9)	47/390 (12.1)	26/97 (26.8)

* Values in parentheses are percentages.
† Significantly different between age groups ($P = 0.001$).
‡ Significantly different between age groups ($P = 0.003$).
§ Based on available information.
(Courtesy of Oehninger S, Maloney M, Veeck L, et al: Intracytoplasmic sperm injection: Achievement of high pregnancy rates in couples with severe male factor infertility is dependent primarily upon female and not male factors. *Fertil Steril* 64:977–981, 1995. Reproduced with permission of the publisher, the American Society for Reproductive Medicine [The American Fertility Society].)

► With the use of ICSI, it is now possible to achieve a pregnancy for couples in whom there are few normal motile sperm in the ejaculated semen. It appears that with the technique of ICSI, the probability of achieving a viable pregnancy is inversely correlated with the age of the woman. The fertilizability of human ova decreases with advancing age and increasing levels of circulating follicle-stimulating hormone. Use of donor eggs should be considered in women older than 40 years and/or those with elevated circulating levels of follicle-stimulating hormone who are candidates for ICSI.

D.R. Mishell, Jr., M.D.

Percutaneous Epididymal Sperm Aspiration and Intracytoplasmic Sperm Injection in the Management of Infertility Due to Obstructive Azoospermia

Craft I, Khalifa Y, Tsirigotis M, Hogewind G, Bennett V, Nicholson N, Taranissi M (London Gynaecology and Fertility Centre)
Fertil Steril 63:1038–1042, 1995   6–5

Background.—In the past, results obtained from in vitro fertilization (IVF) using sperm aspirated from the epididymis have been poor. Micro-epididymal sperm aspiration with scrotal exploration and general anesthesia, which has been used to retrieve sperm for conventional IVF or in assisted fertilization cycles with better results, involves some trauma and postoperative morbidity. The recovery rate of spermatozoa from the epididymis and/or testes using a percutaneous aspiration method and the fertilization rate obtained with intracytoplasmic sperm injection were assessed.

Methods and Findings.—Twenty patients with obstructive azoospermia were enrolled in the study. In 16 patients, the sperm used for intracytoplasmic sperm injection was retrieved by percutaneous epididymal sperm aspiration. Microepididymal sperm aspiration was also done in 1 patient because the quality of the sperm acquired by percutaneous epididymal sperm aspiration was inadequate for microinjection. Neither percutaneous epididymal sperm aspiration nor microepididymal sperm aspiration led to sperm recovery in the remaining 3 patients. In 1 of those patients, sperm was obtained by testicular biopsy. One hundred fifty-seven of 179 collected eggs were microinjected. In 22 oocytes, or 14%, normal fertilization occurred. Altogether, 30 embryos were cleaved. Three of 12 patients undergoing embryo transfer became pregnant, for a rate of 25% per transfer. The implantation rate was 10%. Fertilization failed in 4 cycles.

Conclusions.—In men with obstructive azoospermia, percutaneous epididymal sperm aspiration can be successful in recovering sperm for use in assisted fertilization IVF cycles. Compared with an open microsurgical procedure, this technique is simple and effective and causes less trauma.

Systematic Examination of Immobilizing Spermatozoa Before Intracytoplasmic Sperm Injection in the Human
Fishel S, Lisi F, Rinaldi L, Green S, Hunter A, Dowell K, Thornton S (Nottingham Univ, England; BIOGENESI, Rome)
Hum Reprod 10:497–500, 1995
6–6

Objective.—Intracytoplasmic sperm injection (ICSI) is the most effective procedure for dealing with male infertility and, in extreme cases of male infertility, the only procedure available. The fact that a number of clinics fail to achieve high pregnancy rates suggests that considerable experience with the technique is necessary to achieve success. A systematic study of features necessary to achieve a high fertilization rate was conducted.

Methods.—Patients with severe male fertility problems and their partners were referred for treatment. A drop of sperm suspension in Eagle's minimal essential medium containing HEPES next to a drop of polyvinyl pyrrolidone (PVP) was overlayed with light liquid paraffin. One spermatozoon was transferred to the PVP droplet. In group I the slowest moving spermatozoon was injected into a corona-denuded oocyte; in group II the tail was touched, inhibiting motion; in group III, the tail was broken; and in group IV only nonmotile sperm were injected.

Results.—In the 35 couples, all males were severely oligoteratozoospermic, and 26 were asthenozoospermic. From 839 oocytes, 236 zygotes developed, 204 with 2 pronuclei and 32 with 3 pronuclei. There were significantly more pregnancies in the groups with tail-damaged or nonmotile sperm with a trend to even higher fertilization rates using already nonmotile sperm compared to those made temporarily nonmotile. There was a significant decline in the number of degenerate oocytes when the sperm tail was nonmotile. There was significantly more cytoplasmic fragmentation in groups I and II, and a significant increase in the number of embryos in groups with $\geq 25\%$ cytoplasmic fragmentation. All 6 men who were 100% asthenozoospermic achieved fertilization. Fifty of 112 injected oocytes were fertilized.

Conclusion.—Permanently immobilized spermatozoa and effective penetration of the ooplasm significantly increased the incidence of fertilization. Cytoplasmic fragmentation appeared to be related to the degree of motility of the sperm tail.

Intracytoplasmic Sperm Injection: A Novel Treatment for All Forms of Male Factor Infertility
Palermo GD, Adler A, Cohen J, Rosenwaks Z, Alikani M (New York Hosp-Cornell Med Ctr, New York)
Fertil Steril 63:1231–1240, 1995
6–7

Purpose.—For couples with male factor infertility, the intracytoplasmic sperm injection technique has become an increasingly popular treatment because of its high fertilization rates. The results of assisted fertilization by intracytoplasmic sperm injection in 227 couples were evaluated.

Methods.—The couples underwent 227 consecutive cycles of intracytoplasmic sperm injection. All had either male factor or idiopathic infertility, the latter group including couples in whom a previous attempt at in vitro fertilization (IVF) had failed and others with severely compromised sperm parameters. The primary clinical indication was the male partner's subnormal semen parameters in 150 cases. A total of 322 IVF cycles had failed in 117 couples. The analysis sought to determine the cutoff limits between the frequency of motile spermatozoa in the semen sample; the efficiency of intracytoplasmic sperm injection in achieving fertilization, cleavage, and implantation; and the predictability of success once the sperm is inserted into the ooplasm.

Results.—About 72 hours after intracytoplasmic sperm injection, 653 embryos were transferred in 217 cycles. Before replacement, 79% of embryos were micromanipulated for assisted hatching. A positive human chorionic gonadotropin was noted in 124 patients, including 19 with biochemical pregnancies, 10 patients with a blighted ovum, and 1 with ectopic pregnancy. Ultrasound detected a fetal heart beat in 94 patients. Ongoing pregnancy rate was 37% per oocyte retrieval and 39% per replacement. The pregnancies were 47 singletons, 30 twins, 6 triplets, and 1 quadruplet. Sac formation rate was 25% per embryo. No single sperm parameter correlated with the outcome.

Conclusions.—In couples with male factor infertility, intracytoplasmic sperm injection can achieve fertility despite problems with motility and concentration of normal motile spermatozoa. Fertilization rates are high— 59% overall and 64% in intact oocytes—independent of semen charac-

---

TABLE 3.—Semen Parameters, Fertilization, and Pregnancies Obtained With Intracytoplasmic Sperm Injection According to the Origin of the Semen Sample

Semen origin	Density	Motility	Morph-ology	No. of cycles	Fertilization*		No. of positive hCG	No. of ongoing pregnancies*
	$\times 10^6/mL$	%						
1. Fresh	21.6	34.4†	2.2‡	193	972/1,484	(65.5)§	105	73 (37.8)
2. Frozen	23.9	9.4†	1.6‡	13	75/113	(66.4)§	6	2 (15.4)
3. Electro-ejaculation	27.0	10.3†	3.8‡	4	23/34	(67.6)§	1	0
4. Epididymal	13.4	16.2†	4.2‡	17	72/156	(46.2)§	12	9 (52.9)

* Values in parentheses are percentages.

† 1–4: Single factor analysis of variance, 3 df; differences between sperm motility among different semen origin, $P < 0.001$.

‡ 1–4: Single factor analysis of variance, 3 df; differences between sperm morphology among different semen origin, $P = 0.009$.

§ 1–4: χ^2, 2 × 4, 3 df; differences within semen origin on fertilization, $P < 0.001$. Post hoc comparison using the Bonferroni adjustment shows no significant difference in motility between groups 2 and 3, and no significant difference between groups 1 and 4. For morphology, groups 1, 2, and 3 show no significant difference, whereas group 4 is significantly different from groups 1, 2, and 3. For fertilization percentage, groups 1, 2, and 3 are not significantly different from each other, whereas the group 4 percentage is significantly different from the other 3 rates.

(Courtesy of Palermo GD, Adler A, Cohen J, et al: Intracytoplasmic sperm injection: A novel treatment for all forms of male factor infertility. *Fertil Steril* 63:1231–1240, 1995. Reproduced with permission of the publisher, the American Society for Reproductive Medicine [The American Fertility Society].)

---

teristics (Table 3). The results compare favorably to those of standard IVF in couples with no sperm abnormalities. Intracytoplasmic sperm injection should be studied for patients with other causes of infertility.

Pregnancy Obtained With Human Testicular Spermatozoa in an *In Vitro* Fertilization Program
Schoysman R, Vanderzwalmen P, Nijs M, Segal L, Segal-Betin G, Geerts L, van Roosendaal E, Schoysman-Deboeck A (van Helmont Ziekenhuis, Vilvoorde, Belgium)
J Androl 15:10S–13S, 1994   6–8

Purpose.—Previous studies in animals have demonstrated the fertilizing ability of testicular spermatozoa. In the present study, the fertilizing ability of human testicular spermatozoa and the outcomes of in vitro fertilization were investigated.

Patients and Methods.—Six men with obstructive and inoperable azoospermia were included in the study. Routine testicular biopsies were performed, during which 4- × 4-mm samples were obtained. Samples were divided into fragments of tissue measuring 1 mm in diameter, and were then dissected under the microscope. The end result was a fluid suspension packed with multiple spermatogenic cells and spermatozoa. On average, 150,000 to 300,000 spermatozoa typically were obtained. Isolated spermatozoa were then injected into the perivitelline space or directly into the cytoplasm of oocytes.

Results.—A fertilization rate of 45% was achieved using testicular sperm. Normal cleavage was observed. Replacement of 10 embryos in 6 patients led to 1 biochemical and 1 ongoing pregnancy. In the ongoing pregnancy, 2 pronuclei were observed in 2 of 7 oocytes that had been microinseminated with testicular sperm. A 4-cell grade A embryo and a 2-cell grade B embryo were transferred after 44 hours.

Conclusions.—In men with obstructive azoospermia, epididymal microsurgery may not always be successful, even when normal spermatogenesis is present. Fertilization by testicular sperm therefore may prove to be a useful approach in such patients. Further studies evaluating this technique are recommended.

Pregnancies After Intracytoplasmic Injection of Sperm Collected by Fine Needle Biopsy of the Testis
Bourne H, Watkins W, Speirs A, Baker HWG (Royal Women's Hosp, Carlton, Victoria, Australia; Univ of Melbourne, Australia)
Fertil Steril 64:433–436, 1995   6–9

Background.—The use of intracytoplasmic sperm injection for in vitro insemination has improved the fertilization rate for couples with male genital tract obstruction. The low number of sperm needed for this type of insemination permits sufficient sperm to be isolated by fine-needle biopsy

TABLE 1.—Patient Histories and Outcome of Intracytoplasmic Sperm Injection Cycles Using Sperm Collected by Fine-Needle Biopsy of the Testis

	Case I	Case II
Female age (y)	30	36
Previous IVF*		
Cycles	—	2
Embryos developed per oocytes inseminated†	—	
First cycle		1/6 (17)‡
Second cycle		0/4 (0)
Intracytoplasmic sperm injection results		
Oocytes injection	13	9
Normally fertilized†	9 (69)	5 (56)
Fresh transfers	1	1
Pregnancies	—	1
Single intrauterine fetal heart		1
Frozen transfers	4	—
Pregnancies	2	—
Biochemical	1	
Single intrauterine fetal heart	1	

* Oocytes inseminated by standard IVF using epididymal sperm collected from the husband by microsurgery.
† Values in parentheses are percentages.
‡ Oocyte cleaved to a 4-cell embryo 51 hours after insemination but without pronuclei observed the previous day.
Abbreviation: IVF, in vitro fertilization.
(Courtesy of Bourne H, Watkins W, Speirs A, et al: Pregnancies after intracytoplasmic injection of sperm collected by fine needle biopsy of the testis. *Fertil Steril* 64:433–436, 1995. Reproduced with permission of the publisher, the American Society for Reproductive Medicine [The American Fertility Society].)

of the testis. This procedure is less costly and less invasive than microsurgical epididymal sperm aspiration and can also be used in men with intratesticular blockage. The first 2 cases of intracytoplasmic sperm injection using sperm collected by fine-needle biopsy were reviewed.

Methods.—The 2 couples received diagnoses of intratesticular genital tract obstruction causing infertility. Testicular tissue was collected by fine-needle biopsy. The sperm was immobilized and injected into oocyte cytoplasm.

Results.—In the first case, 14 oocytes were collected. Of those, 13 were mature and they were injected with sperm. Nine oocytes fertilized normally. Two were transferred and the rest frozen. On the fourth transfer, a singleton uterine fetal heartbeat was detected by ultrasound at 6 weeks. In the second case, 9 mature oocytes were collected and injected with sperm. Five oocytes fertilized normally. Two were transferred fresh and a single intrauterine fetal heartbeat was detected by ultrasound at 6 weeks (Table 1).

Conclusions.—Fine-needle biopsy of the testis is a less invasive and less expensive alternative to sperm collection by microsurgical aspiration. It can also be used for patients with intratesticular blockage. The collection of sperm by fine-needle biopsy of the testis combined with intracytoplasmic sperm injection provides a good fertilization rate, even for patients with intratesticular blockage. It may be a preferred option for any patients with genital tract obstruction.

High Fertilization Rate With Intracytoplasmic Sperm Injection in Mosaic Klinefelter's Syndrome

Harari O, Gronow M, Bourne H, Johnston I, Baker G (Royal Women's Hosp, Melbourne, Victoria, Australia)
Fertil Steril 63:182–184, 1995   6–10

Introduction.—Most adults with Klinefelter's syndrome are azoospermic. As many as 12% of azoospermic patients and a smaller proportion of those who are oligospermic may have constitutional chromosomal abnormalities, most often sex chromosome anomalies such as 47,XXY. There are, however, reports of motile sperm and rare reports of fertility and proven paternity. Oocytes were fertilized in vitro in 2 stimulated cycles using the technique of intracytoplasmic sperm injection (ICSI) with sperm from a man with Klinefelter's syndrome.

Case Report.—Man, 35, was seen because of primary infertility after 7 years of marriage. He was a tall, thin man with poorly developed body hair and small, firm testes. The follicle-stimulating hormone level was elevated but levels of testosterone and luteinizing hormone were normal. Karyotyping of peripheral blood cells revealed a predominant 47,XXY pattern, but a few cells were 46,XY or 48,XXXY. Sperm concentrations were less than 1,000/mL and motile sperm were practically absent.

After ovarian stimulation and ICSI, 1 of 4 injected oocytes developed into a good-quality 2-cell embryo that subsequently was transferred to the uterine cavity. Conception did not take place. In a second attempt, 2 good-quality embryos were transferred but there was no evidence of conception.

Conclusion.—This experience shows that ICSI is a potentially useful means of managing extreme male infertility that previously would have been viewed as untreatable.

Fertilization and Pregnancy Achieved by Intracytoplasmic Injection of Sperm Retrieved From Testicular Biopsies

Abuzeid MI, Basata S, Chan Y-M, Beer M, Sasy MA (Hurley Med Ctr, Flint, Mich; Genessee Urological Ctr, Flint, Mich)
Fertil Steril 64:644–646, 1995   6–11

Background.—The number of sperm obtained by microsurgical aspiration of the epididymis is unpredictable, and some of the sperm that are recovered may be poorly motile. If spermatogenesis is adequate, it should be possible to retrieve some sperm from testicular biopsies for use in intracytoplasmic sperm injection (ICSI).

Two Cases.—Intracytoplasmic sperm injection was carried out successfully in 2 instances in which microsurgical epididymal aspiration had failed. Both patients had undergone vasectomy, and in 1, attempted reversal had failed. Both the men had fathered children in a previous marriage before undergoing vasectomy. After testicular biopsy and follicular stimulation for oocyte retrieval, ICSI was carried out without further processing the sperm prepared from the biopsy. Fertilization ensued in both cases, resulting in embryos. The spouse of 1 of the patients conceived and delivered triplets.

Conclusion.—It is possible to achieve conception through ICSI using testicular sperm from a man who has undergone vasectomy some time in the past. Apparently sperm retrieved from an obstructed environment are able to decondense within the oocyte, form pronuclei, and produce a pregnancy.

Using Ejaculated, Fresh, and Frozen-Thawed Epididymal and Testicular Spermatozoa Gives Rise to Comparable Results After Intracytoplasmic Sperm Injection

Nagy Z, Silber S, Liu J, Devroey P, Cecile J, Van Steirteghem A (Dutch-speaking Brussels Free Univ, Brussels, Belgium; St Luke's Hosp, St Louis)
Fertil Steril 63:808–815, 1995   6–12

Background.—Male factor infertility is commonly treated by the standard in vitro fertilization procedure. However, the outcomes have often been disappointing because of the usually low fertilization rate. Much higher fertilization and pregnancy rates (PRs) have been obtained by intracytoplasmic sperm injection, which requires only one spermatozoon per oocyte. These facts have resulted in the use of the intracytoplasmic sperm injection method in which fresh or frozen-thawed epididymal and testicular sperm are used for insemination. The preparation of fresh or frozen-thawed epididymal and testicular sperm for intracytoplasmic single sperm injection was described, and the fertilization, embryo quality, and PRs obtained after the use of these spermatozoa were compared with the results when freshly ejaculated sperm were used for microinjection.

Methods.—A total of 1,034 consecutive microinjection cycles were analyzed retrospectively. The sperm used for intracytoplasmic injection were ejaculated, fresh epididymal, frozen-thawed epididymal, and testicular.

Findings.—For freshly ejaculated sperm, the median values of total sperm count were 17.6×10^6; total motility, 37%; and normal morphology, 8%. For fresh epididymal sperm, the corresponding values were 46.2×10^6, 12%, and 9%. For frozen-thawed epididymal sperm, they were 0.15×10^6, 0%, and 0%. For testicular sperm, the median value of total sperm count was 0.54×10^6 and the total motility, 0%. Morphologic characteristics were not determined for testicular sperm. After microinjection, the percentage of intact oocytes ranged from 84% to 90%. The normalization fertilization rates were 56%, 56%, and 48%, respectively, when fresh or frozen-thawed epididymal and testicular spermatozoa were used for injection. However, the normal fertilization rate for ejaculated sperm was significantly higher at 70%. The proportion of transferable embryos acquired after ejaculated sperm injection was higher than that after testicular sperm injection. Positive serum hCG was documented in 40% of the cycles using ejaculated sperm, in 58% using fresh sperm, in 33% using frozen-thawed epididymal sperm, and in 46% using testicular sperm. In 26.3% of the conception cycles, initial pregnancy loss occurred.

Conclusions.—When fresh or frozen-thawed epididymal and testicular spermatozoa are used, intracytoplasmic sperm injection can provide high normal fertilization, cleavage, and PRs. However, normal fertilization rates associated with the use of such sperm are significantly lower than those associated with microinjection with ejaculated sperm.

▶ The advent of intracytoplasmic sperm injection (ICSI) has revolutionized the treatment of male factor infertility. This series of articles (Abstracts 6–5 through 6–12) delineates the numerous clinical situations in which ICSI should be considered as a treatment option. Intracytoplasmic sperm injection has specifically provided a potentially successful treatment for men with congenital absence of the vas deferens, patients with severe and otherwise untreatable oligospermia, and patients with evidence of obstruction that may not be amenable to surgical correction (see Abstracts 6–5, 6–8, and 6–10). The combination of fine-needle aspiration of testicular tissue with ICSI further simplifies (for the patient) the acquisition of spermatozoa for fertilization and subsequent pregnancy (see Abstract 6–9). It is, however, important to remember that ICSI is *one* treatment, not the *only* treatment for male factor infertility.

Intracytoplasmic sperm injection should be recommended only after a thorough evaluation of the patient has been completed and the conclusion has been reached that no other therapy is appropriate. All evaluations must include a careful history, physical examination, and at least one semen analysis. The need for appropriate hormonal testing is indicated by the findings at the initial consultation.

Before proceeding on to ICSI, the andrologist needs to determine whether the patient has (1) a reversible cause of infertility, (2) a life-threatening disease that is presenting as infertility, or (3) an inheritable disorder that will require careful genetic counseling. Once the andrologist has determined that ICSI is the treatment of choice, the physician must provide information for informed consent, which includes the probability of the birth of a healthy child after the procedure, increased incidence of multiple gestations and the associated health risks to the mother and child, the cost of the procedure, and perhaps most importantly our ignorance regarding long-term genetic outcomes.

R.Z. Sokol, M.D., F.A.C.P.

Controlled Trial of High Spermatic Vein Ligation for Varicocele in Infertile Men

Madgar I, Karasik A, Weissenberg R, Goldwasser B, Lunenfeld B (Sheba Med Ctr, Tel Hashomer, Israel)
Fertil Steril 63:120–124, 1995

6–13

Background.—Varicocele is more common among patients attending infertility treatment clinics than among the general male population. A World Health Organization (WHO) study reported that men with varico-

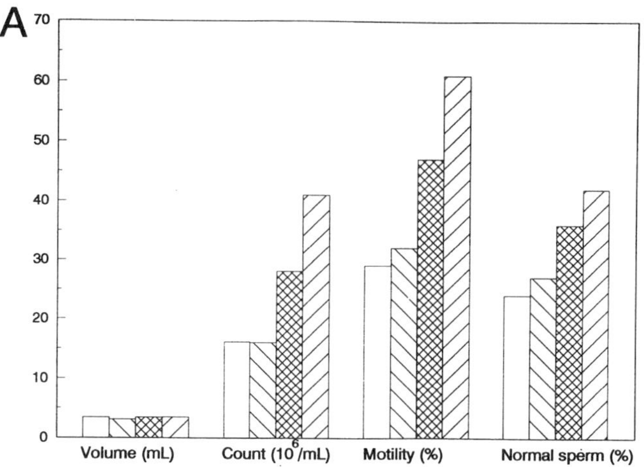
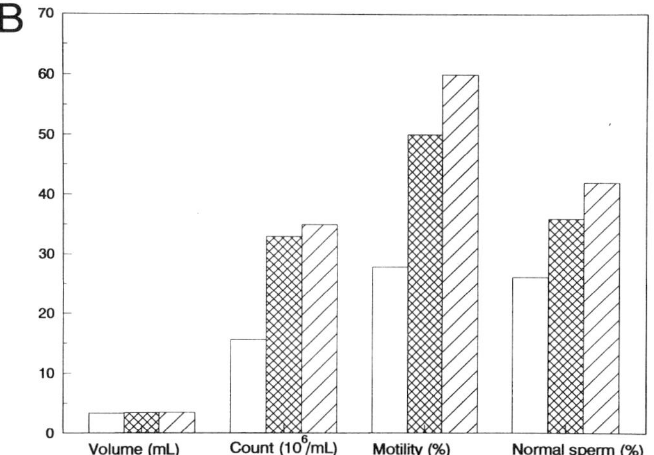

FIGURE 1.—**A,** mean sperm parameters at recruitment (*open bars*), after 12 months of observation (→), and at 12 months after ligation of group A patients who did not achieve pregnancy (*cross-hatched bars*) and of those who did (*striped bars*). **B,** the same for group B but without the observation period. (Courtesy of Madgar I, Karasik A, Weissenberg R, et al: Controlled trial of high spermatic vein ligation for varicocele in infertile men. *Fertil Steril* 63:120–124, 1995, Reproduced with permission of the publisher, the American Society for Reproductive Medicine [The American Fertility Society].)

cele showed a deterioration in sperm concentration and motility. The relationship between varicocele and infertility remains unclear, however. The effectiveness of ligation of the left spermatic vein, an established therapy for varicocele in infertile men, was examined in a randomized, controlled trial.

Patients and Methods.—Study participants were men aged 21–45 years who had been infertile for at least 1 year and whose female partner had no demonstrable cause of infertility. All had a palpable left varicocele only, with no other conditions or medications that might affect fertility. In addition, all exhibited abnormal semen analysis, according to WHO criteria, on 2 different occasions. Twenty men (group A) did not receive any treatment for 12 months after study entry. High ligation of the left spermatic vein was performed if no pregnancy had occurred after the year of observation. These patients were then followed for an additional 36 months. Twenty-five men (group B) underwent high ligation of the left spermatic vein within 45 days of study entry and were observed for a further 36 months.

Results.—Groups A and B were similar in mean age, period of infertility, hormonal status, and seminal parameters. Two pregnancies (10%) were achieved among group A couples during the first year of observation. The number of pregnancies increased to 8 (44.4%) in the year after high ligation, and 4 more pregnancies occurred in the following year. Group B couples had 15 pregnancies (60%) in the first year after high ligation, 3 pregnancies in the second year, and 1 in the third year. Semen parameters significantly improved after ligation in all patients, regardless of whether pregnancy was achieved (Fig 1).

Conclusion.—The association of varicocele with infertility was confirmed, as were the beneficial effects of high ligation. Correction of varicocele by high spermatic vein ligation had a highly significant effect on sperm parameters and pregnancy rate. In both groups, the highest rate of pregnancy was achieved in the first year after operation.

Treatment of Varicocele: Counselling as Effective as Occlusion of the Vena Spermatica

Nieschlag E, Hertle L, Fischedick A, Behre HM (Inst of Reproductive Medicine of the Univ, Münster, Germany)
Hum Reprod 10:347–353, 1995   6–14

Objective.—Surgical ligation and radiologic embolization of the spermatic vein have all been used to treat varicocele. Both techniques are equally effective in achieving pregnancy. Because men with varicocele are not necessarily infertile, the effect of surgical or radiologic occlusion of the spermatic vein was compared with no treatment in a prospective study.

Methods.—A total of 120 couples entered the study and 95 completed it. Patients were randomly assigned to 3 treatment groups: 23 patients were treated by surgical ligation, 24 by radiologic embolization, and 48 with counseling. Doppler sonography, semen analysis, and hormone determinations were performed twice with each patient. Other causes of male and female infertility were ruled out. Patients were counseled every 3 months for a year.

Results.—Sperm concentration increased significantly in the treated groups from 16.6×10^6/mL to 25.1×10^6/mL but not in the control group (Fig 2). There was a significant decrease in percentage of normal sperm

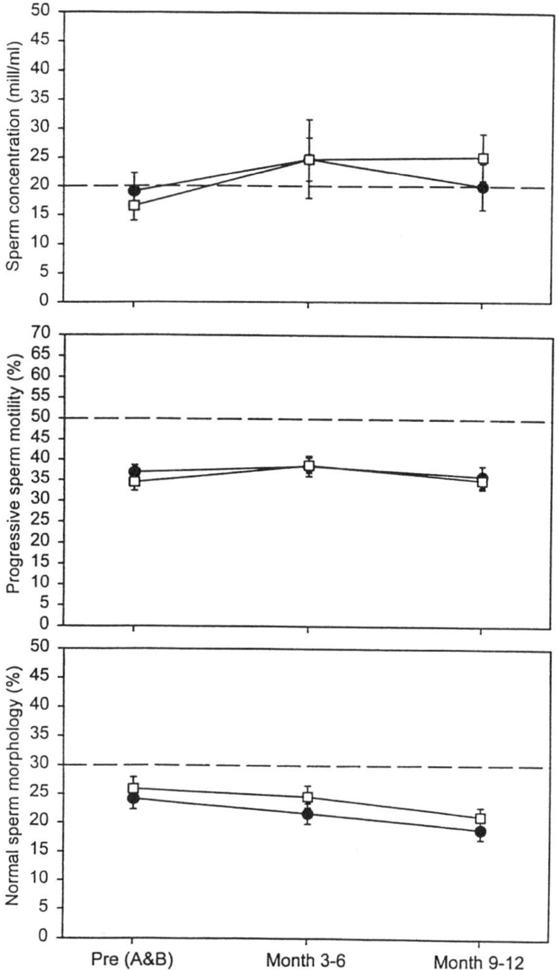

FIGURE 2.—Seminal parameters (mean ± SE) in the untreated (*filled symbols*) and treated (*open symbols*) patients. *Pre (A&B)*: mean of the 2 pre-study baseline examinations; *Month 3–6*: mean of the examinations at months 3 and 6; *Month 9–12*: mean of the examinations at months 9 and 12. The *dashed lines* indicate the lower limits of normal for the different seminal parameters. **Upper panel,** sperm concentration; **middle panel,** sperm progressive motility; **lower panel,** normal sperm morphology. (Courtesy of Nieschlag E, Hertle L, Fischedick A, et al: Treatment of varicocele: counselling as effective as occlusion of the vena spermatica. *Hum Reprod* 10:347–353, 1995, by permission of Oxford University Press.)

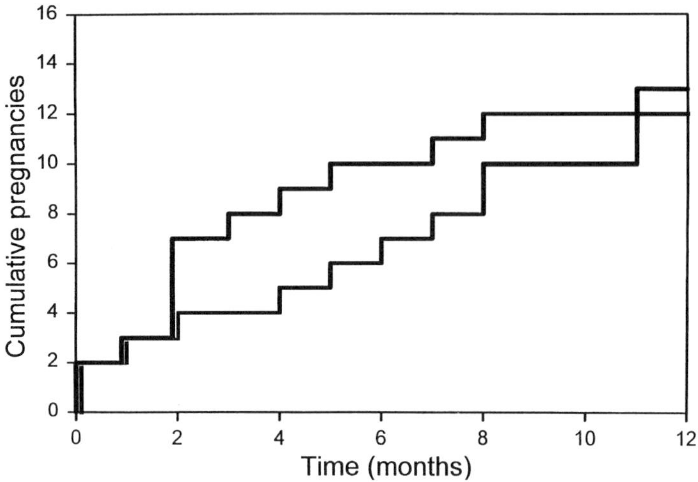

FIGURE 4.—Cumulative pregnancy rates over 12 months in the 48 untreated patients (*black line*) and the 47 treated patients (*gray line*). (Courtesy of Nieschlag E, Hertle L, Fischedick A, et al: Treatment of varicocele: Counselling as effective as occlusion of the vena spermatica. *Hum Reprod* 10:347–353, 1995, by permission of Oxford University Press.)

morphology in all groups but not between groups. There were no significant changes in serum luteinizing hormone, follicle-stimulating hormone (FSH), or testosterone during the study. During the follow-up year, there were 25 pregnancies (26.3%), 12 in the treatment group and 13 in the control group (Fig 4). These results agree with those of previous studies (Table 2). Multifactor analysis of variance showed that significant predictors of pregnancy were partner's age, higher pre-study combined testicular volume, and lower serum FSH. There was no change in testicular volume or FSH during treatment. Those who achieved pregnancy had an average age of 28.4 years, whereas those who did not achieve pregnancy had an average age of 31.2 years.

Conclusion.—Surgical treatment of varicocele is no more effective than counseling in achieving pregnancy. Recommendations for treatment of male infertility should be tested in properly controlled clinical trials.

TABLE 2.—Pregnancy Rates in Couples Participating in the Current and the Previous Study (1993) on the Treatment of Varicocele

	No. pregnancies/no. couples	Percentage
Counselling	13/48	27.1
Intervention	34/118	28.8
Ligation	19/61	31.1
Embolization	15/57	26.3
Total	47/166	28.3

(Courtesy of Nieschlag E, Hertle L, Fischedick A, et al: Treatment of varicocele: Counselling as effective as occlusion of the vena spermatica. *Hum Reprod* 10:347–353, 1995.)

▶ The controversy persists. These 2 studies (Abstracts 6–13 and 6–14), both randomized and controlled, reach opposite conclusions. Why? Perhaps the answer lies in the biases of the investigators. Were the groups truly randomized? Were the investigators really blinded? If the groups in the Madgar et al. paper were truly randomized, then the only statistical comparison that can be made is between groups A and B in the first year. Of interest is the finding in both studies of an increase in sperm concentrations after surgery.

R.Z. Sokol, M.D., F.A.C.P.

In Vitro Fertilization Outcome in the Presence of Severe Male Factor Infertility
Ben-Chetrit A, Senoz S, Greenblatt EM, Casper RF (Toronto Hosp, Ont, Canada)
Fertil Steril 63:1032–1037, 1995   6–15

Purpose.—For couples undergoing in vitro fertilization (IVF), fertility and pregnancy rates are lower when subnormal spermatozoa are used for insemination. Micromanipulation techniques were developed to overcome the low fertilization rate associated with severe male factor infertility; however, few laboratories offer micromanipulation, and not all methods of micromanipulation carry a high monospermic fertilization rate. The results of standard IVF, without micromanipulation, for couples with severe male factor infertility were assessed.

Methods.—The retrospective study included 672 cycles in patients who underwent successful oocyte retrieval in an IVF program. Based on the total motile sperm number recovered using standard swim-up, the cycles were classified into 4 groups: group 1, total motile sperm number 0.50 $\times$ 10^6; group 2, 0.51 to 1.00 $\times$ 10^6; group 3, 1.01 to 1.50 $\times$ 10^6; and group 4, 1.51 $\times$ 10^6 or greater. Couples in group 1 were regarded as having severe male factor infertility. The same controlled ovarian hyperstimulation protocol—consisting of a GnRH analogue flare-up followed by parenteral menotropins—was used in all 4 groups. The groups were compared for their clinical and cycle characteristics and outcomes.

Results.—Clinical and cycle characteristics were comparable among the 4 groups, justifying analysis of their outcome. Couples in group 1 had a fertilization rate of 21.5%, compared with 39.8% for group 2, 59.5% for group 3, and 63.5% for group 4. Number of embryos transferred also increased directly with total motile sperm number, from 0.9 in group 1 to 2.4 in groups 3 and 4. Implantation rate per embryo was not significantly different between groups. Pregnancy rate increased from 7.8% in group 1 to 22.4% in group 4. Failure to fertilize decreased gradually from 47.3% in group 1 to 10.1% in group 4, showing a significant correlation with the increase in total motile count (Table 2).

Conclusions.—A trial of conventional IVF should be offered to couples with severe male factor infertility. This recommendation holds even when

TABLE 2.—In Vitro Fertilization Outcome in Relation to Fertilization

	Group			
	1	2	3	4
Total motile sperm number ($\times 10^6$)	<0.50	0.51 to 1.00	1.01 to 1.50	>1.51
No. of patients with fertilization of at least one oocyte	20	51	39	461
Fertilization in couples with at least one embryo (%)*	40.8 ± 6.4 †	56.5 ± 4.2‡	71.8 ± 4.2	69.6 ± 1.1
No. of embryos transferred	1.8 ± 0.2§	2.2 ± 0.1‖	2.9 ± 0.1	2.6 ± 0.04
Pregnancy rate per ET¶**	3/20 (15)	11/51 (21.5)	10/39 (25.6)	115/461 (24.9)
Implantation rate (%)††	7.9± 5.8	9.9 ± 3.9	14.8 ± 4.6	11.3 ± 1.1
No. of patients with no fertilization	18	23	8	52
Failed fertilization¶‡‡	18/38 (47.3)	23/74 (31.0)	8/47 (17)	52/513 (10.1)

* Values are means ± SEM.
† Group 1 vs. groups 2, 3, and 4, $P < 0.001$.
‡ Group 2 vs. groups 2, 3, and 4, $P < 0.001$.
§ Group 1 vs. groups 2, 3, and 4, $P < 0.001$.
‖ Group 2 vs. groups 2, 3, and 4, $P < 0.001$.
¶ Values in parentheses are percentages.
** Not statistically significantly different, $P = 0.7$.
†† Not statistically significantly different, $P = 0.8$.
‡‡ Groups 1 and 2 vs. groups 3 and 4, $P < 0.01$.
Abbreviation: ET, embryo transfer.
(Courtesy of Ben-Chetrit A, Senoz S, Greenblatt EM, et al: In vitro fertilization outcome in the presence of severe male factor infertility. *Fertil Steril* 63:1032–1037, 1995. Reproduced with permission of the publisher, the American Society for Reproductive Medicine [The American Fertility Society].)

total motile sperm number is less than 0.5×10^6, as long as sufficient motile spermatozoa can be recovered for insemination. The results compare favorably with reported monospermic fertilization rates using partial zone dissection and subzonal insertion, although they are not as good as the results of intracytoplasmic sperm injection.

► Because many clinics that perform IVF do not have individuals who have had sufficient training or experience with the micromanipulation techniques necessary to perform intracytoplasmic sperm injection, the couple who has male factor infertility should be made aware of the prognosis for pregnancy after standard IVF. The results of this study provide information regarding the prognosis for pregnancy with different degrees of abnormalities in the concentration of total motile sperm following the swim-up technique. Pregnancy rates certainly vary among individual clinics, but with a sufficient concentration of motile sperm, standard IVF has a reasonable chance of achieving pregnancy.

D.R. Mishell, Jr., M.D.

Comparison Between a Two-Layer Discontinuous Percoll Gradient and Swim-Up for Sperm Preparation on Normal and Abnormal Semen Samples

Chen S-U, Ho H-N, Chen H-F, Chao K-H, Lin H-R, Huang S-C, Lee T-Y, Yang Y-S (Natl Taiwan Univ, Taipei, Republic of China)
J Assist Reprod Genet 12:698–703, 1995   6–16

Background.—The relative value of the Percoll gradient and swim-up method for sperm preparation is unknown. The effects of these 2 treatments on the percentage of progressive motility, motile sperm recovery, debris removal, percentage of normal forms according to strict criteria, and movement characteristics of sperm using computer-assisted velocity analysis were investigated.

Methods.—Fifty semen samples were obtained from 50 patients attending an infertility clinic. These samples were analyzed and placed into groups. The normal group consisted of 27 samples with normal parameters, and the abnormal group included 23 samples with abnormal findings.

Results.—In both groups, the sperm concentration in the Percoll samples was significantly higher than that in the swim-up samples. The percentage of progressive motility was greater in the swim-up samples than in the Percoll samples. However, the number of motile sperm, indicating the percentage of motile sperm recovery, was greater in the Percoll samples. The 2 methods were comparable in removal of semen debris. The percentage of normal forms was also comparable in samples treated by gradient and swim-up techniques. Compared with the Percoll samples, the swim-up samples had significantly greater curvilinear velocity and straight-line velocity of sperm.

Conclusions.—The Percoll gradient method resulted in a significantly greater final concentration of sperm than the swim-up technique. However, the percentage of motility was lower and the velocity smaller with the Percoll gradient method. Because the gradient method allows recovery of more numerous motile sperm than the swim-up method, the former may be useful in preparing sperm for oligospermic samples. The 2 techniques increased the percentages of normal forms equally. The swim-up method, by virtue of its simplicity and recovery of sperm with superior motility, may continue to be the standard technique for preparing normal semen from which sufficiently motile sperm are obtained for insemination.

▶ It appears that there are no major differences between the 2 techniques currently used to obtain a sufficient number of motile, normally shaped spermatozoa for performing intrauterine insemination or in vitro fertilization. Controlled ovarian hyperstimulation followed by intrauterine insemination is now being performed in many private offices to treat unexplained infertility. Use of the Percoll gradient is somewhat faster and does not necessitate incubation of the semen specimen. Therefore, use of the Percoll gradient may be more convenient than using the swim-up technique.

D.R. Mishell, Jr., M.D.

Successful Use of Pentoxifylline in Male-Factor Infertility and Previous Failure of In Vitro Fertilization: A Prospective Randomized Study
Rizk B, Fountain S, Avery S, Palmer C, Blayney M, MacNamee M, Mills C, Brinsden P (Bourn Hall Clinic, Cambridge, England; Univ of Cambridge, England)
J Assist Reprod Genet 12:710–714, 1995   6–17

Background.—A plethora of basic science research has confirmed the positive effect of pentoxifylline (PF) on sperm function tests. However, relatively few studies of the clinical application in in vitro fertilization (IVF) have appeared. The studies that do exist have yielded conflicting results, with some authors reporting significantly improved fertilization rates and others finding no benefit. The role of PF in IVF for couples with male factor infertility was assessed in a prospective, randomized study.

Methods.—Forty-nine couples were enrolled in the study. All had previous failed fertilization in vitro that was attributed to male factor or male factor infertility with no previous IVF attempts. Controlled ovarian hyperstimulation involved the use of gonadotropin-releasing hormone agonist and human menopausal gonadotropin. Spermatozoa treated with PF and untreated spermatozoa were used to inseminate oocytes of the same grade and maturity. Up to 3 embryos were replaced after 48 hours, and the remainder was cryopreserved.

Findings.—The group in which oocytes were inseminated with PF-treated spermatozoa had a significantly greater fertilization rate than the control group did. Overall, fertilization occurred in 92% of the 49 cycles.

In 4 couples, neither oocytes inseminated with PF-treated spermatozoa nor control spermatozoa fertilized. In 7 cycles, only the oocytes inseminated with PF-treated spermatozoa fertilized, compared with 1 cycle in which only oocytes inseminated with control spermatozoa fertilized. Fifty-seven PF and 31 control embryos were replaced, resulting in 11 clinical pregnancies. Seven pregnancies occurred in the 37 cycles in which both PF and control embryos were replaced, and 3 occurred in the 7 cycles in which only PF embryos were replaced. None of the infants born showed any evidence of congenital malformations.

Conclusions.—Pentoxifylline appears to improve the fertilization rate and outcomes in couples with male factor infertility and poor fertilization rates. There was no evidence of increased teratogenicity or congenital deformities in the pregnancies after IVF cycles in which PF-treated spermatozoa were used for fertilization.

▶ Many centers in which IVF is being performed do not have individuals who have received the necessary training to perform intracytoplasmic sperm injection into the oocyte. If couples with male factor infertility or unexplained infertility have failure of fertilization occur after incubation of the sperm and oocyte, it may be helpful to try the technique described in this report.

D.R. Mishell, Jr., M.D.

Oral Steroid Therapy for Subfertile Males With Antisperm Antibodies in the Semen: Prediction of the Responders
Sharma KK, Barratt CLR, Pearson MJ, Cooke ID (Jessop Hosp for Women, Sheffield, England)
Hum Reprod 10:103–109, 1995   6–18

Objective.—The value of steroid treatment was studied in a prospective series of 48 subfertile couples in which the male partner had 20% or more motile spermatozoa with bound IgG and/or IgA antibodies. Infertility had been present for at least 2 years, or for a year or longer in the 8 men with a history of vasovasostomy. Most of the female partners were ovulating regularly and spontaneously.

Treatment.—The male partners received 20 mg of prednisolone twice daily on the first 10 days of the cycle, and a dose of 5 mg on days 11 and 12. Treatment was repeated each month for as long as 9 months.

Results.—Twelve of the 48 couples achieved pregnancy. The cumulative conception rate after 9 months of treatment was 30%. Side effects were minimal and never required withdrawal from the study. In successful cases steroid treatment significantly suppressed those isotypes that are directed chiefly against the sperm head, and grade I motility became significantly more frequent. Motility also improved when pregnancy was not achieved, and isotypes in seminal plasma that are directed mainly against the head of donor sperm were significantly suppressed. Pregnancy was associated with elevated levels of IgG antibody directed against the spermatozoa tail.

Conclusion.—Antisperm antibodies may disrupt fertilization in subfertile couples by affecting a number of distinct sperm functions. Steroid therapy improves sperm mobility but has variable effects on antisperm antibodies. Treatment appears indicated when high levels of IgG antibody directed against the sperm tail are present, provided that the sperm are adequately mobile.

Intra-Uterine Insemination Versus Cyclic, Low-Dose Prednisolone in Couples With Male Antisperm Antibodies

Lähteenmäki A, Veilahti J, Hovatta O (Infertility Clinic, The Family Federation of Finland, Helsinki; Univ of Helsinki)
Hum Reprod 10:142–147, 1995   6–19

Objective.—Although autoantibodies to spermatozoa are known to impair fertility, their effects on fertility remain unclear. Corticosteroid immunosuppression has been used with various regimens of infertility treatment, with inconclusive results. The results of oral, low-dose cyclic prednisolone were compared with those of intrauterine insemination (IUI) in infertile couples in which the male partners had various levels of sperm-bound antibodies in their semen.

Methods.—The study included 46 couples who had been trying to achieve pregnancy for at least 1 year. The mean duration of infertility was 5 years. The men all had a positive mixed antiglobulin reaction (MAR) to immunoglobulin G (IgG) in their semen. They also had at least 1×10^6 spermatozoa, with a mean progressive motility of 72%. Thirty-eight couples had abnormal postcoital test results. The couples were randomly divided into 2 groups: 1 group received up to 3 attempts at IUI and the other received oral prednisolone therapy for the men combined with timed intercourse in 3 consecutive menstrual cycles. If pregnancy did not occur in the first stage, the couples were crossed over to the other treatment.

The prednisolone treatment consisted of a 20 mg dose once daily on days 1–10 of the woman's menstrual cycle, then 5 mg on days 11 and 12. For most cycles in both groups, clomiphene citrate was used. Couples in the prednisolone group were instructed to have intercourse in each cycle in the evening of the day of the luteinizing hormone rise; IUI was performed the day after the luteinizing hormone surge began. Motile spermatozoa were initially collected by a swim-up technique. However, the discontinuous Percoll gradient technique was found to yield better results and so was used in the latter part of the study.

Results.—There were 10 pregnancies, 9 in IUI cycles and 1 with the prednisolone/timed intercourse regimen. Pregnancy rate before crossover was 17% with 3 cycles of IUI, whereas no pregnancies occurred in 63 timed intercourse cycles. The IgG-MAR and tray agglutination test (TAT) values were no different before and after 3 cycles of IUI. Steroid therapy reduced serum TAT values, but there was no change in IgG-MAR.

Conclusions.—For infertile couples in which the man has sperm-associated IgG and/or IgA immunoglobulins, IUI appears to be superior to low-dose cyclic prednisolone therapy with timed intercourse. The prednisolone regimen used in this study did not cause any significant fluctuation in sperm-bound antibody levels. Well-timed IUI is an effective treatment that achieves rapid results and avoids the side effects of steroids.

▶ The relation between the presence of antibodies to spermatozoa in semen or blood of the male partner or blood of the female partner and the presence of infertility is not clearly defined. Although some studies have shown that corticosteroid treatment of the male partner who has autoantibodies to sperm in the semen results in a greater pregnancy rate than placebo therapy, other studies do not. The study by Sharma et al. (Abstract 6–18) did not have a control group. At this time, the value of performing antibody testing of infertile couples has not been proven, and such diagnostic tests should not be part of the infertility investigation. It is not necessary to perform an expensive diagnostic test if the treatment will not be changed according to the result of the test. Whether sperm antibodies are present or absent, the best initial treatment for couples with unexplained infertility is ovarian hyperstimulation and IUI. The majority of couples who have a male partner with an adequate number of active motile sperm, more than 1 million, in semen and a female partner who ovulates and has a patent oviduct have subfertility, not sterility. If autoantibodies to sperm are found in the seminal fluid, these couples should be treated with a few cycles of controlled ovarian hyperstimulation and washed IUI instead of with corticosteroids as was demonstrated so convincingly in the randomized study by Lähteenmäki et al. (Abstract 6–19). If pregnancy does not occur with controlled hyperstimulation and insemination, then in vitro fertilization, not corticosteroid treatment, should be advised.

D.R. Mishell, Jr., M.D.

Fertilization Rates Using Intracytoplasmic Sperm Injection Are Greater Than Subzonal Insemination But Are Dependent on Prior Treatment of Sperm

Catt J, Ryan J, Pike I, O'Neill C (Royal North Shore Hosp, St Leonards, NSW, Australia)
Fertil Steril 64:764–769, 1995   6–20

Objective.—Both subzonal sperm insertion (SUZI) and intracytoplasmic sperm injection (ICSI) have been used to treat male factor infertility. Fertilization rates of sibling oocytes when inseminated using SUZI or ICSI were compared, and the need for micromanipulative treatment of sperm was evaluated.

Methods.—A total of 99 patients underwent 99 stimulation cycles. Sibling oocytes were inseminated after pretreatment. Trial 1 had no pretreatment for either SUZI or ICSI; trial 2 had no pretreatment for SUZI but for ICSI, sperm were resuspended in polyvinyl pyrrolidone and immobilized before injection; trial 3 had no pretreatment for ICSI but for SUZI, sperm were treated as in trial 2 for SUZI; and trial 4 had the same treatment as for trial 2.

Technique.—For the SUZI technique, sperm are transferred via injection pipette into the perivitelline space of the oocyte oriented so that the polar body is between 9 and 12 o'clock. Insertion takes less than 2 minutes. For the ICSI technique the sperm is immobilized by incising the tail. The cytoplasm of the oocyte, oriented at 12 o'clock, is sucked into the pipette containing the sperm. Insertion takes less than 1 minute. Pregnancy rates are determined.

Results.—In trial 1, fertilization rates were 19% for ICSI and 25% for SUZI, a nonsignificant difference. In trial 2, rates were 44% for ICSI and 17% for SUZI, and in trial 3, rates were 44% for ICSI and 16% for SUZI. These rates were significantly different. In trial 4, rates were 21% for ICSI and 42% for SUZI. Twice as many embryos were produced by the ICSI procedure as by the SUZI method, a significant difference. The SUZI method produced significantly more multinucleate zygotes than did the ICSI procedure. There were no significant differences in the development rates of zygotes or in the method of cryopreservation. There was significantly more degeneration of presumptive mature metaphase II oocytes after manipulation with the ICSI method.

Conclusion.—The ICSI method results in higher fertilization rates than does the SUZI method provided the sperm are pretreated before injection.

Intracytoplasmic Sperm Injection Facilitates Fertilization Even in the Most Severe Forms of Male Infertility: Pregnancy Outcome Correlates With Maternal Age and Number of Eggs Available
Sherins RJ, Calvo LP, Thorsell LP, Krysa L, Dorfmann A, Coulam CB, Dennison-Lagos L, Schulman JD (Genetics & IVF Inst, Fairfax, Va)
Fertil Steril 64:369–375, 1995   6–21

Introduction.—For the most severe forms of male infertility, intracytoplasmic sperm injection offers a new therapy. In infertile couples with severe male infertility, the fertilization and pregnancy rates were evaluated after intracytoplasmic sperm injection in a prospective study.

Methods.—In 190 couples who did not respond to conventional in vitro fertilization, a series of 229 consecutive in vitro fertilization cycles were studied, using intracytoplasmic sperm injection with the husband's sperm as the only method of egg micromanipulation. The median age of females was 35 years (range, 23–48 years) and the median age of males was 38 years (range 27–65 years). There was no waiting list or other type of patient prioritization. Using gonadotropin-releasing hormone analogue with gonadotropins, multiple follicular development was induced. Under transvaginal ultrasound guidance 34–35 hours after injection of 10,000 IU human chorionic gonadotropin, follicles were aspirated. The intracytoplasmic sperm injection was performed, and 4 hours after oocyte retrieval a single motile sperm was injected into each egg.

Results.—Embryo transfers resulted from 206 cycles with 52 pregnancies initiated, giving an overall pregnancy rate of about 25% per transfer. Clinical pregnancies resulted in 38 of 52 (18% per transfer) with established gestational sacs, were ongoing more than 12 weeks, or delivered. Even in older women pregnancies were achieved; however, they were more readily established in younger women. The fertilization rate was slightly affected by the severity of semen abnormality, and a markedly decreased frequency of embryo formation was associated with actual necrospermia. Fewer than 100 viable sperm in the ejaculate resulted in pregnancy in some cases. In the oldest age group, the fertilization rate was 36%, whereas in the youngest group it was 50%.

Discussion.—For severe male infertility, intracytoplasmic sperm injection is a very powerful new treatment, often succeeding with sperm incapable of zona penetration or egg fusion. Now the main determinants of success in treating male infertility are egg number and probably egg quality. Fertilization rates were far better than expected with intracytoplasmic sperm injection than with conventional in vitro fertilization. A sperm concentration of less than 2 million sperm per milliliter of semen is an indicator for intracytoplasmic sperm injection, as well as semen samples with nearly all sperm having a poor acrosome reaction. More studies are needed to develop criteria for initial treatment by intracytoplasmic sperm injection.

▶ Before the development of intracytoplasmic sperm injection (ICSI), the presence of severe sperm abnormalities was associated with the worst prognosis for conception among infertile couples. Although ICSI is an expensive, meticulous technique, the results achieved in the treatment of severe sperm abnormalities are truly remarkable. Questions remain as to whether ICSI should be tried before or after an attempt of regular in vitro fertilization if abnormalities of sperm number and function exist. The magnitude of sperm abnormalities indicating that the initial fertilization attempt should be performed by ICSI also remains to be determined. Sherins et al. suggest that a sperm concentration of less than 2 million per milliliter of semen is an indication for treatment with ICSI, as well as those semen samples with nearly all sperm having a poor acrosome reaction. More studies are needed to develop criteria for initial treatment by ICSI.

D.R. Mishell, Jr., M.D.

A Comparison of Intrauterine Insemination in Superovulated Cycles to Intercourse in Couples Where the Male is Receiving Steroids for the Treatment of Autoimmune Infertility

Robinson JN, Maciocia LR, Forman RG, Barlow DH, Nicholson SC (John Radcliffe Hosp, Oxford, England)
Fertil Steril 63:1260–1266, 1995

6–22

Objective.—A study was planned to compare 2 approaches to infertile men with antisperm antibodies who were receiving intermediate-dose oral steroid treatment: timed coitus and intrauterine insemination (IUI) of washed spermatozoa in superovulated cycles. Thirty infertile couples in which the male partner was autoimmune to spermatozoa, and in which no female factor was apparent, were enrolled in a prospective, randomized crossover trial.

Methods.—Two 4-month periods of oral steroid treatment combined with either timed natural intercourse or superovulated IUI were separated by a 2-month washout period during which steroid treatment was withheld. Patients took 10 mg of prednisolone orally twice a day during the first 10 days of the cycle and 10 mg on days 11 and 12. Superovulation used clomiphene citrate and human menopausal gonadotropin. Sperm used in IUI were prepared by the swim-up method from unprocessed semen.

Results.—Levels of antisperm antibody in seminal plasma (but not in serum) decreased significantly in posttreatment assessments. Sperm parameters including the total count, percent progressive motility, and motility maintenance improved significantly. Cumulative pregnancy rates in 178 treatment cycles were 14% in the first cycle and 39% in the fourth. The cumulative pregnancy rate after 4 cycles was 4.8%. Intrauterine insemination cycles achieved pregnancy significantly more often than did timed intercourse. Seven of 11 conceptions resulting from IUI culminated in a full-term singleton delivery; there was a single triplet pregnancy. Steroid side effects were infrequent.

Conclusion.—Combining cyclic steroid therapy with superovulated IUI significantly improves the chance of conception in couples in which the male partner possesses antisperm antibodies.

▶ Unfortunately, this study did not include adequate control groups. As the authors themselves point out, the present study design does not allow a conclusion regarding the efficacy of steroid therapy. To answer that question, groups of couples in which the husbands were noted to have antisperm antibodies needed to be monitored for pregnancy after a period of intercourse and a period of IUI without steroid therapy.

R.Z. Sokol, M.D., F.A.C.P.

Comparison of the Effectiveness of Placebo and α-Blocker Therapy for the Treatment of Idiopathic Oligozoospermia

Yamamoto M, Hibi H, Miyake K (Nagoya Univ, Japan)
Fertil Steril 63:396–400, 1995

6–23

Background.—There is no standard method for the treatment of idiopathic male infertility. The use of α-blockers has been reported to be effective in the treatment of male infertility. The effectiveness of α-blocker therapy for patients with idiopathic male infertility was evaluated in a placebo-controlled, double-blind clinical study.

Study Group.—Thirty-one infertile adult men aged 25–42 years participated in this study. These men had sperm densities between 5 and 20×10^6 sperm/mL, normal serum gonadotropins and testoserone, and a fertile partner.

Methods.—After a 3-month control period, patients were randomly and blindly assigned to receive either a placebo or the α-blocker, bunazosin (2 mg/day), for 6 months. Semen and blood samples were collected during the control period and after therapy.

Results.—The therapy was well tolerated. During the entire study period there were no significant differences in hormonal values between the 2 groups. However, after therapy, there was a significant increase in sperm concentration and total motile sperm count in the treated group, as compared with the placebo group. There was no statistical difference in the pregnancy rate between the 2 groups.

Conclusions.—Oral administration of an α-blocker significantly improved sperm concentration and total motile sperm count in patients with idiopathic male infertility but did not improve pregnancy rates. Further studies should be carried out to confirm and extend these findings.

▶ The role that the sympathetic nervous system plays in the transport and storage of spermatozoa in the male reproductive tract remains unclear. Although this study documents some improvement in sperm concentration and total motile sperm count, the data do not support the conclusion that α-blocker therapy improves male infertility.

R.Z. Sokol, M.D., F.A.C.P.

Assisted Fertility Using Electroejaculation in Men With Spinal Cord Injury: A Review of Literature

Chung PH, Sanford EJ, Yeko TR, Maroulis GB, Mayer JC, (Univ of South Florida, Tampa)
Fertil Steril 64:1–9, 1995

6–24

Objective.—Men with spinal cord injury are infertile as a result of anejaculation. Electroejaculation using a rectal probe was developed in an attempt to make these men capable of fathering children. This review of the literature is based on a MEDLINE search of English-language studies reporting pregnancies from electroejaculation and manual scanning of recent journals.

> *Technique.*—Primate studies demonstrated that short postganglionic fibers are necessary for electroejaculation to be effective. Patients are given sodium bicarbonate to neutralize the urine. Nifedipine is given sublingually to prevent autonomic dysreflexia. An insemination medium is instilled into the bladder to minimize the effect of urine on retrograde ejaculate. Sigmoidoscopy then is done to introduce a polyvinyl chloride rectal probe. Sine wave stimulation is carried out incrementally until ejaculation takes place, and the bulbous urethra is milked to direct the semen into a container.

Efficacy.—Success rates of 60% to 90% for semen procurement are reported from different centers. The ejaculates tend to have high sperm counts but low motility and poorly functional sperm. Retrograde ejaculation is a common occurrence. Pregnancies have been achieved using electroejaculates since 1975. Recently, assisted reproductive methods have been used in conjunction with electroejaculation, and the early results are encouraging. These patients are best managed by a team approach encompassing a gynecologist/reproductive endocrinologist, urologist, andrologist, nurses, and psychologists.

▶ Spinal cord injury leads to impotence in 30% to 50% and anejaculation in 90% of affected men. Normal ejaculatory function is primarily a sympathetic nervous system event. Adrenergic neurons stimulate the emission of seminal fluid and sperm into the posterior urethra. Tight closure of the bladder neck prevents retrograde ejaculation into the bladder. The level and extent of the spinal cord injury determines the severity of seminal compromise in injured men. Electroejaculation allows for semen procurement in those cases where the man is unable to ejaculate. Ejaculation success rate reported in the literature is variable because there is no strict definition for success. Poor semen quality in electroejaculated samples is a common finding.

The combination of electroejaculation and intracytoplasmic sperm injection (ICSI) should improve pregnancy rates. However, electroejaculation is not without side effects. Autonomic dysreflexia characterized by paroxysmal hypertension, bradycardia, headache, sweating, piloerection, facial flushing, anxiety, and malaise occurs more frequently in patients with spinal cord injury above T5. Prophylactic nifedipine lowers the incidence of this complication. In those instances in which inadequate semen is collected or side effects cannot be prevented, fine-needle aspiration and ICSI should be considered.

R.Z. Sokol, M.D., F.A.C.P.

Choosing Among Different Technical Variations of Percoll Centrifugation for Sperm Selection
Ruiz-Romero J, Antich M, Bassas LI (Fundación Puigvert, Barcelona)
Andrologia 27:149–153, 1995   6–25

Objective.—Ideally a method of sperm selection should concentrate the greatest possible number of morphologically normal spermatozoa that have rapidly progressive motility in a desired volume, and should eliminate seminal plasma, round cells, bacteria, and debris. Five variations of Percoll gradient centrifugation (PC) were examined using 14 semen specimens of varying quality obtained by masturbation from men being evaluated for couple infertility. Five aliquots of each specimen were processed simultaneously.

Findings.—Total sperm concentration was higher after selection with a conventional 4-layer Percoll technique, but slightly more motile spermatozoa were obtained with the 2- and 3-gradient variants. A layer volume of 0.5 mL tended to produce more motile spermatozoa. The concentration of recovered spermatozoa that were optimally motile was highest when samples were centrifuged through 2-layer Percoll gradients, regardless of their volume. When analyzing oligozoospermic and asthenozoospermic samples, Percoll gradients prepared with two 0.5-mL layers yielded the best results. All methods resulted in similar progressive velocity and straightness of recovered spermatozoa. Most techniques effectively removed cellular contaminants.

Conclusion.—Sperm selection by centrifugation through discontinuous Percoll gradients is improved by limiting the number of gradients and by including a layer of 90% Percoll.

▶ The Percoll sperm preparation technique separates sperm via centrifugation through discontinuous Percoll gradients. The gradients are prepared by adding successive layers of each selected Percoll gradient, with the more concentrated layer at the bottom of the tube. Reducing the number of gradients improves the recovery of motile spermatozoa. When sperm are retrieved by fine-needle aspiration of the testicle or by microsurgical or transepididymal aspiration, blood contamination is common. Exposure of sperm to red blood cells can interfere with sperm function. A 2-gradient mini-Percoll preparation harvests a maximal number of motile sperm while preventing the passage of red blood cells to the lower layer of Percoll, thus enhancing the sperm population obtained by microaspiration.

R.Z. Sokol, M.D., F.A.C.P.

Fertility in Cases of Hypergonadotropic Azoospermia

Hauser R, Temple-Smith PD, Southwick GJ, de Kretser D (Monash Univ, Clayton, Victoria, Australia)
Fertil Steril 63:631–636, 1995

6–26

Background.—Azoospermia with normal testicular volume and follicle-stimulating hormone (FSH) levels suggests obstruction and is an indication for testicular biopsy. A series of patients in whom azoospermia was associated with high serum FSH levels was recently reviewed. The outcomes of hypergonadotropic azoospermic patients who underwent scrotal exploration and bypass microsurgery were analyzed.

Methods.—Thirty-one hypergonadotropic azoospermic men undergoing vasoepididymostomy or vasovasostomy were included. All had evidence of spermatogenesis on testicular biopsy. Main outcome measures were intraoperative aspirated sperm, postoperative ejaculated sperm, fertilizations, and pregnancies.

Findings.—In all patients, sperm were aspirated intraoperatively. Sperm were detected in postoperative ejaculations in 87%. Long-term follow-up data were available on 14 patients. Six men successfully impregnated their partners, resulting in 8 births. Another 3 men demonstrated the ability to fertilize at in vitro fertilization.

Conclusions.—A high serum FSH level in men with azoospermia does not exclude the possibility of obstruction and the capacity for fertilization. Caution is needed, especially when unilateral testicular atrophy is present. A testicular biopsy should be done to detect possible spermatogenesis. If it is present, a microsurgical bypass can result in successful pregnancy.

▶ This study reminds all of us to continually reassess our diagnostic criteria for various fertility interventions. However, this study does not allow the conclusion that all men with elevated FSH levels should undergo testicular biopsy. As the authors point out in their discussion, the present study does not provide data regarding how commonly high FSH levels occur simultaneously with active spermatogenesis in azoospermic men. Nor do the data provide an indication of the proportion of men in whom a high level of FSH accurately reflects irreversible testicular damage. In this small number of men in whom follow-up was available, only 5 of 14 fathered spontaneous pregnancies. The size of testes, testicular histologic findings, and FSH values of those men before surgery would be of interest.

R.Z. Sokol, M.D., F.A.C.P.

Effectiveness of Crossover Transseptal Vasoepididymostomy in Treating Complex Obstructive Azoospermia
Sabanegh E Jr, Thomas AJ Jr (Cleveland Clinic Found, Ohio)
Fertil Steril 63:392–395, 1995   6–27

Background.—Obstructive azoospermia can often be corrected by conventional vasovasostomy or vasoepididymostomy. A "crossover" procedure connecting the normal testis and epididymis to the contralateral vas deferens may be effective in patients with an irreparable, unilateral ductal obstruction or agenesis with a normal testis combined with contralateral testicular damage and a normal ductal system.

Methods.—The cases of 10 men undergoing crossover transseptal end-to-side vasoepididymostomies were reviewed. Infertility was primary in 9 men and secondary in 1. Seven men had azoospermia, and 3 had severe oligospermia. All men had irreparable ipsilateral ductal obstruction or agenesis combined with a normal testis and a poorly functional or absent contralateral testis. Atrophy in the contralateral testis was related to previous hernia repair in 3 men, varicocele-induced atrophy in 2, and severe orchitis in 2. Three men had cryptorchidism, testicular torsion, and an unknown cause, respectively. In 5 men, congenital absence of the vas deferens caused the ipsilateral ductal abnormality. In 3 men, vas injury resulted from inguinal surgery in childhood. In 2 men, vas obstruction was idiopathic. A total of 12 microsurgical crossover transseptal vasoepididymostomies were done. Five men had anastomosis to the caput, 2 to the corpus, and 3 to the cauda.

Findings.—Sperm in the ejaculate was found in 8 of 9 men followed for 6 months or more. Pregnancies have occurred in 2 of 7 couples. Total sperm counts ranged from 18 to 201×10^6 with a motility of 5% to 37%. Postoperative total sperm counts were significantly lower in men with congenital absence of the vas deferens (37.8×10^6) than in men with all other causes of ductal abnormality (135×10^6). Postoperative sperm counts were not predicted by infertility type, preoperative semen analysis, cause of testicular abnormality, or site of epididymal anastomosis.

Conclusions.—A crossover transseptal vasoepididymostomy can restore patency in most men with a solitary functioning testis with irreparable excurrent ductal obstruction or agenesis. For experienced microsurgeons, this procedure is easy to perform. No morbidity was associated with it in the current series.

▶ This study reinforces the premise outlined in Abstract 6–26 that surgical intervention should be considered for the patient with azoospermia and unilateral testicular atrophy. The study also serves as a reminder that pediatric inguinal hernia surgery is an important cause of both testicular and ductal damage.

R.Z. Sokol, M.D., F.A.C.P.

7 Ovulation Induction

Corpus Luteum Function and Pregnancy Rates With Clomiphene Citrate Therapy: Comparison of Human Chorionic Gonadotrophin-Induced Versus Spontaneous Ovulation
Agarwal SK, Buyalos RP (Univ of California, Los Angeles)
Hum Reprod 10:328–331, 1995   7–1

Introduction.—Clomiphene citrate, which is used increasingly as infertility therapy along with intrauterine insemination (IUI), has been associated with luteal phase dysfunction. Therefore, the timing of IUI is crucial to its success. A study was undertaken to compare 2 timing methods (triggering ovulation with human chorionic gonadotropin [hCG] vs. using a urinary luteinizing hormone [LH] kit to predict ovulation), to compare the efficacy of clomiphene citrate/IUI therapy in patients with anovulatory vs. ovulatory infertility diagnoses, and to assess corpus luteum function in patients with spontaneous ovulation and in patients with hCG-triggered ovulation after clomiphene citrate/IUI therapy.

Methods.—The records of 233 consecutive patients treated with 508 clomiphene citrate/IUI cycles for infertility were reviewed. Only patients with at least 1 patent fallopian tube and no severe male factor were included. The patients were given 50–150 mg of clomiphene citrate for 5 consecutive days, beginning on days 3–5 of the cycle. Ovulation was triggered with hCG in 247 cycles when the mean follicular diameter was at least 19 mm. Ovulation was predicted with a urinary LH kit in 261 cycles. Intrauterine insemination was undertaken at approximately 36–38 hours after hCG administration or 18–20 hours after the LH surge was detected. Corpus luteum function and pregnancy rates were assessed.

Results.—After adjustment for maternal age, there was no difference in the pregnancy rate between the 2 groups. There were also no differences in the pregnancy rate between patients with ovulatory or anovulatory infertility or within either diagnostic category between the groups defined by the method of ovulation timing. The mean midluteal serum progesterone concentrations and luteal phase lengths did not differ between the 2 groups.

Discussion.—Insemination timed after either a spontaneous surge in urinary LH or ovulation triggered by hCG resulted in similar clinical pregnancy rates after clomiphene citrate therapy. Luteal function was also not affected by the method of timing insemination.

▶ Although this is a retrospective study, the results are of interest. The conclusions reached are that when treating ovulatory or anovulatory infertility with clomiphene citrate, the pregnancy rates are similar when ovulation is induced with hCG or occurs spontaneously and is detected by observing the peak of urinary LH. Thus, women using this therapy can choose to perform daily monitoring of urinary LH or have sonographic monitoring of follicular size followed by an hCG injection. The latter method requires frequent visits to the facility where sonography is performed, so the former method of monitoring is usually more convenient and less expensive. Because monitoring of urinary LH is as effective as sonographic monitoring, patients can be advised to use the former regimen when receiving clomiphene citrate to induce ovulation or for controlled ovarian hyperstimulation.

D.R. Mishell, Jr., M.D.

Clomiphene Citrate and Neural Tube Defects: A Pooled Analysis of Controlled Epidemiologic Studies and Recommendations for Future Studies
Greenland S, Ackerman DL (Univ of California, Los Angeles)
Fertil Steril 64:936–941, 1995   7–2

Objective.—The results of 10 epidemiologic studies that included an internal group were reviewed in an attempt to gauge the extent to which neural tube defects (NTDs) are associated with periconceptional exposure to clomiphene citrate.

The Studies.—Eight case-control studies were reviewed in which the history of clomiphene citrate use was compared in a series of NTD cases and a control series of women treated at clinics and hospitals for infertility. There also were 2 cohort studies in which the proportion of births with defects was compared in pregnancies with and those without periconceptual use of clomiphene citrate. Six of the studies provided data in enough detail to be used directly in pooled analyses.

Findings.—The estimated ratio of prevalence rates of NTD in clomiphene citrate–exposed and nonexposed pregnancies ranged from 0.55 to 5.73 in the various studies. The variation in ratios was consistent with random fluctuation. The summary prevalence ratio was 1.08, with 95% confidence limits of 0.76–1.51. The results were not closely related to the study design used. The only marked subgroup difference was a higher prevalence of NTDs in 3 European studies than in the remaining studies, from the United States and Japan; the respective summary prevalence ratios were 2.85 and 0.94.

Conclusion.—The available evidence neither confirms nor excludes an effect of exposure to clomiphene citrate on the risk of NTD.

▶ Several studies have investigated the risk of an infant being born with an NTD after clomiphene citrate was given around the time of conception. Although several studies suggest that there may be an association between the use of clomiphene citrate and an increased risk for development of an NTD, in only 1 of the studies was the increased risk statistically significant. Furthermore, several other studies have shown that there is no increased risk of NTD associated with periconceptional clomiphene citrate ingestion. The technique of meta-analysis, which pools the results of several studies to determine relative risk, has many limitations. Nevertheless, the fact that the summary relative risk of data published in the scientific literature yields a risk of 1.08 is an indication that no relation exists between the use of clomiphene citrate to induce ovulation or stimulate multiple follicle development and the risk of fetal NTDs if pregnancy occurs.

D.R. Mishell, Jr., M.D.

Visual Disturbance Secondary to Clomiphene Citrate

Purvin VA (Indiana Univ Med Ctr, Indianapolis)
Arch Ophthalmol 113:482–484, 1995
7–3

Introduction.—Most patients tolerate clomiphene well for the treatment of infertility. Vasomotor flushing and abdominal discomfort are the most common side effects. More infrequently, reversible visual symptoms have been reported. However, 3 patients have experienced persistent clomiphene-related visual symptoms, even though results of their neuro-ophthalmologic examinations and electrophysiologic studies were normal.

Case 1.—Woman, 32, took 50 mg/day of clomiphene citrate for 5 days each month for 5 months. She experienced bilateral shimmering vision during each course of treatment, which resolved after treatment cessation. Her dose was doubled for the next 5 months, then halved for 5 months. Her visual symptoms became more severe and persistent when the dose was doubled and persisted even 2½ years after treatment was discontinued.

Case 2.—Woman, 32, was treated with 50 mg/day of clomiphene citrate for 5 days per month. She had peripheral shimmering vision in both eyes after 1 month of treatment. Flickering vision became persistent when her dose was increased to 100 mg/day 2 months later and then 150 mg/day. After 4 months, treatment was discontinued, but she experienced intermittent visual disturbance, including illusory movement in the peripheral vision, prolonged afterimages, and photophobia, for 4 years.

Case 3.—Woman, 36, was initially treated with 50 mg/day of clomiphene citrate; the dose was increased in the second month to 100 mg/day. After 5 months at the increased dose, she reported prolonged afterimages, bilateral blurred vision, flickering vision, and photophobia. The symptoms intensified when encountering brighter light and during menses and have persisted for 7 years after cessation of clomiphene therapy.

Discussion.—The patients reported a distinctive constellation of visual symptoms, which were initially temporary and became persistent. The likelihood of persistent visual disturbance appears to be related to the dose and duration of treatment. It may be that clomiphene-related persistent visual disturbance is underrated. Women should be advised of the possibility of irreversible visual symptoms with continued treatment with clomiphene citrate.

▶ Clomiphene citrate is being used with increasing frequency to treat not only anovulatory infertility but also infertility in ovulatory women. Therefore, it is very important that clinicians be aware of this uncommon but important side effect of clomiphene citrate therapy. Patients receiving this medication should be questioned about the occurrence of visual symptoms. If such symptoms do occur, appropriate management would be to discontinue use of clomiphene citrate and use another agent to induce ovulation or stimulate multiple follicular development.

D.R. Mishell, Jr., M.D.

Ovulation Induction in Premature Ovarian Failure: A Placebo-Controlled Randomized Trial Combining Pituitary Suppression With Gonadotropin Stimulation

van Kasteren YM, Hoek A, Schoemaker J (Vrije Universiteit, Amsterdam)
Fertil Steril 64:273–278, 1995   7–4

Background.—Premature ovarian failure (POF)—the cessation of ovarian function before 40 years of age after normal development—is characterized by secondary amenorrhea with increased gonadotropins and low serum E_2 levels. In most patients, the cause of early menopause is unknown. The hypergonadotropic status itself may play a role in ovarian unresponsiveness. For this reason, several researchers have studied the effect of creating a normogonadotropic status. The efficacy of ovulation induction with gonadotropins preceded by and combined with pituitary suppression with a gonadotropin-releasing hormone agonist (GnRH-a) in patients with POF was investigated.

Methods and Findings.—Thirty patients were enrolled in the placebo-controlled, randomized, 4-phase trial. Fifteen patients were included in each group. Phases 1 and 4 consisted of no intervention; phase 2, a 4-week period in which the patients received either 1,000 µg of intranasal buserelin acetate daily or placebo; and phase 3, a 3-week period in which the patients received human menopausal gonadotropin additionally in weekly augmented doses—2, 4, and 6 ampules daily in the first, second, and third weeks, respectively. Ovulation was induced when the follicular diameter reached 18 mm and/or the total 24-hour estrogen excretion exceeded 140 µg. Luteal support consisted of 5,000 IU human chorionic gonadotropin given every 72 hours. Five patients in the agonist group and 4 in the placebo group showed follicular growth. Ovulation occurred in 3 patients in the agonist group and none in the placebo group, a nonsignificant difference.

Conclusions.—Ovulation rates did not differ significantly between the patients with GnRH-a–induced normogonadotropic status and those with a hypergonadotropic status given placebo. Thus there was not enough evidence to show that pituitary suppression with a GnRH-a improves the success of ovulation induction with exogenous gonadotropins in patients with POF.

▶ Premature ovarian failure may on occasion be attributable to an autoimmune phenomenon, but the etiology is usually unknown and is probably the result of genetic factors. When premature ovarian failure occurs, the condition is usually permanent but on occasion may be transient. The fact that 10% of the women in this study ovulated after therapy with a GnRH agonist and human menopausal gonadotropin (hMG) may be a chance finding. Because ovulation occurred in only 3 of the 33 women treated, the results were not statistically significant. It does not appear to be cost-effective to treat all women with premature ovarian failure with a GnRH agonist and hMG. However, because the only other way to achieve a pregnancy in women with this problem is to perform in vitro fertilization and embryo transfer after oocyte donation if pregnancy is desired, it is certainly less costly to perform a trial of administering the GnRH-a followed by hMG.

D.R. Mishell, Jr., M.D.

Gonadotropin-Releasing Hormone Antagonist Versus Agonist Administration in Women Undergoing Controlled Ovarian Hyperstimulation: Cycle Performance and In Vitro Steroidogenesis of Granulosa-Lutein Cells

Minaretzis D, Alper MM, Oskowitz SP, Lobel SM, Mortola JF, Pavlou SN (Beth Israel Hosp, Boston; Harvard Med School, Boston)
Am J Obstet Gynecol 172:1518–1525, 1995   7–5

Introduction.—Unlike gonadotropin-releasing hormone (GnRH) agonists, which require some time to suppress gonadotropins through pituitary desensitization, GnRH antagonists provide immediate suppression. This effect—the result of receptor antagonism—makes GnRH antagonists ideal for adjuvant treatment during ovarian hyperstimulation.

Objectives.—A GnRH antagonist and a GnRH agonist were compared for their effectiveness in suppressing the spontaneous luteinizing hormone surge during controlled ovarian hyperstimulation in a prospective, case-control study. The effects of in vivo administration of a GnRH antagonist and agonist on granulosa-lutein cell steroidogenesis in vitro was studied as well.

Methods.—The study sample comprised 30 healthy women undergoing ovarian hyperstimulation with human menopausal gonadotropins for in vitro fertilization and gamete intrafallopian transfer. When the lead follicle measured 15 mm or larger and the serum estradiol level was 500 pg/mL or greater, half of the women received the Nal-Glu antagonist, 5 mg IM/day. The remaining women underwent oocyte retrieval on the same day as the study group; they also received the agonist leuprolide acetate, 250 µg/day, beginning on cycle day 1. In addition, granulosa-lutein cells were purified from follicular aspirates from 6 women in each group. Parallel cultures were made to evaluate basal progesterone production, progesterone response to follicle-stimulating hormone or luteinizing hormone, and aromatase activity.

Results.—The 2 groups were similar in the total amount of gonadotropins they received. Mean duration of gonadotropin-releasing hormone antagonist treatment before human chorionic gonadotropin (hCG) administration was 2½ days. On the day of hCG administration, levels of serum luteinizing hormone were 1.0 mIU/mL in the antagonist group vs. 4.2 mIU/mL in the agonist group. On the same day, serum estradiol levels were 820 vs. 1,361 pg/mL, respectively. The 2 groups had similar numbers of oocytes retrieved; however, 82% of oocytes were mature in the antagonist group, compared with 62% in the agonist group. Proportion of good-quality embryos was 70% vs. 44%. In the first 6 hours after retrieval, granulosa-lutein cells from the women in the antagonist group had significantly lower aromatase activity, 18 vs. 31 ng/mL per 6 hours estradiol. However, there were no significant differences in basal and gonadotropin-stimulated progesterone responses.

Conclusions.—In women undergoing ovarian hyperstimulation, GnRH antagonists may offer some important practical advantages over GnRH agonists. Giving a GnRH antagonist during the late follicular phase leads to lower serum luteinizing hormone and estradiol levels, as well as more mature oocytes and better-quality embryos. In addition to their direct effects on ovarian function, GnRH analogues may have differential effects on the activity of aromatase in granulosa-lutein cells. These effects could account for the reduced serum estradiol levels seen in women treated with a GnRH antagonist.

▶ This paper adds new information regarding the use of a GnRH antagonist in controlled ovarian stimulation. We and others have conducted several trials using these agents. The clear advantage of the antagonist is the rapid onset of downregulation and the ease with which it can adjust the cycle. It can be used, for example, just at midcycle to prevent the luteinizing hormone (LH) surge. These data suggest that there are some clinical advantages of the antagonist over the agonist, which is a conclusion we were not able to observe. Nevertheless, they did notice lower levels of estradiol and a more profoundly suppressed LH level. The reduction in aromatase activity in granulosa cells could have been secondary to the abrupt cessation of gonadotropin function. In cycles treated with the GnRH antagonist, there appears to be a disassociation between follicle size and estradiol levels.

Follicles will continue to grow in the presence of the antagonist and exogenous stimulation while the estradiol levels are lower. The criteria, therefore, for monitoring cycles have to be adjusted and recognized as being different from the usual stimulation regimen. However, when it becomes available, the antagonist will really revolutionize our ability to control ovulation and avoid the consequences of premature luteinization.

R.A. Lobo, M.D.

Gonadotrophin-Releasing Hormone Agonist Compared With Human Chorionic Gonadotrophin for Ovulation Induction After Clomiphene Citrate Treatment
Shalev E, Geslevich Y, Matilsky M, Ben-Ami M (Central Emek Hosp, Afula, Israel)
Hum Reprod 10:2541–2544, 1995   7–6

Background.—In patients who respond to clomiphene citrate but do not ovulate, injection of human chorionic gonadotropin (hCG) can induce ovulation. Gonadotropin-releasing hormone analogue (GnRHa) administration also effectively induces ovulation in in vitro fertilization (IVF) as well as in non-IVF settings. The response to GnRHa may be more physiologic, similar to a spontaneous midcycle surge. Hormonal response, luteal phase adequacy, and pregnancy and abortion rates were compared in patients receiving hCG and in those given GnRHa during ovulation cycles stimulated by clomiphene citrate.

Methods.—Two hundred ten anovulatory women were randomly assigned to hCG or GnRHa. One hundred four received 1 subcutaneous dose of tryptorelin, 0.1 mg, and 106 received 1 IM dose of hCG, 10,000 IU, after clomiphene citrate stimulation had induced enlarged ovarian follicles.

Findings.—Twelve hours after GnRHa injection, there was a brief, transitory increase in serum luteinizing hormone and follicle-stimulating hormone. These concentrations returned to baseline levels within 36 hours of the injection. The hCG and GnRHa groups had similar midluteal progesterone levels. The mean luteal phase duration was also not significantly different. The 2 groups had comparable pregnancy and abortion rates. In the GnRHa group, these respective rates were 12% and 18.2%; in the hCG group, they were 12.6% and 12.5%. Neither treatment caused complications.

Conclusions.—A relatively low dose of GnRHa can stimulate a midcycle surge of gonadotropins, similar to that in a natural cycle. It can also induce ovulation and an adequate luteal phase. The pregnancy and abortion rates associated with GnRHa treatment are comparable to those with hCG.

▶ Because GnRH agonists have a much shorter half-life than hCG, use of the former agent for ovulation induction after appropriate follicular development may be associated with a lower incidence of the ovarian hyperstimulation syndrome than occurs when hCG is used. Clinicians may wish to try to induce ovulation with a single subcutaneous injection of a GnRH agonist in women at risk for development of the ovarian hyperstimulation syndrome, such as those with polycystic ovaries.

D.R. Mishell, Jr., M.D.

Cotreatment With Growth Hormone and Gonadotropin for Ovulation Induction in Hypogonadotropic Patients: A Prospective, Randomized, Placebo-Controlled, Dose-Response Study

Shoham F, for the European and Australian Multicenter Study (Kaplan Hosp, Rehovot, Israel)
Fertil Steril 64:917–923, 1995   7–7

Background.—Increasing evidence has implicated growth hormone (GH) in the reproductive process. Uncontrolled studies have shown improved ovarian response during in vitro fertilization (IVF) when GH is incorporated in the treatment regimen. Verification of this effect of cotreatment with GH and human menopausal gonadotropin (hMG) was assessed in a prospective, randomized, double-blind, dose-response, placebo-controlled, multicenter trial.

Methods.—Over a 3-year period, 68 patients, with infertility for 1–15 years, were randomly assigned to receive 1 IVF treatment cycle of hMG with either 4, 12, or 24 IU of human GH or placebo. Serum E_2 concentrations and the ultrasound evidence of follicular development were monitored daily to guide the daily dose of hMG. The 4 treatment groups were compared for the following features: total dose of hMG, days of hMG treatment, daily effective dose of hMG, the number of follicles, and serum follicle-stimulating hormone (FSH) and E_2 concentrations.

Results.—Cotreatment with GH resulted in a statistically significant dose-dependent reduction in the total dose of hMG administered, with patients receiving 24 IU of GH requiring 39% less hMG to induce follicular growth. The number of treatment days needed before ovulation occurred was also reduced in a dose-dependent fashion. The daily effective dose of hMG was reduced similarly in all 3 groups treated with GH, compared with those given placebo. The number and size of follicles and serum E_2 concentrations did not differ significantly in the 4 treatment groups. However, serum insulin-like growth factor I (IGF-I) concentrations increased in a dose-related fashion in patients treated with GH.

Conclusions.—Cotreatment with GH in women with hypogonadotropic hypogonadism significantly enhances the ovarian response to stimulation by gonadotropins. However, it is unclear whether this effect is directly related to GH treatment or is mediated by an increase in IGF-I. Further study is necessary to identify the minimum effective dose of GH.

▶ We always look forward to well-controlled prospective trials, particularly those that are placebo-controlled. This is such a study, looking at the adjunctive benefit, if it exists, of GH used in conjunction with gonadotropins for induction of ovulation in patients who have hypothalamic amenorrhea. The important group of patients that should benefit from this treatment are patients who have reduced hypothalamic pituitary function and perhaps deficiency in GH secretion. This is often difficult to document, and, in some patients, may be merely secondary to hypoestrogenism. Nevertheless, as shown in Figure 1 in the original article, in a dose-response way, the addition of GH significantly reduced the amount of ampules of gonadotropins used. Commensurate with the increase in GH was an increase in IGF-I, which promoted additional action on the ovary. In a practical sense, however, the increase in the dose of GH, which translates into a lower dose of gonadotropins, may actually be a more expensive way to go than just merely increasing the dose of gonadotropins. The number of follicles and estrogen concentration in this instance were not very different. Indeed there is cross-reactivity in the actions of the different types of protein hormones, including perhaps between GH and gonadotropins for the purposes of follicular recruitment. In the way of anecdote, patients treated with Pergonal alone have been able to achieve ovulation even with documented deficiency of GH. Thus, we will need to know whether or not it has any additional benefit in terms of fine-tuning of the process to ascertain the best treatment in the future.

R.A. Lobo, M.D.

Human Menopausal Gonadotropin and the Risk of Epithelial Ovarian Cancer

Shushan A, Elchalal U, Paltiel O, Peretz T, Iscovich J, Schenker JG (Hebrew Univ, Jerusalem, Israel; Israel Cancer Registry, Jerusalem)
Fertil Steril 65:13–18, 1996   7–8

Background.—Several reports, including case-control studies, have raised concern about the possible development of ovarian cancers in women with a history of exposure to ovulation-inducing drugs. It is essential to investigate this link further, especially given the use of newer assisted reproduction techniques involving potent follicle stimulation regimens. Exposure to fertility drugs—particularly human menopausal gonadotropin (hMG)—was compared in women with epithelial ovarian cancer and healthy controls.

Methods.—Data from the Israel Cancer Registry were used to identify 200 living women aged 36–64 years with histologically confirmed primary invasive or borderline epithelial ovarian cancer. Eighty-two percent of the women had invasive cancer; all of which was diagnosed between 1990 and 1993. Four hundred eight control women were studied as well. Both groups were evaluated by interview using a standard questionnaire. The possible link between exposure to fertility drugs and ovarian cancer was assessed by a multivariate logistic model, which controlled for variables identified as significant on univariate analysis.

Results.—Fertility drug use was reported by 12% of women with ovarian cancer and 7% of controls, for an adjusted odds ratio (OR) of 1.31. Twenty-two women with ovarian cancer and 24 controls said that they had used hMG, alone or in combination with clomiphene citrate, adjusted OR 1.42. Eleven women with cancer and 6 controls reported use of hMG alone. A marked increase in risk was noted for the case subjects with borderline ovarian tumors.

Conclusions.—Women exposed to hMG to induce ovulation may be 3 times more likely to have epithelial ovarian tumors than nonexposed women, the findings suggest. Women who have used hMG are also at markedly greater risk of borderline ovarian tumors. Further study is needed, and the data do not yet warrant any change in treatment policy. However, women should be made aware of the possible increased risk of ovarian cancer before they give informed consent to ovulation induction.

▶ This study has to be added to the growing list of papers on the subject and the prospective trials that are currently under way attempting to answer this question more definitively. Infertility itself is associated with an increased risk of ovarian cancer; thus, data like these in isolation, without knowledge of how many patients really have the diagnosis of infertility and those who do not, are difficult to factor in. The study did show with small numbers that the odds ratio was in the range of 1.4, suggesting a 30% to 40% increased risk with the use of fertility drugs and with hMG specifically. The risk also appeared to be higher for borderline tumors. However, the case numbers again were small and the type of infertility and the length of infertility or treatment in the groups were not specified. Therefore, this study raises some question and suggests that we should be cautious about using these drugs indiscriminately but does not allow us to scare our patients into saying there is a definitive association until further studies are completed.

R.A. Lobo, M.D.

Variability in the Immunoreactive and Bioactive Follicle Stimulating Hormone Content of Human Urinary Menopausal Gonadotrophin Preparations

Rodgers M, McLoughlin JD, Lambert A, Robertson WR, Mitchell R (Hope Hosp, Salford, England)
Hum Reprod 10:1982–1986, 1995   7–9

Introduction.—The administration of urinary gonadotropin preparations is crucial in the increasing success of assisted reproduction techniques. However, considerable clinical and biochemical variations have been reported in the response to this treatment, and it has been suggested that this may be the result of variability in the quality of the gonadotropin preparations. To investigate this possibility, the within- and between-batch variations in the follicle-stimulating hormone (FSH) content of Pergonal, Metrodin, and Metrodin–high purity (Metrodin-HP) were compared.

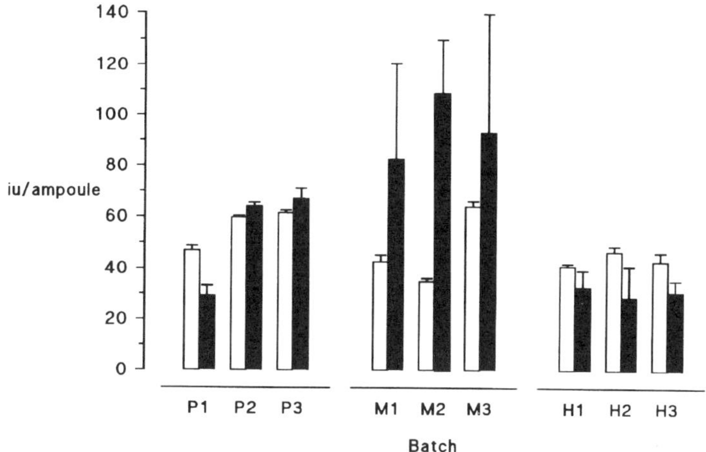

FIGURE 1.—Immunoreactive (*open bars*) and bioactive (*filled bars*) FSH content (mean ± 2 SEM IU/ampule, *n* = 3 assays) for 3 different batches of Pergonal (*P1–P3*), Metrodin (*M1–M3*), and Metrodin-HP (*H1–H3*). Data for M1–M3, P1–P3, and H3 are derived from 3 ampules per batch, whereas H1 and H2 represent single ampules. The mean ± SEM is derived from the 3 assays performed. (Courtesy of Rodgers M, McLoughlin JD, Lambert A, et al: Variability in the immunoreactive and bioactive follicle stimulating hormone content of human urinary menopausal gonadotrophin preparations. *Hum Reprod* 10:1982–1986, 1995, by permission of Oxford University Press.)

Methods.—The immunoreactive FSH potencies (R-FSH) in 3 ampules from each of 3 batches of Pergonal, Metrodin, and Metrodin-HP were measured with a polyclonal antibody radioimmunoassay. In addition, an FSH bioassay (B-FSH) was performed to measure FSH-stimulated estradiol production in cultured rat Sertoli cells.

Results.—No batches of any preparation showed within-batch variation in R-FSH, and only 2 batches of Metrodin had within-batch B-FSH variability of up to 2.4-fold. There was between-batch variation in both R-FSH and B-FSH, which correlated, in the Pergonal batches. All 3 batches of Metrodin had substantial variations in both R-FSH and B-FSH, which were too large to demonstrate clear correlations. There was no significant between-batch variation in either R-FSH or B-FSH with Metrodin-HP (Fig 1). The ratio of FSH bioactivity to immunoreactivity varied considerably among the 3 preparations: 0.9 with Pergonal, 2.2 with Metrodin, and 0.7 with Metrodin-HP.

Conclusions.—Variations in B-FSH and R-FSH are found among human urinary gonadotropin preparations. It appears that bioactivity varies more than immunoreactivity. Metrodin-HP had more tightly controlled FSH content than Pergonal and Metrodin, although it also had the lowest bioactivity potency.

▶ The more experienced clinician who has used gonadotropins for some time will be able to recall anecdotes regarding batch-to-batch variability in the induction of ovulation or in in vitro fertilization. This has been a bone of contention for some time, but there are papers such as that by Bronte Stone and colleagues[1] suggesting great biological variability. Nevertheless, the data at hand suggest that the within-batch variability is minimal and the inter-batch variability, which is what has been suspected to be abnormal, is sometimes quite discrepant and varies according to the preparation used. Figure 1 shows first of all that the difference is primarily in the bioactivity rather than in immunoreactivity and this is also consistent with previous data by Stone, who showed about a 50% variability. The nature of the discrepancy is not a quality control issue but is the result of the nature of the purification process.

That the new ultrapure preparation (Metrodin-HP) has the least variability suggests that the methodology for purification and the amount of foreign protein in the preparation is largely responsible for the variability in biological content. The older products of urinary preparation leading to Metrodin or Pergonal result in a fair amount of foreign protein. This occasionally also leads to reactions in the patients and is the reason IM injections are required. However, Metrodin-HP, which is ultrapurified, is more than 90% pure relative to the older preparations and has a very low protein load and high specific activity. Because of this, theoretically there is less interference with gonadotropin function and there should be less batch variability encountered. With the recombinant products that are soon to be available, we would expect almost no variability.

R.A. Lobo, M.D.

Reference

1. Stone B, Quinn K, Quinn P, et al: Responses of patients to different lots of human menopausal gonadotropins during controlled ovarian hyperstimulation. *Fertil Steril* 52:745, 1989.

8 Disorders of the Fallopian Tube

Correlation Between the American Fertility Society Classifications of Adnexal Adhesions and Distal Tubal Occlusion, Salpingoscopy, and Reproductive Outcome in Tubal Surgery
Marana R, Catalano GF, Rizzi M, Caruana P, Muzii L, Mancuso S
(Universita'Cattolica del Sacro Cuore, Rome)
Fertil Steril 64:924–929, 1995

8–1

Objective.—The American Fertility Society (AFS) classification of tubal disease is based on the degree of distal tubal occlusion and adnexal adhesions. Visualizing the entire extent of the ampullary mucosa by intra-operative salpingoscopy gives additional information about the extent of tubal disease. This examination has by no means been universally carried out, however. For this reason, a prospective study was planned to correlate AFS scores of distal tubal occlusion and adnexal adhesions with salpingoscopic findings and the reproductive outcome in patients having reconstructive surgery.

Study Population.—Fifty-five women having microsurgery or operative laparoscopy for tubal infertility and concomitant salpingoscopy were included in the study. Twenty-nine patients with adnexal adhesions underwent salpingo-ovariolysis, whereas 26 with hydrosalpinx had salpingoneostomy. The patients, whose average age was 30 years, had been infertile for 53 months on average. Infertility was primary in 33 cases and secondary in 22.

Findings.—No immediate or delayed complications resulted from salpingoscopy. The examination required only a few extra minutes. In both groups of patients, the salpingoscopic grade of involvement correlated with the AFS classification, although there were exceptions. Mucosal damage was present in 4 tubes in the minimal AFS class. There were 29 pregnancies; 23 patients carried an intrauterine pregnancy to term. Four of 22 patients evaluated who did not conceive were found to have occluded tubes. Term pregnancy was achieved in 55% of patients having salpingo-ovariolysis and 73% of those with a normal ampullary mucosa. Twenty-seven percent of patients undergoing salpingoneostomy achieved term pregnancy; the rate for those with normal ampullary mucosa was 64%. In

147

the group having salpingo-ovariolysis, term pregnancy was not infrequent in patients with severely affected tubes as judged from AFS scores. In neither group did term pregnancy correlate with the AFS score.

Conclusion.—Salpingostomy contributes significantly to identifying those patients who can be expected to benefit the most from tubal reconstruction, whether performed for adhesions or distal occlusion.

▶ The results of this study demonstrate the importance of determining the extent of alterations to the normal morphology of the tubal mucosa as well as the extent of external adhesions. If there is extensive damage to the endosalpinx, performing an operative procedure to create tubal patency will be unlikely to achieve the goal of enhancing the ability to have an intrauterine pregnancy. If there are large hydrosalpinges, the tubal mucosa—which is necessary for blastocyst development—is extensively damaged. Therefore, in vitro fertilization is the preferred therapeutic regimen, not distal tubal surgery.

D.R. Mishell, Jr., M.D.

Prospective Study of Tubal Mucosal Lesions and Fertility in Hydrosalpinges

Vasquez G, Boeckx W, Brosens I (Univ Hosp Gasthuisberg, Leuven, Belgium)
Hum Reprod 10:1075–1078, 1995   8–2

Background.—In patients with sequelae of pelvic inflammatory disease, tubal mucosal pathology is related to fertility outcome. Endoscopic techniques now permit accurate identification of mucosal lesions, but the prognostic importance of these findings remains to be validated. A prospective, multicenter study was performed to relate the macroscopic and microscopic pathologic findings of the endosalpinx to the fertility outcome in patients with hydrosalpinx.

Methods.—Fifty patients were selected for the study. All were younger than 40 years of age, had bilateral postinflammatory hydrosalpinges or hydrosalpinx in a single tube, and were undergoing salpingoneostomy to restore tubal patency. Patients with other fertility-decreasing conditions were excluded. At salpingoneostomy, macroscopic features, such as peritubal adhesions and the mucosal diameter and quality, were scored. Representative biopsy specimens were evaluated by scanning electron and light microscopy. The findings were related to the fertility outcomes at up to 3 years' follow-up.

Results.—At operation, 37 patients had thin-walled and 13 had thick-walled hydrosalpinges. The thickness of the tubal wall was 1 to 2 mm vs. 2 to 10 mm at the thinnest part and 1.5 to 4 mm vs. 4 to 10 mm at the thickest part, respectively, in these 2 groups. In the patients with thin-walled hydrosalpinges, the mucosa was rated as good—with more than 75% of the newly reconstructed fimbriae being normal—in 13 patients.

Ten patients had a moderately damaged mucosa (50% to 75% normal) and 14 had a severely damaged mucosa (less than 50% normal).

None of the women with thick-walled hydrosalpinges had an intrauterine pregnancy. In the women with thin-walled hydrosalpinges, the mucosal appearance through the operating microscope was the most important factor. The prognosis was significantly better with a small diameter than with a medium or large diameter. The presence of more than 50% damaged mucosa significantly influenced the fertility prognosis, whereas the extent of peritubal adhesions did not. The absence of mucosal adhesions was associated with a pregnancy rate of 58%.

Conclusion.—Thick-walled hydrosalpinges with wall fibrosis are incompatible with intrauterine pregnancy. In contrast, the pregnancy rate is very good for women with thin-walled hydrosalpinges with normal or flattened ampullary mucosal folds but without adhesions. The pregnancy rate falls and the risk of tubal pregnancy rises when mucosal adhesions are present. Women with sequelae of pelvic inflammatory disease have a wide range of tubal pathologic conditions.

▶ Tubal obstruction is present in about one third of infertile couples, and 80% of the obstruction occurs in the distal portion of the oviduct with some degree of hydrosalpinx. Because tubal obstruction is a common cause of infertility, knowledge regarding the best type of treatment is important for both the clinician and the infertile couple. Two types of therapy are used for the treatment of infertility caused by distal tubal obstruction: neosalpingostomy and in vitro fertilization with embryo transfer.

Neosalpingostomy should not be performed if the chances of a subsequent intrauterine pregnancy are small and those of tubal pregnancy are high. The results of this study indicate that if there is a thick-walled hydrosalpinx or a thin-walled hydrosalpinx greater than 1 or 2 cm in diameter, with more than 50% mucosal damage or mucosal adhesions, it is better to perform in vitro fertilization instead of a neosalpingostomy.

D.R. Mishell, Jr., M.D.

Selective Salpingography With an Insemination Catheter in the Treatment of Women With Cornual Fallopian Tube Obstruction

Motta ELA, Nelson J, Batzofin J, Serafini P (Escola Paulista de Medicina, São Paulo, Brazil; Huntington Mem Hosp, Pasadena, Calif)
Hum Reprod 10:1156–1159, 1995   8–3

Background.—About one fifth of women with tubal disease have cornual obstruction of the fallopian tube. Conventional treatment approaches are invasive, costly, and sometimes risky. In many patients, the cause of obstruction is unclear—possibly an accumulation of debris or amorphous and crystalized secretions. Thus, selective tubal cannulation with guide wires and infusion of radiographic contrast under pressure may easily dislodge such obstructive materials. One experience with the use of a commercially available transcervical fallopian tube insemination catheter under fluoroscopic guidance was reported.

Methods.—Twenty-seven infertile patients, aged 26–42 years and with a mean length of infertility of 5.9 years, were treated between 1991 and 1994. Twenty-three patients had bilateral and 4 had unilateral cornual tube blockage as seen on hysterosalpingographic study.

Findings.—Selective fluoroscopic tubal catheterization was achieved in 95% of the patients. Tubal patency resulted in 70% of the procedures. Eight of 23 patients, or 34.8%, became pregnant. Six were delivered of infants at term, and 2 had first-trimester abortions. One woman conceived twice, giving birth to 1 infant after the first recanalization and to twins after the second salpingography. There were no complications.

Conclusion.—Selective salpingography with an insemination catheter is easy to perform, cost-effective, and safe. It can be used in patients with cornual fallopian tube obstruction as the sole treatment or combined with other assisted conception treatment alternatives.

▶ Fallopian tube obstruction is the cause of infertility in about one third of infertile couples. About one fifth of all women with tubal obstruction have proximal disease, with the remainder having distal tubal obstruction. Although distal tubal blockage is nearly always a result of prior salpingitis, proximal tubal obstruction is frequently caused by the presence of plugs of amorphous crystalized secretions.

In the past few years, various transuterine cannulation techniques have been developed to restore tubal patency when proximal tubal obstruction is observed at the time of hysterosalpingostomy. Patency rates after these procedures range from 60% to 85%, with subsequent pregnancy rates in the 20% to 50% range in various series of small numbers of women. These relatively easy outpatient procedures, such as the one described in this paper, whether performed under fluoroscopic or hysteroscopic visualization, should now be considered the initial treatment of choice for proximal tubal obstruction.

D.R. Mishell, Jr., M.D.

Hysteroscopic Cannulation for Proximal Tubal Obstruction: A Change for the Better?
Das K, Nagel TC, Malo JW (Reproductive Health Associates, St Paul, Minn; Univ of Minnesota, Minneapolis)
Fertil Steril 63:1009–1015, 1995   8–4

Introduction.—The surgical management of proximal tubal obstruction has veered away from resection anastomosis and has moved toward transcervical cannulation in the past decade. Although resection anastomosis remains the gold standard in terms of pregnancy, the advantages of cannulation include patient convenience, ease, and decreased cost. The overall results of hysteroscopic tubal cannulation were compared with resection anastomosis for proximal tubal occlusion.

Methods.—Over a 10-year period (1983–1993), 74 women with bilateral or unilateral proximal occlusion of a single remaining tube who were operated on by 1 of 2 surgeons were analyzed in the nonrandomized retrospective study. In the prehysteroscopic tubal cannulation era (between 1983 and 1989), 31 women aged 23–38 years had microsurgical proximal tubal resection anastomosis for proximal tubal obstruction. For 28 women, hysteroscopic tubal cannulation under laparoscopic guidance was performed from 1989 until the end of 1992 (the posthysteroscopic tubal cannulation era), as there was no evidence of proximal tubal disease. During this same period, 20 women with evidence of proximal tubal disease had microsurgical resection anastomosis.

Results.—Excluded from the resection anastomosis and the hysteroscopic tubal cannulation groups were women with clinical evidence of nodularity, thickening of the proximal tubal segment, and associated distal tubal disease (Table 1). In the hysteroscopic tubal cannulation group, there were 21 patients with normal tubes. In the resection anastomosis group, there were 24 patients with normal tubes. In both groups, intrauterine pregnancy rates were similar in patients with normal distal tubes (57% for the cannulation group vs. 50% for the anastomosis group). Ectopic pregnancy rates were lower in the cannulation group (0% for the cannulation group vs. 29% for the anastomosis group). In the anastomosis group, the 1-year patency rate in nonpregnant patients was higher (80% for anastomosis vs. 33% for cannulation).

TABLE 1.—Pregnancy Rates After Successful Hysteroscopic Tubal Cannulation or Resection Anastomosis

Groups	Patient number	Pregnancy* Intrauterine	Ectopic
Hysteroscopic tubal cannulation			
Normal tubes†	21	12 (57.1)	0 (0)‡
Resection anastomosis			
Normal tubes†	24	12 (50)	7 (29.1)
Thickening of the proximal tubal segment§	12	4 (33.3)	2 (16.6)
Bipolar disease‖	17	1 (5.9)	2 (11.8)

Note: Patients in all groups with distal disease are excluded from the analysis.

* Values in parentheses are percentages.

† Patients in these groups had proximal tubal occlusion with normal-appearing tubes at laparoscopy or laparotomy.

‡ $P = 0.007$ using χ^2 analysis between the groups.

§ Patients in this group had proximal tubal occlusion with clinical evidence of thickening of the proximal tubal segment at laparoscopy or laparotomy.

‖ All patients with distal tubal disease whether treated by hysteroscopic tubal cannulation or resection anastomosis are in this group.

(Courtesy of Das K, Nagel TC, Malo JW: Hysteroscopic cannulation for proximal tubal obstruction: A change for the better? *Fertil Steril* 63:1009–1015, 1995. Reproduced with permission of the publisher, the American Society for Reproductive Medicine [The American Fertility Society].)

Conclusion.—The prognosis for intrauterine pregnancy in patients with proximal tubal obstruction has improved significantly with hysteroscopic tubal cannulation. In the management of proximal tubal obstruction in selected women, hysteroscopic cannulation should be the first choice. After successful cannulation or resection anastomosis, hysteroscopic cannulation may be a treatment option for delayed occlusion.

▶ Various transcervical cannulation techniques have been shown to treat proximal tubal obstruction. Success has been reported whether these procedures have been performed using fluoroscopic visualization or, as was done in this study, under direct visualization with the use of hysteroscopy and concurrent laparoscopy. Good success rates have been reported with both techniques. However, because laparoscopy requires general anesthesia whereas fluoroscope-guided cannulation requires only local anesthesia with sedation, it would appear that the latter technique would be safer and more cost-effective.

D.R. Mishell, Jr., M.D.

Differential Impact on Pregnancy Rate of Selective Salpingography, Tubal Catheterization and Wire-Guide Recanalization in the Treatment of Proximal Fallopian Tube Obstruction

Woolcott R, Petchpud A, O'Donnell P, Stanger J (Lingard Fertility Centre, Newcastle, Australia)
Hum Reprod 10:1423–1426, 1995

8–5

Background.—Recently, one team of researchers questioned the benefit of wire-guide cannulation alone in treating patients with proximal tubal obstruction who wish to become pregnant. Although wire guides may achieve patency, they may have no additional therapeutic benefit over tubal catheterization in achieving pregnancy. The impact on pregnancy rates of selective salpingopgraphy, tubal catheterization, and wire-guide cannulation done to achieve patency was investigated.

Methods.—Sixty-six patients with a total of 113 proximal obstructed fallopian tubes were included in the study. Obstruction was diagnosed by laparoscopy and hysterosalpingography. Each patient underwent a transcervical recanalization procedure sequentially using selective salpingography followed, if needed, by tubal catheterization with a soft Teflon 2-French catheter and finally, if necessary, wire-guide cannulation. Once patency was achieved, the procedure was ended.

Findings.—Patency was attained in 34.5% of fallopian tubes by selective salpingography alone, in 46% by tubal catheterization, and in 8.9% by wire guide. Patency could not be achieved in 10.6% of the tubes. During a mean 17-month follow-up, 36.4% of the patients became pregnant without recourse to another treatment. Among the 59 patients in whom patency was achieved, 44.1% of those treated for bilateral obstruction and 31.3% of those treated for unilateral obstruction became pregnant. Pregnancy occurred in 27.3% of the 22 patients in whom selective salpingography was used to produce tubal patency, in 56.7% in whom tubal catheterization was used, and in 14.3% in whom a wire guide was used. The 1 patient becoming pregnant after wire guide use had an ectopic pregnancy. The difference between the ongoing pregnancy rates after tubal catheterization and wire-guide cannulation (50% and 0%, respectively) was significant.

Conclusion.—Although wire-guide cannulation is the most effective way to achieve tubal patency, when it is truly necessary rather than elective the pregnancy prognosis associated with it is poor. Alternative treatments, such as microsurgery or in vitro fertilization should be considered.

▶ The initial treatment for proximal tubal obstruction has changed from surgical reanastomosis through a laparotomy incision to some type of transcervical recanalization procedure performed under fluoroscopic or hysteroscopic guidance. Because the majority of proximal tubal occlusions are caused by debris, mucus, or other materials that block the proximal portion of the oviduct, passage of a small catheter into the oviduct can usually produce tubal patency and can frequently enable pregnancy to occur. The results of this study indicate that if passage of a flexible catheter cannot be undertaken and it is necessary to use a rigid wire guide to produce tubal patency, it is unlikely that intrauterine pregnancy will subsequently occur. When it is necessary to use a wire guide, obstuction is most often caused by tubal pathology such as salpingitis isthmica nodosa. Since the intrauterine pregnancy rates are low after it was necessary to use the wire guide, alternative therapy such as surgical reanastomosis should be considered.

D.R. Mishell, Jr., M.D.

Expanded Polytetrafluoroethylene (Gore-Tex Surgical Membrane) Is Superior to Oxidized Regenerated Cellulose (Interceed TC7) in Preventing Adhesions
Haney AF, Murphy AA, Hesla J, Rock JA, Hurst BS, Rowe G, Kettel LM, Schlaff WD (Duke Univ, Durham, NC; Emory Univ, Atlanta, Ga; Univ of Colorado, Denver; et al)
Fertil Steril 63:1021–1026, 1995   8–6

Introduction.—Pelvic adhesions remain an important problem in women undergoing gynecologic surgery, as they may impair fertility even after attempted lysis. The lack of effective medical measures for preventing postoperative adhesion formation has prompted the use of a mechanical barrier that will allow the injured peritoneal surfaces to heal. Most attempts have used either oxidized regenerated cellulose, a degradable material having procoagulant properties, or expanded polytetrafluoroethylene (PTFE), a permanent material.

Trial.—These materials were contrasted and evaluated in 32 women requiring open reconstructive pelvic surgery who had adhesions between the pelvic side walls and reproductive organs and were candidates for second-look laparoscopy. Pelvic surgery had been done previously in 85% of patients, whereas 16% had a history of pelvic infection.

Management.—Antibiotics were given 1 hour before the initial procedure and continued for at least 24 hours. After adhesions were lysed, 1 pelvic side wall was covered with either PTFE or cellulose, and the opposite side wall with the remaining material. The materials were tailored to overlap the defect by at least 1 cm and were sutured in place with 1 or more 7-0 or 8-0 nylon or polypropylene sutures. A second-look laparoscopy was undertaken 1–6 weeks after reconstructive surgery.

Results.—Both barriers significantly reduced adhesion scores compared with the original side wall scores, but PTFE appeared to be most effective. Analysis of the area of adhesion yielded the same result. Second-look procedures confirmed that cellulose is rapidly degraded, whereas PTFE remains unchanged in appearance. There were no problems in removing the PTFE barrier.

Conclusion.—Polytetrafluoroethylene is an effective means of limiting adhesion formation in women undergoing reconstructive pelvic surgery. It appears feasible to leave it in place and thereby avoid another procedure.

▶ This multicenter study demonstrated that after a reconstructive pelvic surgical procedure is performed to lyse adhesions between the pelvic side wall and the adnexa, the permanent barrier, PTFE, prevented reformation of adhesions to a significantly greater extent than did the absorbable material. Because the permanent material is usually removed after partial healing occurs, its use is associated with the need to perform a second operative procedure. To determine whether the better results with the permanent barrier justify its greater cost and need for a second surgical procedure, fecundity rates with the 2 techniques need to be analyzed. If a much greater pregnancy rate occurs with the permanent barrier, the added expense may be worthwhile.

D.R. Mishell, Jr., M.D.

9 Endometriosis

Clinical Evaluation of CA-125 Concentrations as a Prognostic Factor for Pregnancy in Infertile Women With Surgically Treated Endometriosis
Pittaway DE, Rondinone D, Miller KA, Barnes K (Wake Forest Univ, Winston-Salem, NC)
Fertil Steril 64:321–324, 1995   9–1

Background.—CA-125 is a glycoprotein occurring on the surface of certain normal and some cancerous cells, such as in nonmucinous ovarian cancer. Previous research has suggested that serial CA-125 determinations are of prognostic value in some infertile women with surgically treated endometriosis. The recent development of a second-generation CA-125 assay provided an opportunity to extend and confirm these earlier findings.

Methods.—The new automated enzyme immunoassay was used to determine CA-125 values in 123 women with endometriosis identified during laparoscopy for infertility. Forty-five percent of these women had preoperative CA-125 values of 16 units/mL or greater. Serial CA-125 determinations were performed during the 12-month follow-up.

Findings.—Women who became pregnant did not have mean preoperative CA-125 levels significantly different from those who did not. However, mean postoperative CA-125 values were significantly lower for women achieving pregnancy than for those who did not (Fig 2). In a univariate analysis, preoperative CA-125 values between 16 and 25 units/mL and postoperative CA-125 values of less than 16 units/mL were correlated with significantly greater pregnancy rates. In a multivariate analysis of 10 covariables, postoperative CA-125 concentration was the only factor associated with pregnancy, even after controlling for all covariables.

Conclusion.—This study confirms the previous observation that CA-125 levels are prognostic indicators for pregnancy in infertile women treated surgically for endometriosis. The current findings also provide additional support for the clinical use of CA-125 concentrations in selected women with endometriosis.

▶ The authors have shown that when an infertile woman with endometriosis is treated with conservative reconstructive surgery, if the preoperative serum CA-125 level is ≤ 25 units/mL, the chance of becoming pregnant after

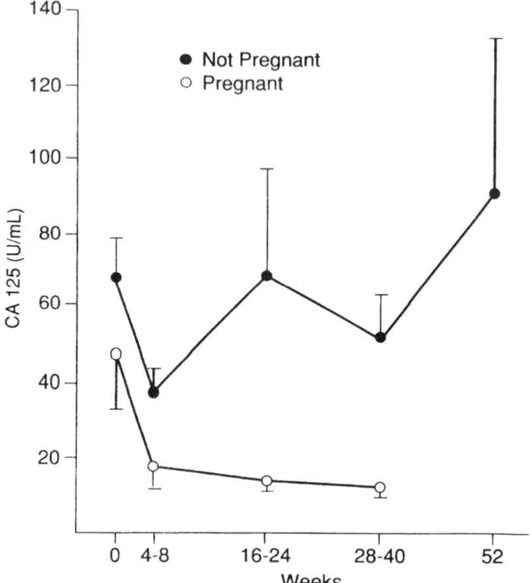

FIGURE 2.—Mean ± standard error preoperative and postoperative CA-125 concentrations for women who conceived and those who did not. (Courtesy of Pittaway DE, Rondinone D, Miller KA, et al: Clinical evaluation of CA-125 concentrations as a prognostic factor for pregnancy in infertile women with surgically treated endometriosis. *Fertil Steril* 64:321–324, 1995. Reproduced with permission of the publisher, the American Society for Reproductive Medicine [The American Fertility Society].)

the operative procedure is greater than if the preoperative CA-125 level is > 25 units/mL. If the postoperative CA-125 levels were < 16 units/mL, 70% of the women conceived, whereas if they were higher than this level, only 15% of the women conceived. Clinicians can measure the CA-125 level before and after surgical treatment of infertile women with endometriosis to help determine (1) whether to perform pelvic surgery in asymptomatic women and (2) whether to proceed more rapidly with additional treatment for the infertility after conservative surgery is performed.

D.R. Mishell, Jr., M.D.

10 Treatment of Unexplained Infertility

Ovulation Induction in 1995: A New Policy
Fanchin R, Fernandez H, Olivennes F, Frydman R (Univ Hosp Antoine Béclère, Clamart, France)
Hum Reprod 10:2224–2225, 1995

10–1

Background.—Although ovulation induction is a successful infertility treatment, the results of ovarian stimulation with human menopausal gonadotropins (hMG) followed by intrauterine insemination (IUI) are disappointing. An in vitro fertilization protocol for ovulation induction followed by IUI was developed. A 7-day regimen of gonadotropin-releasing hormone agonist (GnRHa) is combined with a purified follicle-stimulating hormone (FSH) preparation in the early follicular phase. In theory, this approach should improve oocyte quality by preventing or decreasing the adverse effects of high plasma levels of luteinizing hormone (LH) on oocyte maturation and by allowing a more comfortable and adequate multifollicular development before human chorionic gonadotropin administration.

Methods.—A retrospective study of 580 consecutive ovarian stimulation cycles followed by IUI in 370 subfertile patients was done to verify the practical efficacy of this approach. The patients ranged in age from 20 to 39 years. Three stimulation protocols were used: clomiphene citrate plus hMG, hMG alone, and GnRHa.

Findings.—The prevalence of spontaneous LH surge was significantly greater in cycles treated with clomiphene plus hMG and hMG alone than in those treated with GnRHa plus FSH plus hMG. Patients receiving the latter combination had significantly higher clinical and ongoing pregnancy rates, at 27% and 24%, respectively, than those treated with the first 2 protocols. Those given clomiphene plus hMG had clinical and ongoing pregnancy rates of 16% and 14%, respectively, and those given hMG alone had rates of 13% and 11%, respectively. Multiple pregnancy rates did not differ among the 3 groups. Overall, the incidence of moderate hyperstimulation was 11%.

Conclusion.—Pregnancy rates associated with GnRHa plus FSH plus hMG are significantly higher than those associated with clomiphene citrate plus hMG and hMG alone. The use of GnRHa and purified FSH preparations may be effective, reliable, and safe in improving the outcomes of ovulation induction. Further prospective randomized studies are needed.

▶ The problem with this study, as the authors indicate, was that it was a retrospective analysis, not a prospective randomized trial. In addition, only pregnancy rates, not cycle fecundability rates, were reported. Nevertheless, it is interesting that the pregnancy rates were similar when either clomiphene citrate or hMG was used to stimulate multiple follicular development. Whether the regimen of GnRHa plus FSH is truly superior needs to be determined by prospective studies. This latter regimen is certainly more costly and requires more monitoring—which also increases the cost—than clomiphene citrate. Therefore, clomiphene citrate should be considered the agent of choice to induce ovarian hyperstimulation for at least the first 4 treatment cycles of couples with unexplained infertility.

D.R. Mishell, Jr., M.D.

Gamete Intra-Fallopian Transfer or In-Vitro Fertilization After Failed Ovarian Stimulation and Intrauterine Insemination in Unexplained Infertility?
Ranieri M, Beckett VA, Marchant S, Kinis A, Serhal P (Univ College Hosp, London)
Hum Reprod 10:2023–2026, 1995   10–2

Objective.—The best management for patients with unexplained infertility who fail to conceive after ovarian stimulation and intrauterine insemination (IUI) remains uncertain. To address the question, the first prospective randomized study was planned to compare gamete intrafallopian transfer (GIFT) with in vitro fertilization (IVF) in patients who had failed to conceive in 3 or more cycles of ovarian stimulation and IUI. Sixty-nine couples with unexplained infertility were randomly assigned to one of the two treatments.

Results.—Thirty-five patients treated by GIFT and 34 in the IVF group were evaluated. All patients in the GIFT group received 3 oocytes, and 25 of the 34 IVF patients received 3 embryos. Fertilization rates were comparable in the 2 groups. Although significantly more embryos implanted per embryo transfer in the IVF group than per oocyte transfer in the GIFT group, the difference in clinical pregnancies was not significant (Table 1). Twin pregnancies were significantly more frequent in the IVF group. There were proportionately more deliveries in the IVF group, but the difference was not significant.

Implications.—Both GIFT and IVF/embryo transfer are frequently effective in couples with unexplained infertility who have resisted treatment by ovarian stimulation and IUI. In vitro fertilization/embryo transfer is a less invasive approach, and it may be advantageous to observe the development of all embryos in vitro.

TABLE 1.—Results of Gamete Intrafallopian Transfer and In Vitro Fertilization in Couples With Unexplained Infertility

	GIFT ($n = 35$)		IVF ($n = 34$)		
	Number	Mean/rate	Number	Mean/rate	P value*
Age (years)		32.8 (±3.2)		31.9 (±3.7)	0.3
Retrieved oocytes	275	7.8 (±2.8)	231	6.8 (±2.7)	0.1
Transferred oocytes (GIFT)	105	3.0 (±0.1)	91	2.7 (±0.1)	0.001
% embryos (IVF)					
Inseminated oocytes	170	4.8 (±2.7)	231	6.8 (±2.7)	0.005
Oocytes fertilized *in vitro* (%)	96	57	135	58	0.8
Pregnancies (%)	12	34	17	50	0.28
Implanted embryos (%)	14	13	26	29	0.01
Twin pregnancies (%)	2	17	9	53	0.005
Delivered (%)	9	75	16	94	0.1

* $P < 0.05$ was considered statistically significant.
Abbreviations: GIFT, gamete intrafallopian transfer; *IVF,* in vitro fertilization.
(Courtesy of Ranieri M, Beckett VA, Marchant S, et al: Gamete intra-fallopian transfer or in-vitro fertilization after failed ovarian stimulation and intrauterine insemination in unexplained infertility? *Hum Reprod* 10:2023–2026, 1995, by permission of Oxford University Press.)

▶ Evidence is accumulating that the optimal initial treatment for couples with unexplained infertility (those women with patent oviducts who ovulate and whose male partner has an adequate number of motile sperm) is controlled ovarian hyperstimulation and IUI. Cycle fecundability rates with this treatment are generally reported to range between 10% and 20%. If the couple does not conceive with several cycles of this therapy and they wish to undergo assisted reproduction, the results of this study indicate that satisfactory and comparable pregnancy rates are achieved with both GIFT and IVF. Because IVF is less invasive than GIFT, and because the problem of infertility may be caused by failure of fertilization, IVF should be the assisted reproductive technique that is recommended to couples with unexplained infertility who fail to conceive with several cycles of controlled ovarian hyperstimulation and IUI.

D.R. Mishell, Jr., M.D.

Is There a Role for Ovarian Stimulation and Intra-Uterine Insemination After Age 40?

Frederick JL, Denker MS, Rojas A, Horta I, Stone SC, Asch RH, Balmaceda JP (Univ of California Irvine, Orange)
Hum Reprod 9:2284–2286, 1994   10–3

Purpose.—The treatment of infertility in women over 40 years of age has become a major clinical challenge. Previous studies of assisted reproduction have noted an age-related decline in pregnancy, but there have been few reports on the results of ovarian stimulation and intrauterine insemination (IUI) with respect to age. The results of ovarian stimulation/IUI in 77 women aged 40 years and older were reviewed.

TABLE 1.—Results of Ovarian Stimulation/Intrauterine Insemination in Patients ≥ 40 Years of Age

No. of patients	77
No. of cycles	210
Mean no. of cycles per patient	2.7
No. of patients with LH surge	63 (30%)
No. of patients receiving hCG injection	147 (70%)
No. of pregnancies	11
Pregnancy rate per patient	14.3%
Pregnancy rate per cycle	5.2%
No. of miscarriages	8
Abortion rate	72.7%
Live birth rate per patient	3.9%
Live birth rate per cycle	1.4%

Abbreviations: LH, luteinizing hormone; *hCG*, human chorionic gonadotropin.
(Courtesy of Frederick JL, Denker MS, Rojas A, et al: Is there a role for ovarian stimulation and intra-uterine insemination after age 40? *Hum Reprod* 9:2284–2286, 1994, by permission of Oxford University Press.)

Methods.—The couples underwent 210 cycles of ovarian stimulation/ IUI. The women's mean age was 42 years, and 26% had primary infertility. The couples' mean duration of infertility was 6 years. Intrauterine insemination was selected because of poor postcoital test results in 6% of cases, abnormal semen analyses in 18%, and oligo-ovulatory status in 22%; there was no obvious diagnosis in 54% of cases. Thirty-one percent of cycles used clomiphene citrate alone, 30% used human menopausal gonadotropin (hMG) alone, and 39% used a combination of clomiphene citrate and HMG. Two consecutive IUIs were performed 24 to 48 hours after urinary luteinizing hormone (LH) testing showed a positive surge. If the LH result was negative by day 15 and ultrasonography showed at least 1 follicle of at least 18 mm in diameter, the women received human chorionic gonadotropin (hCG), 5,000 IU IM. They then had IUI over the next 2 days.

Results.—Thirty percent of the 300 cycles initiated were canceled because of poor response. The average number of completed cycles was 2.7 per patient, and the average number of follicles per cycle with ovarian stimulation was 5.3. The cycle outcomes were unaffected by the type of ovarian stimulation used or by the administration of hCG. Although 11 pregnancies were achieved, there were 8 spontaneous abortions. The live birth rate was only 3.9% per patient and 1.4% per cycle (Table 1).

Conclusion.—For infertile couples in which the woman is 40 years of age or older, ovarian stimulation/IUI yields a very poor live birth rate. The findings will be an important part of patient counseling and suggest that assisted reproductive treatment should be offered as soon as ovarian responsiveness is documented.

▶ Controlled ovarian hyperstimulation and IUI is being widely used for the treatment of unexplained infertility with pregnancy rates in the range of 10% to 15% per cycle. However, fecundability rates normally decline after age 39 years and decrease dramatically after age 40 years. Pregnancy rates with IVF also decrease substantially after the female partner is older than 40 years of age. In this report, the pregnancy rate per cycle with ovarian hyperstimulation and IUI in women over age 40 years was only 5.1% compared with 10% to 15% in younger women. The low live birth rate of 1.4% per cycle was mainly the result of the extremely high abortion rate of 72.6%.

Whether the more expensive in vitro fertilization procedure should be offered to these patients is debatable because live birth rates with in vitro fertilization of < 10% have been reported in women over age 40.[1] The best chance for a live birth in infertile women over age 40 is in vitro fertilization with the use of donor eggs. It is useful to have data such as those obtained in this report to adequately counsel infertile couples when the woman is older than 40 years of age because the various treatments differ with respect to cost and chance of successful life birth.

D.R. Mishell, Jr., M.D.

Reference

1. Piette C, de Mouzon J, Bachelot A, et al: In-vitro fertilization: Influence of women's age on pregnancy rates. *Hum Reprod* 5:56–59, 1990.

A New System for Fallopian Tube Sperm Perfusion Leads to Pregnancy Rates Twice as High as Standard Intrauterine Insemination
Fanchin R, Hazout A, Olivennes F, Schwab B, Righini C, Frydman R (Hôpital Antoine Béclère, Clamart, France)
Fertil Steril 64:505–510, 1995   10–4

Background.—To overcome the limitations of standard intrauterine insemination (IUI), several authors have focused on new IUI methods that are able to ensure the presence of higher sperm densities in the fallopian tubes at the time of ovulation. One device specifically adapted for fallopian tube sperm perfusion—the Fallopian Sperm Transfer (FAST) System—was tested.

Methods.—Seventy-four infertile women aged 20–38 years were enrolled in a prospective, randomized comparison of fallopian tube sperm perfusion using the FAST System and standard IUI. The patients underwent 100 cycles of controlled ovarian hyperstimulation (COH) between December 1993 and May 1994. Exclusion criteria were obstructed or severely damaged fallopian tubes, estradiol levels per mature follicle of less than 250 pg/mL on the day of human chorionic gonadotropin (hCG) administration, spontaneous luteinizing hormone surge, and marked sperm abnormalities. Three types of ovarian stimulation protocols were used to achieve COH: clomiphene citrate and human menopausal gonadotropin (hMG) in 35 patients, hMG alone in 35, and gonadotropin-releasing hormone agonist and follicle-stimulating hormone and hMG in 30. Thirty-six hours after hCG was administered, 50 patients were assigned to IUI, designated group A, and 50 to fallopian tube sperm perfusion, designated group B. The FAST System ensures a good cervical seal and allows a pressurized injection of 4 mL of sperm suspension.

Findings.—Ten clinical pregnancies occurred in group A (20% per cycle). Seven of these pregnancies were ongoing. Twenty clinical pregnancies occurred in group B (40% per cycle). Seventeen (34%) were ongoing. The group B rate was significantly higher than the group A rate. The 2 groups were comparable in the prevalence of twin and 3 or more sac pregnancies. None of the patients experienced moderate or severe ovarian hyperstimulation syndrome.

Conclusion.—The pregnancy rates associated with fallopian tube sperm perfusion are significantly better than those obtained with standard IUI. The FAST System is not invasive or traumatic. None of the patients had cervical bleeding, vasovagal episodes, or pelvic infections after this new procedure.

A Randomized Prospective Comparison Between Intrauterine Insemination and Fallopian Sperm Perfusion for the Treatment of Infertility
Karande VC, Levrant S, Rao R, Morris R, Pratt DE, Dudkeiwicz A, Balin M, Gleicher N (Ctr for Human Reproduction, Chicago; Found for Reproductive Medicine, Chicago)
Fertil Steril 64:638–640, 1995   10–5

Introduction.—Previous reports suggested that fallopian sperm perfusion resulted in higher pregnancy rates than intrauterine insemination (IUI), now considered standard infertility therapy. In IUI, pretreated semen is concentrated in small volume and deposited into the uterine cavity by catheter. With fallopian sperm perfusion, the sperm is diluted in a larger volume of media. A prospective randomized study was designed to determine whether fallopian sperm perfusion resulted in higher pregnancy rates than IUI.

Methods.—Consecutive infertile women had ovulation induction with clomiphene citrate or gonadotropins. On 2 consecutive days after human chorionic gonadotropin (hCG) administration, 120 women had IUI and 120 women had fallopian sperm perfusion performed. Semen for both procedures had 3 routine sperm washes. During fallopian sperm perfusion, the sperm was suspended in 4 mL of media, whereas for the IUI, the sperm volume was less than 0.5 mL. The fallopian sperm perfusion was carried out over 4 minutes, whereas the IUI was conducted by rapid plunger action of a syringe.

Results.—Consecutive ovarian stimulation cycles were performed in 240 women. In the IUI group, 44 had clomiphene citrate and 76 had gonadotropin. In the fallopian sperm perfusion group, 44 had clomiphene citrate and 76 had gonadotropin. The overall pregnancy rate per cycle for both groups was 10.8%. When compared for ovulation induction, the pregnancy rates were also similar (6.8% for the IUI group vs. 9.1% for the fallopian sperm perfusion group with clomiphene citrate; 13.2% for the IUI group vs. 11.8% for the fallopian sperm perfusion group with gonadotropin).

Conclusion.—No advantage is seen with fallopian sperm perfusion over IUI. Fallopian sperm perfusion is also more time consuming and more costly because of the increased media use. It should not replace IUI.

▶ The techniques for COH and IUI are being used frequently for the treatment of unexplained infertility as well as by couples with mild degrees of sperm abnormalities and tubal damage. Most reports indicate that these techniques result in cycle fecundability rates of 10% to 15%. The results of these studies (Abstracts 10–4 and 10–5) indicate that insemination of a greater volume of sperm suspension to place a portion of the sperm directly in the oviduct does not result in increased pregnancy rates, unless some technique is used to create a cervical seal so that most of the inseminated fluid is directed toward the oviduct.

In the study reported in Abstract 10–4, gonadotropins were used to stimulate the ovaries, with a high incidence of multiple pregnancy. Other studies need to be undertaken, with use of the system that creates a cervical seal in which clomiphene is used to stimulate the ovaries, to determine whether cycle fecundability can be increased with this simple method of hyperstimulation combined with IUI. The cervical seal technique is promising and, if found by others to be more effective than routine IUI, deserves increased use for the treatment of the infertile couple.

D.R. Mishell, Jr., M.D.

Controlled Ovarian Hyperstimulation With or Without Intrauterine Insemination for the Treatment of Unexplained Infertility

Gregoriou O, Vitoratos N, Papadias C, Konidaris S, Gargaropoulos A, Louridas C (Univ of Athens, Greece)
Int J Gynaecol Obstet 48:55–59, 1995   10–6

Objective.—As many as 15% of cases of infertility are unexplained, despite thorough assessment. These couples are managed empirically. Their pregnancy rate is no better than the spontaneous rate for untreated infertile couples. Whether intrauterine insemination (IUI) is preferable to timed intercourse (TI) in ovulated cycles for couples with long-standing infertility of unknown origin was determined.

Patients and Management.—Forty-six couples who had been infertile for a median of 6 years and for as long as 12 years were included in the study. In a crossover design, the couples began treatment with either controlled ovarian hyperstimulation (COH) in conjunction with IUI or COH with TI. After 2 consecutive treatment cycles and a rest cycle, they changed to the alternative regimen. Ovarian stimulation used human menopausal gonadotropin (hMG) and human chorionic gonadotropin.

Results.—The couples completed 141 cycles of COH/TI and 74 cycles on COH/IUI. The respective pregnancy rates were 17% and 45%, a significant difference. Cycle fecundity rates were 9% in patients receiving COH/TI and 26% in those receiving COH/IUI. There were no significant differences in follicle numbers, endometrial thickness, or sperm parameters between conception and nonconception cycles. In no case did COH/IUI lead to pelvic infection or significant cramping. Two of 19 pregnancies aborted spontaneously after IUI. The rate of multiple gestation in this group was 9%.

Conclusion.—The results to date suggest that combined treatment with hMG and IUI is an effective approach to unexplained infertility.

Ovuluation Induction With Gonadotropins as Sole Treatment in Infertile Couples With Open Tubes: A Randomized Prospective Comparison Between Intrauterine Insemination and Timed Vaginal Intercourse

Melis GB, Guerriero S, Paoletti AM, Depau GF, Ajossa S, Mais V (Univ of Cagliari, Italy)
Fertil Steril 64:1088–1093, 1995   10–7

Objective.—Pregnancy rates are higher in women who have undergone intrauterine insemination (IUI) after ovulation induction with gonadotropins than in women who have undergone IUI in spontaneous cycles. Pregnancy rates were compared for couples with mild male factor–related or unexplained infertility treated with ovulation induction and vaginal intercourse vs. couples treated with IUI after ovulation induction.

Methods.—Two hundred couples with mild male factor–related infertility (group 1) and unexplained infertility (group 2) were randomized to receive either 3 consecutive cycles of ovulation induction with gonadotropins and timed intercourse (TI) (group A) or 3 consecutive cycles of ovulation induction with gonadotropins and IUI (group B). Pregnancy rates were measured.

Results.—Eleven of 100 group 1 couples and 5 of 100 group 2 couples were excluded from the study. There were 41 couples in group 1 (group 1A) and 52 couples in group 2 (group 2A) treated with ovulation induction and TI and 40 couples in group 1 (group 1B) and 51 couples in group 2 (group 2B) treated with ovulation induction and IUI. The numbers of cycles performed were 110 in group 1A, 126 in group 2A, 103 in group 1B, and 123 in group 2B. There were 12 pregnancies in group 1A (29% per patient; 11% per cycle), 11 in group 1B (28% per patient; 11% per cycle), 23 in group 2A (44% per patient; 18% per cycle), and 22 in group 2B (43% per patient; 18% per cycle). There were no significant differences between groups 1A and 1B and groups 2A and 2B. The pregnancy rate was significantly lower in couples with mild male-related infertility than for couples with unexplained infertility.

Conclusion.—Ovulation induction with gonadotropins and TI appears to be as effective as ovulation induction and IUI in couples with unexplained and mild male factor infertility. This approach can be used as the initial treatment.

▶ The results of these 2 studies (Abstracts 10–6 and 10–7) yield conflicting results despite the fact that they were both randomized clinical trials. The different results could be the result of several factors. The design of the studies differed, as did the techniques of sperm preparation and the time when sexual intercourse was advised after the injection of human chorionic gonadotropin to induce ovulation. Because the separation of motile sperm and IUI is a relatively easy process without complications, this technique is usually used in combination with ovarian hyperstimulation to treat couples with unexplained infertility. However, if the couple wishes to attempt natural intercourse in combination with ovarian hyperstimulation for a few cycles, their chances of pregnancy success may not be greatly reduced, provided there is no problem with in vivo sperm cervical mucus penetration.

D.R. Mishell, Jr., M.D.

The Results of In Vitro Fertilization-Embryo Transfer in Couples With Unexplained Infertility Failing to Conceive With Superovulation and Intrauterine Insemination
Gürgan T, Urman B, Yarali H, Kisnisci HA (Univ of Hacettepe, Ankara, Turkey)
Fertil Steril 64:93–97, 1995   10–8

Objective.—Although superovulation and/or intrauterine insemination (IUI) are commonly used as treatment for couples with unexplained and prolonged infertility, some couples still fail to conceive. The prognosis for these couples is unknown. To determine if failure to conceive after 4–6 cycles of superovulation and IUI represented a decreased chance of conception, 157 in vitro fertilization (IVF) cycles in 117 couples with unexplained infertility were retrospectively analyzed and compared with 250 tubal factor cycles in 194 couples.

Methods.—Unexplained infertility was defined as failure to conceive after 2 or more years of unprotected intercourse. Couples with tubal factor infertility were recruited for IVF–embryo transfer (ET) treatment after conventional methods of conception had failed.

Results.—In couples with unexplained infertility, the 20.4% total infertility failure rate was significantly higher than in couples with tubal factor infertility, who had a failure rate of 7.6%. Couples with unexplained infertility tended to have repetitive fertilization failures whereas couples with tubal factor infertility did not. When fertilization did occur, cleavage rates were 89.2% and 87% for couples with unexplained infertility and couples with tubal cycle infertility, respectively. Pregnancy rates per cycle and per ET, abortion rates, and cumulative conception rates were similar for the 2 groups. When couples with total fertilization failure were excluded from the analysis, the cumulative conception rate of 55.3% for couples with unexplained infertility exceeded, albeit insignificantly, the cumulative conception rate of 46.5% for couples with tubal cycle infertility.

Conclusion.—Couples with unexplained infertility who have failed to conceive after 4–6 cycles of superovulation and IUI have higher total fertilization failure rates compared with couples with tubal factor infertility. However, they have a relatively good chance of conceiving in subsequent IVF-ET cycles.

▶ The results of this study indicate that one of the reasons for unexplained or undiagnosed infertility is failure of the sperm to fertilize the ovum. Therefore, if couples fail to conceive after several cycles of controlled ovum hyperstimulation and IUI, they should be advised to attempt at least 1 cycle of IVF to determine whether failure of fertilization is the cause of the infertility. If this cause of infertility is found to be present, the couples can be advised to use intracytoplasmic sperm injection in an attempt to achieve fertilization.

D.R. Mishell, Jr., M.D.

11 Assisted Reproductive Technologies

Assisted Reproductive Technology in the United States and Canada: 1993 Results Generated From the American Society for Reproductive Medicine/Society for Assisted Reproductive Technology Registry
Society for Assisted Reproductive Technology, American Society for Reproductive Medicine (Birmingham, Ala)
Fertil Steril 64:13–21, 1995   11–1

Introduction.—The assisted reproductive technology (ART) activities carried out in 1993 were described. The report reflects voluntarily reported information from 267 ART programs.

Findings.—The programs initiated a total of 43,975 cycles of ART treatment during 1993: 31,900 were standard in vitro fertilization (IVF). 1,397 were IVF with oocyte micromanipulation, 4,992 were gamete intrafallopian transfer (GIFT), 1,792 were zygote intrafallopian transfer (ZIFT), and 882 were combinations of IVF and tubal transfer. Also reported were 2,766 donor oocyte cycles and 246 cycles of IVF for host uterus, as well as 6,869 frozen embryo transfer (ET) procedures. In the IVF cycles, overall the cancellation rate was 14%, and 89% of retrievals led to a transfer. Delivery rates were 16% per initiated cycle, 19% per retrieval, and 21% per transfer. Sixty-six percent of deliveries were singletons and 28% were twins. The defect rate was 2.3 per 100 neonates. Four hundred eighty-one cycles were unstimulated, with a 32% cancellation rate. Sixty-two percent of retrievals resulted in a transfer; the delivery rate was 4% per retrieval. For women aged 40 years or less with no diagnosed male factor, the success rate in unstimulated cycles was 6% deliveries per retrieval.

For stimulated cycles, the success rate of deliveries per initiated cycle was 19% for women less than 40 years of age with no male factor diagnosis vs. 7% for women 40 years of age or older with no male factor diagnosis. Abortion rates were 19% and 34%, respectively. Eighty percent of male factor stimulated cycles proceeded to transfer. The clinical pregnancy rate was 18% per cycle for women less than 40 years of age with male factor.

Data on oocyte micromanipulation were reported as well. Clinical pregnancy rates were 10% per initiated cycle, 11% per retrieval, and 15% per ET. In contrast, delivery rates were 8%, 8%, and 12%, respectively. Eighty-four percent of cycles of GIFT alone resulted in retrievals. Clinical pregnancy rates were 30% per initiated cycle, 35% per retrieval, and 36% per gamete transfer. Seventy-nine percent of clinical pregnancies proceeded to delivery. Four percent of pregnancies were ectopic. The delivery rates with ZIFT were 21% per initiated cycle, 24% per retrieval, and 29% per zygote transfer.

With donor oocytes, overall clinical pregnancy rates were 32% per initiated cycle, 38% per retrieval, and 36% per ET. The delivery rate was 29% per transfer. In host uterus cycles, clinical pregnancy rates were 38% per initiated cycle, 41% per retrieval, and 41% per ET. The delivery rate was 34% per transfer. With transfer of cyropreserved embryos, clinical pregnancy occurred in 15% and 16% of transfer procedures. Delivery rates were 12% per thaw and 13% per transfer.

Summary.—This 1993 report of ART activities suggests that success rates for standard IVF and GIFT increased over the previous year. The findings confirm the importance of age and male factor diagnosis; couples with a younger woman and a man with no identified sperm problems are more likely to succeed. Ectopic pregnancy rates for IVF and tubal transfer remain in the range of 1% to 2% per transfer. More and more families are benefiting from oocyte donation and embryo cryopreservation.

▶ The data in this report are of interest when counseling couples regarding their likelihood of taking home an infant after receiving some type of ART. The likelihood of delivering a term infant is greater among couples undergoing the GIFT procedure than those having IVF and is lessened with both techniques if the woman is 40 years of age or older or if there is a decreased number of sperm or percentage of motile sperm in the semen samples. These data were collected from summary sheets submitted by each clinic. In 1994, individual case forms from each treatment cycle will be sent to a central agency for analysis. It will be interesting to see whether the 1994 results will remain similar to those found when the clinics performed their own analyses or whether they will show a decreased rate of deliveries of infants after ART.

D.R. Mishell, Jr., M.D.

Results of IVF in Patients With Endometriosis: The Severity of the Disease Does Not Affect Outcome, or the Incidence of Miscarriage
Geber S, Paraschos T, Atkinson G, Margara R, Winston RML (Royal Postgraduate Med School, London)
Hum Reprod 10:1507–1511, 1995   11–2

Purpose.—Previous reports have suggested that the outcomes of in vitro fertilization (IVF) for patients with endometriosis are influenced by the stage of endometriosis. Patients with more severe disease are believed to have a higher IVF failure rate, and women treated for endometriosis are believed to have a higher miscarriage rate. The results of IVF in patients with endometriosis were assessed.

Methods.—The analysis included 140 patients with endometriosis who underwent IVF. None received any treatment during or after diagnostic laparoscopy, which was performed 2–4 years before IVF was attempted. The patients underwent a total of 182 cycles of IVF with gonadotropin-releasing hormone analogues. Patients with endometriosis only and those with endometriosis with associated severe tubal disease were considered separately. The results of the patients with endometriosis only were compared with those of 3 other groups of patients: 44 couples with male factor infertility only, 161 couples with unexplained infertility, and 3 couples with tubal factor infertility only.

Results.—There was no difference between groups in number of oocytes retrieved. The fertilization rate was significantly lower only for the couples with male factor infertility; all of the other groups had comparable fertilization rates. The groups were comparable in number of transferred embryos and implantation rates. Pregnancy rates per transfer were 39% in couples with male factor infertility, 48% in those with unexplained infertility, 45% in those with tubal factor infertility, and 40% in those with endometriosis only.

Within the endometriosis group, there were 100 cycles in patients with revised American Fertility Society (AFS) stage I–II endometriosis and 29 in those with revised AFS stage III–IV endometriosis. Although the stage III–IV patients had a greater fertilization rate, number of embryos, and transfer rate per cycle, the difference was not significant. The implantation and overall pregnancy rates per transfer were also nonsignificantly higher in the stage III–IV group.

Conclusion.—The largest study to date of IVF in patients with endometriosis suggests that the results are similar to those of other patients. The presence or degree of endometriosis does not appear to affect pregnancy outcomes, including pregnancy rate or incidence of spontaneous abortion. In contrast to previous reports, this study found no cases of miscarriage in patients with endometriosis.

▶ This very large study of couples undergoing IVF indicates that neither the presence of endometriosis nor the severity of endometriosis affects the pregnancy rate after IVF treatment when compared with the rate among couples with tubal disease or unexplained infertility. These findings suggest that the presence of endometriosis does not cause problems of fertilization or implantation nor increase the rate of abortion. It is probable that endometriosis is a result of infertility and repeated episodes of retrograde menstruation but does not cause infertility unless it produces tubal adhesions or endometriomas that interfere with ovum pickup.

D.R. Mishell, Jr., M.D.

Pregnancies and Births Resulting From In Vitro Fertilization: French National Registry, Analysis of Data 1986 to 1990

French In Vitro National (Universitaire de Bicêtre, France)
Fertil Steril 64:746–756, 1995

11–3

Background.—Any assessment of the cost-benefit ratio of in vitro fertilization (IVF) must include the evaluation criteria of pregnancy outcome and infant characteristics. In 1986, a French collaborative survey began collecting individual data on patients undergoing assisted reproductive technology (ART) techniques. These data were used to examine the outcomes of pregnancy and birth after IVF.

Methods.—The analysis included prospective registry data on each recovery attempt performed at most French IVF centers since 1986. Up to 1990, the registry received more than 76,000 IVF cycle forms and about 8,000 obstetric and pediatric forms regarding all ART techniques. The report abstracted here included IVF pregnancies and resulting newborns only, excluding thawed embryo transfers. A total of 7,024 clinical pregnancies, 5,371 deliveries, and 6,879 newborns were analyzed (Table 1).

Results.—Miscarriage occurred in 18% of clinical pregnancies and ectopic pregnancy occurred in 6%. The multiple delivery rate increased from 20% in 1986 to 29% in 1990. Nearly half of the infants were the result of multiple pregnancies, 34% being twins and 10% triplets. Preeclampsia occurred in 6% of pregnancies and diabetes in 1%. The rate of induced labor increased during the study period. Ninety-two percent of singleton pregnancies had a cephalic presentation. Although 57% of deliveries were vaginal, 13% required forceps. One third of cesarean sections were performed before labor. Eighty-eight percent of multiple pregnancies were

TABLE 1.—Outcomes of Clinical Pregnancies From 1986 to 1990*

	Clinical pregnancies	Miscarriages† Early, <12 weeks of amenorrhea	Late, >12 weeks of amenorrhea <6th month	Ectopic pregnancies†‡	Voluntary abortions†	Therapeutic abortions†	Deliveries†§
1986	665	93 (14.0)	16 (2.4)	48 (7.2)	0	0	508 (76.4)
1987	1,455	233 (16.0)	51 (3.5)	92 (6.3)	0	5 (0.3)	1,074 (73.9)
1988	1,397	199 (14.2)	33 (2.4)	83 (5.9)	2 (0.1)	7 (0.5)	1,073 (76.9)
1989	1,617	250 (15.5)	39 (2.4)	82 (5.1)	1 (0.1)	7 (0.4)	1,238 (76.6)
1990	1,890	262 (13.9)	60 (3.2)	78 (4.1)	2 (0.1)	10 (0.5)	1,478 (78.2)
Total	7,024	1,037 (14.8)	199 (28)	383 (5.4)	5 (0.1)	29 (0.4)	5,371 (76.5)

* Clinical pregnancies are defined as the detection of a gestational sac by ultrasound scan or a very high level of human chorionic gonadotropic (> 1,000 mIU/mL).

† Values are number of incidences with percentages in parentheses.

‡ In addition, 21 ectopic pregnancies associated with an intrauterine pregnancy (i.e., heterotopic pregnancies) are included. Thus, total percentage of both ectopic and heterotopic pregnancies was 5.8% of the clinical pregnancies and 7.5% of the deliveries.

§ Includes simple deliveries and heterotopic pregnancies ($n = 21$) or therapeutic abortion ($n = 1$) terminated with deliveries.

(Courtesy of French In Vitro National: Pregnancies and births resulting from in vitro fertilization: French National Registry, analysis of data 1986 to 1990. *Fertil Steril* 64:746–756, 1995. Reproduced with permission of the publisher, the American Society for Reproductive Medicine [The American Fertility Society].)

delivered by cesarean section, mainly for prophylactic reasons. Just 39% of births were uncomplicated vaginal deliveries; the rate was lower for multiple pregnancies.

Twenty-nine percent of the infants were born prematurely; the rate was higher for multiple pregnancies. Multifetal pregnancies were unassociated with variation in the sex ratio. The overall mean Apgar score was 9, with less than one third of the infants being underweight. Ninety-four percent of infants were found to be in good health, with no complications or malformations at birth. The perinatal mortality rate was 27%; it was higher for multiple births.

The congenital malformation rate was 2.8% (1.2% for major and 1.6% for minor malformations) with no change from 1986 to 1990. The malformation rate was 3.3% when interrupted pregnancies were included. The most common major malformations in live-born infants were cardiopathies. Twelve infants had chromosomal defects, including 7 with Down syndrome. Down syndrome accounted for 3.4% of malformations in live-born infants and 8.2% of malformations when interrupted pregnancies were included.

Conclusion.—In this French experience, more than three fourths of clinical pregnancies induced by IVF result in a delivery. Rates of ectopic pregnancy, prematurity, stillbirth, and perinatal mortality are all higher with IVF than in the general population. However, for singleton IVF pregnancies, stillbirth and perinatal mortality rates are very similar to those of the general population. Malformations appear to be no more common after IVF than after natural conception.

▶ It is estimated that, to date, more than 100,000 children have been born throughout the world by IVF or other ART. The data reported from this large French study are in agreement with surveys of pregnancy outcome after ART obtained in other countries. The data regarding a similar prevalence of congenital malformations after assisted reproduction and natural conception are reassuring. However, the higher rates of spontaneous abortion, ectopic pregnancy, multiple gestation, preterm birth, and perinatal mortality with assisted reproduction remains a problem caused by this expensive method of human procreation.

D.R. Mishell, Jr., M.D.

***In Vitro* Fertilization in Women Age 40 and Older: The Impact of Assisted Hatching**
Schoolcraft WB, Schlenker T, Jones GS, Jones HW Jr (Ctr for Reproductive Medicine, Englewood, Colo; Jones Inst for Reproductive Medicine, Norfolk, Va)
J Assist Reprod Genet 12:581–584, 1995   11–4

Background.—A maternal age of 40 years or older continues to be a barrier to the success of in vitro fertilization (IVF). There were no significant advances in this age group until the introduction of assisted hatching, which involves drilling a hole with an acidic solution in the zona pellucida of a 3-day-old embryo to promote embryonic hatching. This procedure has proved most beneficial. The impact of assisted hatching on IVF outcomes in women aged 40 years and older was investigated.

Methods.—Twenty-eight cycles of IVF without assisted hatching were compared retrospectively with 38 cycles of IVF with assisted hatching. The mean ages of the assisted hatching and control groups were 41.2 and 41.3 years, respectively.

Findings.—In women in the assisted hatching group, the delivery rate per oocyte retrieval was 48%, significantly greater than the 11% rate in the control group. The implantation rate of hatched embryos was 22% in the assisted hatching group and only 6% in the control group. The 2 groups were comparable in fertilization rate and the number of oocytes and embryos per patient.

Conclusion.—Assisted hatching markedly increases embryonic implantation and term pregnancy rates in women aged 40 years and older having IVF. There are several mechanisms by which drilling a hole in the zona pellucida may improve older women's pregnancy prognosis. For example, it may rescue the embryo from an abnormally hard or thick zona by promoting hatching. Because assisted hatching leads to earlier embryonic implantation, embryo-endometrial synchrony may be improved in stimulated cycles. Also, creating an artificial gap may lower the energy needed for hatching.

▶ Ongoing pregnancy rates after IVF in women older than 40 years are significantly lower than when IVF is performed in younger women. The technique of drilling the zona pellucida of a 3-day-old embryo is called assisted hatching. The results of this study indicate that this technique is beneficial in achieving pregnancy in women over 40 years of age who undergo IVF. However, the study was retrospective and was performed at 2 different time intervals, and the authors transferred up to 6 embryos among the women in the older age group. Randomized clinical trials comparing older women undergoing assisted hatching with controls must be performed before the technique can be considered truly beneficial for older women.

D.R. Mishell, Jr., M.D.

Hydrosalpinges in In-Vitro Fertilization: An Unfavourable Prognostic Feature
Vandromme J, Chasse E, Lejeune B, Van Rysselberge M, Delvigne A, Leroy F (Free Univ Brussels, Belgium)
Hum Reprod 10:576–579, 1995   11–5

Introduction.—Of 37 patients with unilateral or bilateral hydrosalpinges, 22 had surgical correction by salpingectomy or salpingoplasty, and 15 were left untreated by surgery. Comparisons were drawn between these

TABLE 1.—Pregnancy Rates in Hydrosalpinx Patients, Other Tubal Patients (Controls), and Operated Patients

	Hydrosalpinges	Controls	Operated*
No. of patients	37	41	22
Total no. of oocyte retrievals	78	67	46
Oocyte retrieval failure	2	2	0
Fertilization failure	7	4	4
No. of successful retrievals	69	61	42
No. of embryos transferred	190	154	115
No. of pregnancies			
Single	6	11	9
Twin	1	1	4
Triplet	0	1	0
Abortion	0	1	3

* Patients in operated group were included in hydrosalpinx group before they were operated upon.

(Courtesy of Vandromme J, Chasse E, Lejeune B, et al: Hydrosalpinges in in-vitro fertilization: An unfavourable prognostic feature. *Hum Reprod* 10:576–579, 1995, by permission of Oxford University Press.)

2 groups and a control group of 41 surgically sterilized patients in regard to the success of in vitro fertilization (IVF). Patients were studied retrospectively and restricted to those of less than 40 years of age having had an embryo transfer and stimulated by human menopausal gonadotropin under nasal buserelin desensitization. Two of the 22 patients operated on for hydrosalpinges received a unilateral salpingectomy, 14 had bilateral salpingectomies, and 6 had bilateral salpingoplasties. The diagnosis of hydrosalpinx was made based primarily on hysterosalpingogram or laparoscopy; clinical pregnancy was defined by serum β–human chorionic gonadotropin and confirmed by ultrasound.

Results.—Although cases of fertilization and retrieval failures were evenly distributed among the 3 groups (Table 1), clinical and ongoing pregnancy rates were significantly lower in the group with uncorrected hydrosalpinges. The pregnancy rates, both by oocyte retrieval and by implantation rate, were more than twice as high in controls and more than 3 times as high in the operated group as they were in the group with hydrosalpinges.

Discussion.—Not only is the presence of hydrosalpinx associated with a poor success rate for IVF treatment, but surgical correction of this defect appears to restore the likelihood of success. The fact that patients in the operated group had failed previous IVF attempts before surgery makes their improved success rate even more significant, as in general IVF success rates tend to drop as the number of IVF trials increase. The mechanism accounting for the poor IVF success rates in patients with hydrosalpinges remains unclear.

▶ Several studies have revealed the same conclusions found in this retrospective review indicating that the presence of hydrosalpinges decreases

the prognosis for a successful pregnancy outcome after IVF. It is therefore
advisable to remove the diseased oviducts, if hydrosalpinges are present,
before performing IVF.

D.R. Mishell, Jr., M.D.

Effect of Uterine Leiomyomata on the Results of In-Vitro Fertilization Treatment

Farhi J, Ashkenazi J, Feldberg D, Dicker D, Orvieto R, Rafael ZB (Tel Aviv Univ, Israel)
Hum Reprod 10:2576–2578, 1995

11–6

Background.—Authorities disagree on whether uterine leiomyoma affects infertility. Gamete transport obstruction and impaired implantation are the 2 main mechanisms that have been proposed for the association of leiomyomata and infertility. The effects of uterine leiomyomata on the results of in vitro fertilization (IVF) were reported.

Methods.—Forty-six women with documented uterine leiomyoma undergoing a total of 172 IVF treatment cycles were included in the retrospective study. These patients were compared with a control group of women with mechanical infertility. Implantation rates and pregnancy outcomes were analyzed.

Findings.—The patients with uterine leiomyoma had implantation rates of 22.1% per transfer and 6.8% per embryo. The abortion rate in this group was 36%. These rates were comparable to those in the control group. When hysteroscopic pretreatment findings were considered, it was found that impaired implantation was associated with leiomyoma only when uterine intracavitary abnormalities co-existed.

Conclusion.—Only uterine leiomyomata that cause uterine cavity deformation impair implantation rates and pregnancy outcomes. Uterine cavity assessment is, therefore, mandatory in patients with uterine leiomyomata. Surgery may be needed before IVF in patients with leiomyomata and an abnormal uterine cavity to improve implantation rates.

▶ In the presence of submucosal uterine leiomyomata, the implantation rate per embryo transfer was only 9%, compared with an implantation rate of 30% per transfer when leiomyomata were present in the uterus but did not alter the surface of the endometrial cavity. Therefore, if submucus leiomyomata are present, it would be best to resect them before performing IVF.

D.R. Mishell, Jr., M.D.

Six Year Follow-Up of Cryopreserved Human Embryos
Lornage J, Chorier H, Boulieu D, Mathieu C, Czyba JC (Hôpital Edouard Herriot, Lyon, France)
Hum Reprod 10:2610–2616, 1995   11–7

Introduction.—The ability to preserve supernumerary embryos by freezing, in conjunction with in vitro fertilization (IVF), has lent hope to sterile couples, but the status of these embryos and their destiny remain in doubt. The practice has limited the number of operative procedures required and reduced the financial and personal costs of IVF. What happens to cryopreserved embryos is determined essentially within the context of a parental plan.

Objective.—The fate of cryopreserved embryos was examined in 145 of 407 couples who had adopted this practice but who had not used the embryos to fulfill a parental plan within 1 year. Successive questionnaires were sent to these couples at annual intervals between 1987 and 1992. Ultimately, 82.5% of the original couples had used their embryos in a parental plan.

Observations.—Pregnancy was achieved by 79% of the 145 couples questioned after a year of embryo cryopreservation. Of 72 couples who had initially chosen to preserve embryos for later transfer, 39% subsequently conceived after a cycle of IVF and reconsidered. Of 52 couples who did not initially adopt a parental plan but, instead, gave away their embryos or destroyed them, 27% achieved pregnancy after an IVF cycle. When final intentions were analyzed, 51% of couples had undertaken embryo transfer or were planning to do so. Another 43% decided to abandon their parental plans. Twenty-four couples elected to give their supernumerary embryos to another couple, whereas 28 chose to destroy them. In all, 28% of couples changed their intentions in the course of follow-up.

Implications.—When couples decide to cryopreserve their extra embryos, it seems necessary to maintain contact with them to provide a structure within which they can fulfill their intention or modify it appropriately. At times it may be helpful to interrupt contact to allow time to achieve pregnancy, resolve marital problems, or effect adoption.

▶ The fate of cryopreserved embryos involves many ethical concerns. When a couple achieves their desired family size or decides not to undergo embryo transfer, they need to decide what to do with the cryopreserved embryos containing their own genetic material. More studies such as this one are needed to understand what happens to cryopreserved embryos over time in various countries and cultures. Couples who have cryopreserved embryos need to take some responsibility for deciding their outcome over time.

D.R. Mishell, Jr., M.D.

Cocultured Blastocyst Cryopreservation: Experience of More Than 500 Transfer Cycles

Kaufmann RA, Nicollet B, Menezo Y, DuMont M, Hazout A, Servy EJ (Augusta Reproductive Biology Associates, Ga; Institut Rhonalpin Fondation Merieux, Lyon, France; Clinique Pierre Cherest, Paris)
Fertil Steril 64:1125–1129, 1995   11–8

Background.—A recent report suggested that in vitro fertilization (IVF) is more successful when pre-embryos are transferred after coculture and at the blastocyst stage. The use of cryopreserved blastocysts for infertile patients undergoing IVF-embryo transfer (ET) was evaluated retrospectively at 3 different centers in the largest series reported to date.

Methods.—Between January 1991 and April 1995, 563 IVF cycles with blastocyst cryopreservation were studied. Patients underwent ovarian stimulation; follicle growth was followed by sonography and assessment of estradiol blood levels. All IVF procedures were done in B2 medium, and pre-embryos were cocultured on Vero cells. Supernumerary pre-embryos were frozen on days 5–7 after insemination at the expanded blastocyst stage. Patients were prepared for transfer either by hormonal replacement or in natural cycles.

Results.—The proportion of the transfer cycles was high (92%; 516 of 563 cycles thawed). From the 516 transfer cycles, 112 clinical pregnancies resulted. After adjustment for the 8 miscarriages, the ongoing pregnancy rate per transfer was 19%. The post-thaw viability was high (83%; 1,033 transferred of 1,239 thawed blastocysts). Of the 1,033 pre-embryos, 138 implanted—an implantation rate of 13.4%. The implantation rate was significantly higher in cycles prepared with exogenous steroids (26.2%) than in those with spontaneous cycles (12%).

Conclusion.—Freezing at the blastocyst stage is a reliable IVF method. Although fewer pre-embryos may be available to cryopreserve, those remaining appear to be of superior quality. Their implantation ability approaches that of a fresh transfer.

▶ The results of this study indicate that it may be preferable to perform blastocyst freezing on days 5–7 after fertilization rather than earlier. Randomized studies in which embryo freezing is performed at different stages of development should be undertaken to determine whether freezing at the later stage truly results in greater rates of implantation.

D.R. Mishell, Jr., M.D.

Cryopreservation of Human Oocytes and Fertilization by Two Techniques: In-Vitro Fertilization and Intracytoplasmic Sperm Injection
Kazem R, Thompson LA, Srikantharajah A, Laing MA, Hamilton MPR, Templeton A (Aberdeen Maternity Hosp, Scotland)
Hum Reprod 10:2650–2654, 1995   11–9

Background.—The human oocyte seems to be particularly susceptible to freeze-thaw damage. Even in those embryos that survive freeze-thawing, fertilization is reduced or aberrant. The effects of intracytoplasmic sperm injection (ICSI) on both the fertilization rate and the number of normal fertilizations in human oocytes that survive cryopreservation were investigated.

Methods.—Sixteen volunteers underwent ovarian stimulation using the "flare-up" short protocol. Morphologically normal oocytes were cryopreserved using a slow freeze–rapid thaw method. Oocytes that survived cryopreservation were randomly allocated to either fertilization by conventional in vitro fertilization (IVF) or by ICSI. In the insemination procedures, frozen-thawed spermatozoa from a single donor of proven fertility were used. Intracytoplasmic sperm inspection was performed only with oocytes that had extruded their first polar body.

Results.—Most (94%; 220 of 234) of the oocytes obtained for research were suitable for cryopreservation. Of the 220 cryopreserved oocytes, 215 were recovered on thawing. After 3 hours of culturing, 74 of the oocytes (34%) survived. Of the 74, 37 were randomized to be fertilized by conventional IVF and 37 by ICSI. The rate of fertilization was significantly higher in the ICSI group (46%) than in the IVF group (14%). Only 1 oocyte in the IVF group exhibited normal fertilization vs. 16 (43%) in the ICSI group. About 32% of the oocytes in the ICSI group did not survive the ICSI procedure. The 1 oocyte fertilized by IVF underwent cleavage with asynchronous cell division. Sixteen of the 17 oocytes fertilized by ICSI had synchronous cleavage to the 4-cell stage. Six of the donors used half their oocytes for treatment. Those oocytes were fertilized by convention IVF technique using sperm from different donors. Of the 57 oocytes obtained for treatment, 61% underwent fertilization. Five embryo transfers resulted in 2 pregnancies.

Conclusion.—In oocytes surviving cryopreservation, intracytoplasmic sperm injection significantly improves fertilization rates. These findings are consistent with the hypothesis that cryopreservation causes some damage at the zona pellucida that interferes with normal sperm attachment or penetration. Intracytoplasmic sperm injection effectively overcomes this barrier to normal fertilization.

▶ Cryopreservation of oocyte for use in IVF and embryo transfer at a later date has not proven to be successful because of damage to the oocyte during the freezing-thawing process. The results of this study indicate that with the use of ICSI, the chances of fertilization and embryo development are enhanced. If this technique results in pregnancies that produce normal infants, it can be used for women who are experiencing ovarian destruction as a result of chemotherapy as well as those having surgical removal of their ovaries for disease.

D.R. Mishell, Jr., M.D.

Two Instead of Three Embryo Transfer in In-Vitro Fertilization
Tasdemir M, Tasdemir I, Kodama H, Fukuda J, Tanaka T (Akita Univ, Japan)
Hum Reprod 10:2155–2158, 1995   11–10

Background.—It has been proposed that, when attempting in vitro fertilization (IVF), 3 or even 4 embryos be transferred to maximize the pregnancy rate and limit multiple pregnancies. Transferring 3 embryos, however, sometimes results in a triplet pregnancy that may end very prematurely. For this reason, some IVF units now prefer to electively transfer 2 embryos.

Objective.—Double and triple embryo transfers were compared in 287 couples having a total of 486 IVF treatment cycles. The 1,224 embryos transferred were judged as being good (A) or poor (B) on the basis of fragmentation rate and morphology.

Results.—When only good-quality embryos were transferred, the result-ant pregnancy rates for double (AA) and triple (AAA) transfers were 40.5% and 43%, respectively, not a significant difference. When only poor-quality embryos were used, the respective pregnancy rates were 11% (BB) and 23% (BBB). When embryos of mixed quality were transferred, the pregnancy rate was 37% for double (AB) transfers and 40% for triple (AAB or ABB) transfers. Multiple pregnancies were significantly more frequent after triple embryo transfers (32% vs. 14%), but there was no difference in the number of abortions.

Implications.—Double embryo transfer is adequate for IVF if at least 1 good-quality embryo is available. If only poor-quality embryos are transferred, triple embryo transfer will maximize the chance of achieving a pregnancy.

▶ All centers performing IVF attempt to achieve the highest pregnancy rate per embryo transfer that can be achieved. However, when more than 2 embryos are transferred, the chance of multiple gestation, with its accompanying risk of pregnancy complications, is markedly increased. Therefore, to reduce the risk of triplets or a higher number of gestations, it has been proposed that when several good-quality embryos are found after fertilization, no more than 2 of them be transferred. The results of this study indicate that limiting the number of embryos transferred to 2 when an embryo of good quality is present will reduce the risk of multiple gestation without affecting the pregnancy rate.

D.R. Mishell, Jr., M.D.

Gamete Intrafallopian Transfer: Prospective Randomized Comparison Between Hysteroscopic and Laparoscopic Transfer Techniques
Seracchioli R, Fabbri R, Porcu E, Colombi C, Ciotti P, Flamigni C (Univ of Bologna, Italy)
Fertil Steril 64:355–359, 1995   11–11

Background.—At the authors' center, hysteroscopy is preferred as an alternative to the traditional gamete intrafallopian transfer (GIFT) by laparoscopy. The efficacies of hysteroscopy and laparoscopy were prospectively compared in a randomized study of patients undergoing GIFT.

Methods.—One hundred thirty-three couples with tubal patency documented at a previous diagnostic laparoscopy were enrolled. Fifty-seven were randomly assigned to hysteroscopic GIFT and 60 to laparoscopic GIFT. All women were younger than 38 years. The duration of infertility was 3 years or more. Laparoscopic GIFT was done with patients under general anesthesia 34–36 hours after administration of human chorionic gonadotropin (hCG). Transvaginal ultrasonography (US)-guided retrievals were scheduled 34–36 hours after administration of hCG in hysteroscopic GIFT. In both techniques, 2–4 mature oocytes with 200,000 to 300,000 motile spermatozoa were transferred.

Findings.—In the hysteroscopic group, 547 oocytes were recovered and 205 mature oocytes transferred, compared with 522 and 229, respectively, in the laparoscopic group. There were no complications during or just after either procedure. The mean duration of the procedures, including US oocyte recovery, was 28 minutes in the hysteroscopic group and 33 minutes in the laparoscopic group. Patients undergoing hysteroscopic GIFT were discharged after 3 hours, whereas those undergoing laparoscopic GIFT were hospitalized for 24 hours. The pregnancy and implantation rates in the hysteroscopic group were 29.8% and 9%, respectively. These rates were not significantly different from those in the laparoscopic group, which were 43.3% and 14%, respectively.

Conclusion.—Hysteroscopic GIFT is a safe procedure that can be done quickly and easily. Because it requires no hospitalization, general anesthesia, or operating room, costs are reduced and psychophysical involvement is low.

▶ Even though the pregnancy rate with hysteroscopic GIFT was only 30% compared with 43% with laparoscopic GIFT, it appears that the cost saving of the former technique made it an attractive alternative to the latter. Hysteroscopic GIFT can be performed in an office setting, thus not requiring the use of an operating room and general anesthesia as does laparoscopic GIFT. Further experience with transfer of sperm and eggs into the oviduct transcervically instead of transperitoneally is certainly warranted as hysteroscopic transfer appears to be safe and effective.

D.R. Mishell, Jr., M.D.

In-Vitro Fertilization in Completely Natural Cycles

Fahy UM, Cahill DJ, Wardle PG, Hull MGR (Univ of Bristol, England)
Hum Reprod 10:572–575, 1995   11–12

Background.—Although assisted conception techniques are well established, concerns exist regarding the risks associated with ovulation induction therapy. Recently, there has been renewed interest in in vitro fertilization (IVF) during unstimulated, natural ovarian cycles. The feasibility of IVF during natural ovarian cycles as a fertility treatment was examined.

Methods.—A prospective study was undertaken of 39 fully investigated couples who were patients at the Reproductive Medicine Unit, St. Michael's Hospital, Bristol, England. There were 26 couples with a diagnosis of tubal disease and 13 with a diagnosis of unexplained infertility. Patients were monitored by daily capillary blood sampling and vaginal ultrasonography, followed by midcycle vaginal oocyte recovery under sedation. Outcome measures included fertilization, implantation, and pregnancy.

Results.—The 39 couples had 79 cycles of IVF during natural ovarian cycles. Oocyte recovery was attempted in 65 cycles. The overall fertilization rate was 80% and the implantation rate was 14% (Table 1). There were 6 clinical pregnancies, with a rate of 9% per attempted egg recovery. The implantation rate in the tubal infertility group was 16% per embryo, and in the unexplained infertility group it was 8% per embryo.

Conclusion.—Natural cycle IVF and embryo transfer offers an acceptable chance for pregnancy in selected patients, as well as an opportunity for in-depth investigation of follicular and ovarian function in infertile couples. The results presented in this paper should encourage further research and development of this technique for assisting infertile couples.

TABLE 1.—Results of In Vitro Fertilization in Unstimulated Cycles Analyzed by Category of Infertility and in Total

	Tubal disease (n = 26)		Unexplained infertility (n = 13)		Total (n = 39)	
Age (years)*	32.5	(26–38)	34	(25–39)	33	(25–39)
Duration of infertility (years)*	4.5	(1.5–12)	6	(3–10)	5.5	(1.5–12)
Primary infertility	3	(11%)†	11	(85%)†	14	(36%)
Cycles	59		20		79	
Cancelled/ovulated (per cycle)	13	(22%)	1	(5%)	14	(17%)
Attempted oocyte recovery (per cycle)	46	(78%)	19	(95%)	65	(83%)
Successful oocyte recovery (per attempt)	39	(85%)	15	(79%)	54	(83%)
Fertilization rate (per oocyte)	31	(79%)	12	(80%)	43	(80%)
Clinical pregnancy (per cycle/embryo transfer)	5	(8.5%/16.1%)	1	(5.0%/8.3%)	6	(7.6%/14.0%)

* Results are expressed as median (range).
† Significantly different by Fisher's exact test. *P* = 0.01.
(Courtesy of Fahy UM, Cahill DJ, Wardle PG, et al: In-vitro fertilization in completely natural cycles. *Hum Reprod* 10:572–575, 1995, by permission of Oxford University Press.)

Natural Cycles for In-Vitro Fertilization: Cost-Effectiveness Analysis and Factors Influencing Outcome

Daya S, Gunby J, Hughes EG, Collins JA, Sagle MA, YoungLai EV (McMaster Univ, Hamilton, Ont, Canada)
Hum Reprod 10:1719–1724, 1995   11–13

Background.—Although initial success with in vitro fertilization (IVF) was achieved during unstimulated menstrual cycles, ovarian stimulation soon became routine practice in the hope of enhancing the yield of oocytes. The chance of conceiving was increased as a result, but there is still a risk of hyperstimulation, and multiple pregnancies are reported in perhaps one third of deliveries. There is also concern over a possible increase in the long-term risk of ovarian tumors. Stimulated IVF is quite expensive.

Objective.—The outcome of IVF was examined for infertile patients treated in 240 natural menstrual cycles. All patients had regular cycles at 25- to 35-day intervals and had achieved fertilization in a previous, stimulated IVF cycle but had not conceived.

Results.—Excluding cancelled cycles and cycles in which a luteinizing hormone surge was noted, 156 cycles progressed to oocyte retrieval. No oocytes were obtained in 17% of these cycles. A majority of the remaining cycles yielded a single oocyte. The oocyte yield was significantly improved when a double-bore needle was used. Embryos suitable for transfer were available in 92 instances. Eleven clinical pregnancies were achieved (12%). The chance of pregnancy was greater, although not significantly so, when embryos containing 4 or more blastomeres were transferred. No factors could be found that significantly predicted the achievement of clinical pregnancy.

Conclusion.—It is feasible to plan IVF in natural cycles as an alternative to ovarian stimulation. This approach offers a less costly alternative and will avoid the adverse consequences of ovarian hyperstimulation.

► The results of these 2 studies (Abstracts 11–12 and 11–13) indicate that the pregnancy rate per treatment cycle is about twofold to threefold less when a single oocyte is retrieved for IVF during an unstimulated cycle than when ovulation-inducing agents are used to allow several oocytes to be retrieved, fertilized, and transferred. Nevertheless, there are many advantages to performing IVF after an unstimulated cycle. These include greater patient convenience, much lower cost, avoidance of multiple gestation with its accompanying high rate of obstetric complications, and elimination of the risk of ovarian hyperstimulation syndrome. Thus, for some infertile couples when the woman is younger than 40 years of age and the man has normal results of semen analysis, natural cycle IVF might be offered as an alternative to the routine ovarian stimulation protocol.

D.R. Mishell, Jr., M.D.

Satellite In Vitro Fertilization: The Oregon Experience
Kaplan PF, Gorrill MJ, Burry KA, Vos KL, Sherrill GM, Hollander JC (Women's Health Care Fertility Ctr, Eugene, Ore; Oregon Health Sciences Univ, Portland)
Am J Obstet Gynecol 172:1823–1829, 1995   11–14

Introduction.—Although in vitro fertilization (IVF) has proven very successful, it is still an expensive and time-consuming approach. Ten or more visits are necessary for each treatment cycle, and many participants find it difficult, at best, to attend consistently. The problem is compounded for those who live some distance from the program site. Satellite systems consequently have been developed to stimulate and monitor IVF patients away from the main program site.

Objective.—The results of IVF were compared in 222 treatment cycles completed at the main campus of Oregon Health Sciences University and 54 others in which oocyte retrieval cycles took place at a satellite location. The participants had at least 1 patent tube, and they generally completed 2–3 cycles of ovarian hyperstimulation with gonadotropin plus intrauterine insemination before starting IVF.

Results.—There were no significant differences between the 2 sites in the number of embryos achieved, the number of fresh embryos transferred, or the number of embryos frozen. All retrieval cycles at the satellite center yielded at least 2 embryos and at least 1 transfer. In 14 cycles for couples with male factor infertility at the main campus site, no fertilization or embryo transfer took place. The rate of clinical pregnancies per retrieval cycle was 39% at the satellite location and 23% at the main campus site. The respective live birth rates were 33% and 21%. Multiple gestations were more prevalent at the central site.

Conclusion.—In vitro fertilization may be carried out at satellite sites, using community services and a team approach, without compromising the outcome.

Results of Decentralized In-Vitro Fertilization Treatment With Transport and Satellite Clinics
Roest J, Verhoeff A, van Lent M, Huisman GJ, Zeilmaker GH (Zuiderziekenhuis, Groene Hilledijk, Rotterdam, The Netherlands; Univ Hosp, Rotterdam, The Netherlands; Erasmus Univ, Rotterdam, The Netherlands)
Hum Reprod 10:563–567, 1995   11–15

Background.—No more than 12 in vitro fertilization (IVF) laboratories are permitted in The Netherlands. Because the laboratory's capacity is usually greater than the achievable treatment volume, aspirated oocytes are carried from a transport IVF clinic to a central laboratory. The transport clinic has facilities for complete clinical management of IVF. It has proven possible to transport oocytes for up to 1 hour without any loss of fertilizability.

Objective.—In a retrospective study, the results of IVF performed at a university center were compared with those achieved after transporting oocytes over 15 to 40 minutes from a transport IVF clinic to the central laboratory. In 3,333 cycles, the clinical and laboratory phases of IVF were completed at the central IVF laboratory. Another 2,207 cycles were managed clinically at the transport site, after which oocytes were taken to the central laboratory for embryo transfer. In this group, 1,637 cycles were stimulated and monitored at the transport clinic. In the remaining 570 cycles, these functions took place at 1 of 6 satellite clinics.

Results.—Fewer embryo transfers took place at the transport clinic than at the central university laboratory. Cryopreservations were more prevalent in the transport clinic population. There were more multiple gestations in the central laboratory group. Embryo implantation rates were similar in the 2 main groups. Pregnancy rates were similar for treatment cycles monitored at the transport clinic and those monitored at the satellite clinics. Rates of severe ovarian hyperstimulation were also comparable.

Implications.—Good communication between treatment sites and the use of standard protocols will enhance the success of a decentralized IVF program. In large urban areas, a decentralized program including a central laboratory is preferable to the use of several small laboratories with less experienced staff, and it is also more cost-effective.

▶ The results of these 2 studies (Abstracts 11–14 and 11–15) indicate that it is cost-effective and feasible to use satellite sites to perform many of the preliminary functions of IVF in combination with a central core clinic in which the actual fertilization procedure and embryo transfer takes place. Even in urban areas with 1 or more IVF laboratories, it may be more convenient to have multiple follicular development and monitoring taking place at peripheral sites; this includes physicians' offices before oocyte retrieval is performed.

D.R. Mishell, Jr., M.D.

***In Vitro* Fertilization: A Cost-Effective Alternative for Infertile Couples?**
Trad FS, Hornstein MD, Barbieri RL (Harvard Med School, Boston)
J Assist Reprod Genet 12:418–421, 1995   11–16

Objective.—The United States has one of the lowest rates of use of in vitro fertilization (IVF) in the industrialized world; this is primarily the result of the high cost of the procedure. Results of a retrospective review of the cost of an in IVF birth and of the cost variations according to the clinical characteristics of a particular population were presented.

Methods.—Records of 182 infertile couples were reviewed for a maximum of 3 IVF cycles, and each woman was followed until she gave birth or had a successful pregnancy. Women were divided into 3 groups depending on their probability of achieving a successful pregnancy: group A (women 32 years of age or younger who had IVF for any reason other than male infertility or abnormal sperm count); group B (women under 40 years of age who had IVF for severe male factor infertility); and group C (women over 40 years of age with the same indications as group A). The cost per delivery was calculated by dividing the average cost of an IVF cycle ($8,000) by the number of cycles each woman required to achieve pregnancy. The cost per pregnancy was determined by multiplying the average cost of IVF by the total number of cycles performed divided by the number of successful pregnancies.

Results.—Fifty women had successful pregnancies after their first IVF cycle. There were 78 pregnancies established after 308 cycles in patients with a maximum of 3 IVF cycles. After 1 IVF cycle, the cost per pregnancy for groups A, B, and C were $22,857, $34,000, and $42,666, respectively, and after a maximum of 3 cycles, the costs were $26,800, $34,666, and $74,666, respectively. These costs compare with costs of tubal surgery and adoption. Pregnancy is 50% to 70% cheaper in the group with the highest probability of pregnancy than for the group with the lowest probability. The cost of pregnancy was stable after 3 IVF cycles in groups A and B.

Conclusion.—In vitro fertilization could become the second or third line of treatment, particularly for those infertile couples with the highest probability of pregnancy. Additional prospective studies need to be conducted to determine the cost-effectiveness of this strategy.

▶ This study provides useful data regarding the actual estimated cost of achieving a pregnancy with IVF in the United States among couples with women of different ages and men with and without abnormalities in the semen analysis. This information should prove useful when counseling couples with tubal disease as to whether they should attempt tubal reconstructive surgery or IVF.

D.R. Mishell, Jr., M.D.

Intravenous Albumin Does Not Prevent the Development of Severe Ovarian Hyperstimulation Syndrome in an In-Vitro Fertilization Programme

Ng E, Leader A, Claman P, Domingo M, Spence JEH (Univ of Ottawa, Ontario, Canada)
Hum Reprod 10:807–810, 1995

11–17

Background.—Ovarian hyperstimulation syndrome is a recognized sequel to ovulation induction and is occurring increasingly as assisted reproduction is more broadly applied. In its most severe form, the syndrome causes significant morbidity—including thromboembolism, adult respiratory distress syndrome, and renal failure—and it may be fatal. No way has been found of consistently preventing severe ovarian hyperstimulation syndrome, but Asch et al. recently reported promising results when 5% human albumin solution was given IV before and just after transvaginal oocyte retrieval to patients at very high risk.

Objective.—The effects of human albumin solution and Ringer's lactate were compared in 207 women who had serum estradiol values greater than 10,000 pmol/L and/or more than 15 follicles over 10 mm in diameter on the day of human chorionic gonadotropin (hCG) injection.

Methods.—Lactated Ringer's solution was given in a volume of 500 mL before egg retrieval and in the same volume afterward to 158 women. The remaining 49 women received the same volume of 5% human albumin in normal saline. Women whose estradiol levels exceeded 10,000 pmol/L at the time of hCG injection received progesterone IM for luteal support.

Results.—In each treatment group, about three fourths of women had tubal infertility. The average number of follicles present at the time of oocyte retrieval did not differ significantly, and similar estradiol levels were present. Severe (grade 4/5) ovarian hyperstimulation syndrome developed in 4% of albumin-treated women and 6.3% of control women, not a significant difference.

Conclusion.—Administering 5% human albumin solution at the time of oocyte retrieval does not prevent severe ovarian hyperstimulation syndrome in women at risk, although it may lessen the severity of stimulation.

Decreased Incidence of Severe Ovarian Hyperstimulation Syndrome in High Risk In-Vitro Fertilization Patients Receiving Intravenous Albumin: A Prospective Study

Shalev E, Giladi Y, Matilsky M, Ben-Ami M (Central Emek Hosp, Afula, Israel)
Hum Reprod 10:1373–1376, 1995   11–18

Background.—Human serum albumin administration reportedly prevents severe ovarian hyperstimulation syndrome in patients at risk for this syndrome undergoing ovarian stimulation for in vitro fertilization (IVF). The effect of IV albumin on the incidence of ovarian hyperstimulation syndrome in high-risk IVF patients was determined.

Methods.—A single IV dose of 20 g of human serum albumin was given immediately after oocyte retrieval to 22 women in this prospective, randomized trial. Eighteen women not receiving the treatment served as the control group. All women in the IVF program received the long gonadotropin-releasing hormone agonist triptorelin and an individually adjusted human menopausal gonadotropin. Ultrasound was performed every 3 days after treatment.

Findings.—Four cases of severe ovarian hyperstimulation syndrome occurred in the control group, compared with none in the treatment group. This difference was significant. When analysis included only patients with an estradiol concentration exceeding 15,000 pmol/L, the difference between treatment and control groups was highly significant (Table 1).

TABLE 1.—Comparison Between Treatment and Control Groups of In Vitro Fertilization Data and Incidence of Ovarian Hyperstimulation Syndrome

	Treatment group	Control group	Significance
No. patients	22	18	
Oestradiol (pmol/l)	15,051 ± 5650*	14,064 ± 3594†	NS†
(range)	(9293–26,220)	(9568–23,920)	
No. of oocytes	21 ± 5.7*	19.3 ± 4.3*	NS†
(range)	(15–36)	(14–34)	
Fertilization rate (%)	56.7 ± 31.0*	60.4 ± 27.0*	NS†
Cleavage rate (%)	89.5 ± 10.5*	88.1 ± 11.5*	NS†
No. of embryos transferred	19	17	NS†
No. of pregnancies	6	2	NS‡
Pregnancy rate/ embryo transfer (%)	31.6	11.8	NS‡
No. of OHSS cases	0	4	$P = 0.35$‡
OHSS rate (%)	0	23.5	

* Mean ± standard error of the mean.
† Unpaired *t*-test, 2-tailed.
‡ Fisher's exact test, 2-tailed.
Abbreviations: NS, not significant; *OHSS*, ovarian hyperstimulation syndrome.
(Courtesy of Shalev E, Giladi Y, Matilsky M, et al: Decreased incidence of severe ovarian hyperstimulation syndrome in high risk in-vitro fertilization patients receiving intravenous albumin: A prospective study. *Hum Reprod* 10:1373–1376, 1995, by permission of Oxford University Press.)

Conclusion.—Albumin administration appears to be safe, effective, and inexpensive for preventing ovarian hyperstimulation syndrome in patients undergoing ovarian stimulation in IVF programs. This treatment does not interfere with the stimulation cycle. It was recommended for IVF patients with estradiol concentrations of more than 15,000 pmol/L.

▶ The ovarian hyperstimulation syndrome occurs infrequently in ovulating women who receive human menopausal gonadotropin and subsequently become pregnant. Nevertheless, this syndrome, in its severe form, can be life threatening and requires aggressive therapy. The results of these 2 papers (Abstracts 10–17 and 10–18) suggest that administration of IV human serum albumin may reduce the severity and frequency of this syndrome. Because the severity of the syndrome is related to the number of follicles and estradiol levels achieved during hyperstimulation, it may be beneficial to administer human serum albumin if estradiol levels are high (above 5,000 pg/mL) in an attempt to prevent this serious complaint.

D.R. Mishell, Jr., M.D.

12 Early Pregnancy

Obstetric Outcome in Singleton Pregnancies After Assisted Reproduction
Tanbo T, Dale PO, Lunde O, Moe N, Åbyholm T (Univ of Oslo, Norway)
Obstet Gynecol 86:188–192, 1995   12–1

Introduction.—Worldwide, the number of births resulting from various techniques of assisted reproduction may exceed 10,000 per year. Some studies have linked infertility to increased risks of low birth weight, small for gestational age, and preterm birth; however, others have failed to confirm these results. The obstetric and neonatal outcomes of singleton pregnancies achieved with assisted reproduction were studied.

Methods.—The retrospective study examined the maternal and perinatal outcomes of 355 assisted-reproduction singleton pregnancies lasting 140 days or more, all resulting from infertility treatment at 1 university hospital. The obstetric and neonatal outcomes were compared with those of a control group of 643 pregnant women, matched for age and parity with delivery in the obstetric department of the same hospital.

Findings.—The median age was 33 years in the study group and 32 years in the control group. More than three fourths of the women in both groups were nulliparous. The women who had assisted reproduction had a greater frequency of pregnancy-induced hypertension than did the controls (11% vs. 6%). They were also more likely to have placenta previa (2.8% vs. 0.5%). Six percent of patients in the study group had elective cesarean section, compared with less than 2% of the control group. The duration of pregnancy was significantly shorter than in the control group (278 vs. 280 days), and the incidence of preterm birth was significantly greater (14.9% vs. 9.5%). The median birth weight was 3,360 g in the study group compared with 3,460 g in the control group. The infants resulting from assisted-reproduction pregnancies were also more likely to be sent to the neonatal ICU.

Conclusion.—Obstetric risk appears to be increased for singleton pregnancies resulting from various techniques of assisted reproduction. The differences in complication rates noted in this study appear to be unrelated to maternal age and parity, representing instead an inherent adverse effect resulting from infertility or assisted reproduction. As such, and because the pregnancy will likely be their only one, women who have undergone assisted reproduction should receive special attention during pregnancy.

▶ A pregnancy resulting from in vitro fertilization entails a great amount of emotional and financial expenditure. It is known that pregnancy complications are markedly increased after in vitro fertilization because of the high incidence of multiple births associated with ovarian stimulation. The results of this study indicate that pregnancy complications such as preterm birth, placenta previa, and need for neonatal intensive care are also increased in singleton births after in vitro fertilization. Because it is likely that a pregnancy after in vitro fertilization will be the woman's only pregnancy, careful antenatal monitoring of the pregnancy is essential.

D.R. Mishell, Jr., M.D.

The Prediction of Ectopic Pregnancy After In-Vitro Fertilization and Embryo Transfer

Marcus SF, Macnamee M, Brinsden P (Bourn Hall Clinic, Cambridge, England)
Hum Reprod 10:2165–2168, 1995

12–2

Background.—Four and one half percent of pregnancies resulting from in vitro fertilization (IVF) and embryo transfer are ectopic. Early diagnosis of this condition is essential. The use of the discriminant function of history of pelvic inflammatory disease (PID), plasma progesterone concentration, and plasma human chorionic gonadotropin (hCG) concentration in predicting ectopic pregnancy by the 23rd day after embryo transfer was reported.

Methods.—Between 1983 and 1993, 135 ectopic pregnancies occurred after IVF and embryo transfer at 1 center. Data on these women were compared with data on 135 randomly selected women who progressed to singleton deliveries after IVF and embryo transfer during the same period. Twenty ectopic pregnancies were heterotopic, 8 were ovarian, and 6 were bilateral tubal. The rest were singleton tubal pregnancies.

Findings.—The mean plasma level of hCG and progesterone was significantly lower in the women with ectopic pregnancies than in those who delivered. However, because the overlap was so great, a cutoff concentration useful for predicting ectopic pregnancy could not be identified for either hormone. Using the discriminant function analysis of these data together with a history of PID, 90% of ectopic pregnancies could be identified by the 23rd day after embryo transfer, long before ultrasonographic imaging would be of value diagnostically.

Conclusion.—A prediction value for ectopic pregnancies of up to 90% can be obtained by calculating the discriminant function value of PID; progesterone levels on day 13; and hCG levels on days 13, 18, and 23. Larger IVF centers may use their own data on hCG and progesterone concentrations in a similar model, improving their ability to diagnose ectopic pregnancy early after IVF and embryo transfer.

▶ Nearly 5% of pregnancies occurring after IVF and embryo transfer are ectopic. Furthermore, about 15% of these are heterotopic pregnancies and 5% of the ectopic pregnancies are bilateral. It is important to establish the presence of these tubal gestations early in pregnancy to effect prompt treatment. Measurement of serum progesterone and hCG levels early in gestation aids in the prediction of the presence of an ectopic gestation before an embryo can be visualized in the uterine cavity sonographically.

D.R. Mishell, Jr., M.D.

Antibodies to Oxidized Low-Density Lipoprotein and to Cardiolipin in Nonpregnant and Pregnant Women With Habitual Abortion

Tulppala M, Ailus K, Palosuo T, Ylikorkala O (Univ Central Hosp of Helsinki; Natl Public Health Inst, Helsinki)
Fertil Steril 64:947–950, 1995

12–3

Objective.—Because titers of circulating antibody against oxidized low-density lipoprotein (LDL) are elevated in preeclamptic women, a study was planned to identify these antibodies in nonpregnant women and in expectant women with a history of habitual abortion.

Study Population.—Forty-two women who had had 3–7 consecutive miscarriages, occurring at a median gestational age of 8 weeks, formed the study group. Half of them had never been delivered of a child. All these women conceived during a median follow-up of 7 months. Twelve of the 39 initially viable pregnancies ended in miscarriage, whereas 27 led to the

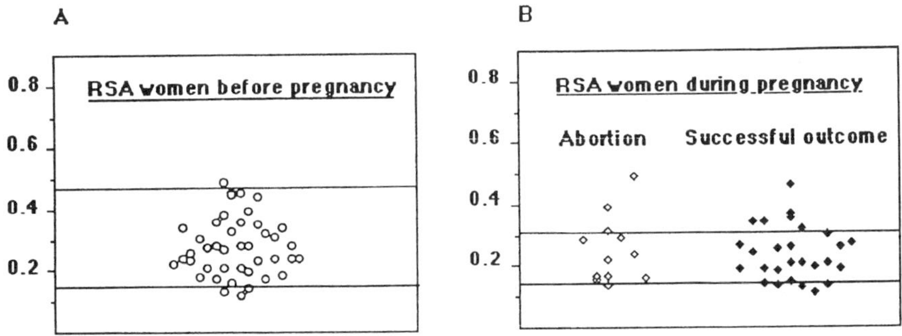

FIGURE 1.—Distribution of IgG antibodies to oxidized low-density lipoprotein (*LDL*) in patients with a history of habitual abortion. Results are expressed as optical density values calculated by subtracting binding to native LDL from binding to malondialdehyde-LDL. **A,** habitual aborters before pregnancy. *Lines* indicate 10th and 90th percentiles of concentrations observed in nonpregnant control women. **B,** habitual aborters during pregnancy. *Lines* indicate 10th and 90th percentiles of concentrations observed in pregnant control women. (Courtesy of Tulppala M, Ailus K, Palosuo T, et al: Antibodies to oxidized low-density lipoprotein and to cardiolipin in nonpregnant and pregnant women with habitual abortion. *Fertil Steril* 64:947–950, 1995. Reproduced with permission of the publisher, the American Society for Reproductive Medicine [The American Fertility Society].)

birth of a healthy child. Twenty-three healthy nonpregnant women and 22 pregnant women with no past abortions were also studied.

Methods.—A solid-phase enzyme-linked immunosorbent assay was used to measure immunoglobulin G antibodies to malondialdehyde-modified LDL. Anticardiolipin antibodies were also estimated.

Results.—Both groups of pregnant women had relatively low median titers of antibody to oxidized LDL. Nine of the habitual aborters with initially viable pregnancies (23%) had increased antibody titers during pregnancy, regardless of whether the pregnancy continued or ended in miscarriage (Fig 1). The same proportion of habitual aborters had detectable anticardiolipin antibody when pregnant, but increased titers were more frequent in those who miscarried in their current pregnancies. Three of the 27 ongoing pregnancies were complicated by preeclampsia, and fetal growth retardation was noted in 5 instances.

Conclusion.—These findings do not support a role for antibody against oxidized LDL in determining the outcome of a current pregnancy in habitually aborting women.

▶ The results of this study indicate that in addition to the presence of lupus anticoagulant and anticardiolipin and thyroid antibodies being risk factors for recurrent abortion, elevation of levels of antibodies to oxidized LDLs may be found during early pregnancy in about one fourth of women with recurrent abortion. Whether elevated antibodies to oxidized LDL have a causal relationship to recurrent abortion remains to be determined. However, the fact that a similar percentage of women with recurrent abortion and elevated levels of this antibody carried their pregnancy to viability or aborted their pregnancy suggests that a causal relationship is unlikely.

D.R. Mishell, Jr., M.D.

Antiphospholipid Antibodies and β_2-Glycoprotein-I in 500 Women With Recurrent Miscarriage: Results of a Comprehensive Screening Approach

Rai RS, Regan L, Clifford K, Pickering W, Dave M, Mackie I, McNally T, Cohen H (St Mary's Hosp Med School, London; Central Middlesex Hosp, London; Univ College Hosp, London)

Hum Reprod 10:2001–2005, 1995   12–4

Objective.—The prevalence of antiphospholipid antibodies (APA), the lupus anticoagulant (LA), and anticardiolipin antibodies (ACA) was determined in 500 consecutive women 19–45 years of age who had had 3 or more consecutive miscarriages. The median number of miscarriages was 4 but the range was 3 to 16. Two thirds of women had had only early miscarriages in the first trimester.

Methods.—Both the IgG and IgM forms of ACA were determined by enzyme-linked immunosorbent assays. Lupus anticoagulant was estimated using 3 coagulation tests: the activated partial thromboplastin time, the kaolin clotting time, and the dilute Russell viper venom time. Values of β_2-glycoprotein-I and antinuclear factor were also determined.

Findings.—More than one fourth of women (26.4%) tested positive for LA or ACA on initial sampling. Fifteen percent of these women were LA positive, 9% had IgG ACA, and 6% had IgM ACA. Lupus anticoagulant was detected much more consistently by the dilute Russell viper venom time test than by the other coagulation tests. Only 3.3% of all women tested persistently positive for IgG ACA and 2.2% for IgM ACA when tested again at least 8 weeks after initial evaluation. Sixty-one women (12%) were persistently APA positive. No woman with an initially negative ACA test later was found to be positive.

Conclusion.—In this, the largest series of women with recurrent miscarriage to be comprehensively evaluated for APA, many women were only transiently positive. No more than 10% of women were persistently positive for LA, and fewer than 5% were positive for either form of ACA. A huge majority of initially negative women remained negative on repeat testing. Those who are found to be positive should have a confirmatory test after at least 8 weeks. The dilute Russell viper venom time assay is the best screening measure for LA.

▶ Study results of this very large series of women with recurrent abortion help to further clarify the association between 2 ADAs—LA and ACA—and recurrent abortion. The finding that a positive antibody test may be transient indicates that the test should be repeated after an interval of more than 2 months to determine whether the antibody is permanently present. The finding that the dilute Russell viper venom time (dRVVT) was more sensitive than the kaolin clot time or the activated partial thromboplastin time in detecting LA indicates that the dRVVT is the best test for women with recurrent abortion in determining whether LA is present.

About 15% of women with recurrent abortion of undetermined cause will have 1 of these antibodies present. If antibodies are present, the abortion occurs more frequently in the first trimester than in the second. Whether therapy with prednisone, heparin, or aspirin or a combination of these agents yields a greater incidence of viable pregnancies than placebo in women with these antibodies remains to be determined, but treatment with heparin and aspirin is now the recommended therapeutic regimen for women with recurrent abortion who have either of these antibodies present.

D.R. Mishell, Jr., M.D.

13 Basic Investigations

Exaggerated Effects of Progestogen on Uterine Artery Pulsatility Index in Turner's Syndrome Patients Receiving Hormone Replacement Therapy
Biljan MM, Garden AS, Taylor CT, Fraser WD, Matijevic R, Diver MJ, Jones SV, Kingsland CR (Univ of Liverpool, England)
Fertil Steril 64:1104–1108, 1995   13–1

Introduction.—Women with Turner's syndrome fail to produce estrogen, and the resultant lack of sexual maturation is accompanied by sequelae of estrogen deficiency including atherosclerotic coronary heart disease, osteoporosis, and breast atrophy. These patients require lifelong hormone replacement therapy (HRT), but the reduced risk of coronary heart disease documented in postmenopausal women receiving HRT has not been confirmed in patients with Turner's syndrome. A majority of premature deaths result from coronary disease.

Objective and Methods.—The effects of HRT on cardiovascular function were studied by measuring pulsatility indices in 5 patients with Turner's syndrome, 6 women castrated surgically for nonmalignant conditions, and 5 women with idiopathic primary ovarian failure. Patients received 2 mg of estradiol valerate and, for 10 days of each cycle, 500 µg of norgestrel. The pulsatility of the uterine arteries was studied using a pulsed color Doppler system and transvaginal probe.

Results.—Pulsatility indices decreased, indicating less resistance to blood flow, in all 3 groups. The effect of estrogen was partly negated when progestogen was added. Patients with Turner's syndrome had significantly higher pulsatility indices on day 9 of progestogen therapy than did the surgically castrated group (Fig 2). Study patients also had consistently higher indices than women with idiopathic ovarian failure, but the difference was not significant.

Conclusion.—The uterine arteries of women with Turner's syndrome are especially sensitive to the tonic effect of progestogen. If the cardiac arteries are similarly affected, this may help account for the increased risk of cardiovascular disease in Turner's syndrome. These patients may benefit from specially tailored HRT.

▶ In postmenopausal women receiving estrogen, there is an increase in blood flow reflected in the reduction of the pulsatility index. It has been

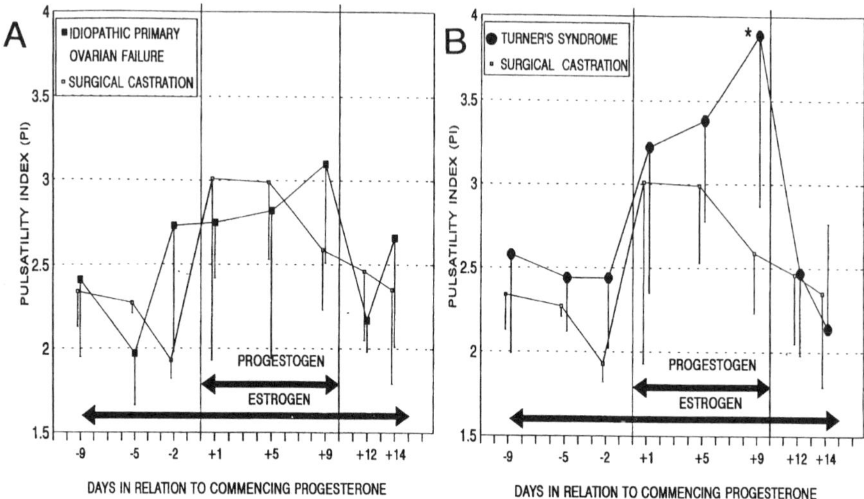

FIGURE 2.—Pulsatility index relative to ingestion of progestogen. **A,** no significant difference between the group with idiopathic primary ovarian failure and the patients who had surgical removal of ovaries was observed. **B,** the difference between the group with Turner's syndrome and the patients who had surgical removal of ovaries reached the level of significance at the end of the period of progestogen administration ($P = 0.028$; confidence interval = 0.17 to 2.42). *Vertical bars* represent 95% confidence intervals. (Courtesy of Biljan MM, Garden AS, Taylor CT, et al: Exaggerated effects of progestogen on uterine artery pulsatility index in Turner's syndrome patients receiving hormone replacement therapy. *Fertil Steril* 64:1104–1108, 1995. Reproduced with permission of the publisher, the American Society for Reproductive Medicine [The American Fertility Society].)

known that with progestins, the production of the pulsatility index is somewhat attenuated by 20% to 25%. This is a provocative study because, for the first time, it was noted that the progestin response is different in patients with Turner's syndrome. These young women were treated with HRT. Patients with Turner's syndrome are known to be at great risk for atherosclerotic heart disease, and discovery of a difference in the way these patients are affected by sex steroid may be a clue to other high-risk profiles.

The benefits of HRT in these patients in terms of overall mortality and cardiovascular risk are not known. Whereas estrogen reduced the pulsatility index as expected in these patients, the addition of progestin was different. As shown in the figure, this attenuation was exaggerated in Turner's syndrome, as opposed to other forms of hypogonadism. This, therefore, constitutes a potential risk for patients with Turner's syndrome who appear to be more susceptible to the effects of progestin.

It is not known, and it would be of interest to know, whether there are other differences, such as in lipoproteins, Until we have more clinical data to go on, it may be beneficial in treating patients with Turner's syndrome to limit the progestin exposure as long as the endometrium is protected.

R.A. Lobo, M.D.

Soluble Interleukin-6 (IL-6) Receptor in the Sera of Pregnant Women Forms a Complex With IL-6 and Augments Human Chorionic Gonadotropin Production by Normal Human Trophoblasts Through Binding to the IL-6 Signal Transducer

Matsuzaki N, Neki R, Sawai K, Shimoya K, Okada T, Sakata M, Saji F, Koishihara Y, Ida N (Osaka Univ, Japan; Chugai Pharmaceutical Co Ltd, Gotemba-shi, Japan; Toray Industries Inc, Kamakura, Japan)
J Clin Endocrinol Metab 80:2912–2917, 1995   13–2

Background.—Cytokines including interleukin (IL)-1 help regulate the placental production of human chorionic gonadotropin (hCG). Previous studies have shown that IL-6 receptor (IL-6R) is expressed on trophoblast membrane, and that activation of the IL-6R complex induces the production of hCG.

Objective.—The role of soluble IL-6R during pregnancy was studied by estimating serum levels throughout pregnancy in 80 healthy pregnant women at 7–40 weeks' gestation. Forty-five healthy nonpregnant women with normal menstrual function were also studied.

Findings.—Pregnant women had significantly higher serum levels of soluble IL-6R than did control women at any phase of the menstrual cycle,

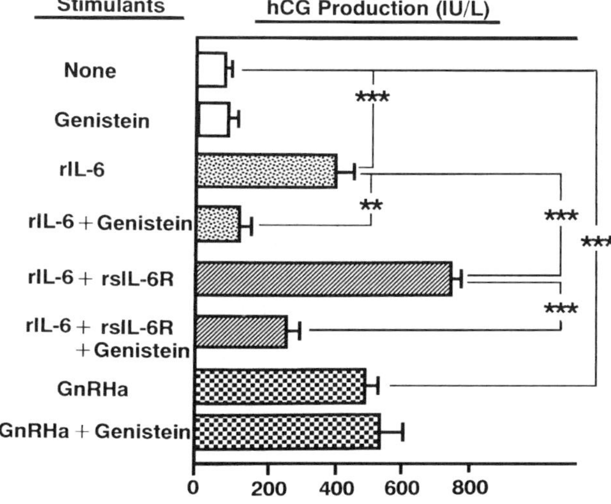

FIGURE 4.—Blocking by genistein of recombinant interleukin-6 (*rIL-6*) and recombinant soluble interleukin-6 receptor (*rsIL-6R*)–induced human chorionic gonadotropin (*hCG*) production by the enriched trophoblasts. The enriched trophoblasts were cultured in the presence or absence of 20 mg/L of genistein for 30 minutes and then stimulated with control medium (*open bars*), 4 µg/L of rIL-6 (*lightly stippled bars*), 4 µg/L of rIL-6 and 1 µg/L of rsIL-6R (*slant-lined bars*), or 10^{-6} mol/L of gonadotropin-releasing hormone (*heavily strippled bars*). Each bar represents the mean ± standard error of the mean hCG value determined in triplicate. **, P < 0.01; ***, P < 0.001. (Courtesy of Matsuzaki N, Neki R, Sawai K, et al: Soluble interleukin-6 (IL-6) receptor in the sera of pregnant women forms a complex with IL-6 and augments human chorionic gonadotropin production by normal human trophoblasts through binding to the IL-6 signal transducer. *J Clin Endocrinol Metab* 80:2912–2917, Copyright 1995, The Endocrine Society.)

but levels remained unchanged throughout pregnancy. Serum levels of IL-6 at all stages of pregnancy were comparable to those in nonpregnant women. Recombinant soluble IL-6R increased the production of hCG by trophoblasts stimulated by recombinant IL-6 in vitro in a dose-dependent manner. It had no such effect on unstimulated trophoblasts. Induced hCG production was blocked by antibodies against IL-6R and antisignal transducing glycoprotein, as well as by genistein, a tyrosine kinase inhibitor (Fig 4).

Interpretation.—Complexed serum soluble IL-6R and trophoblast membrane-bound IL-6R may act together through binding to glycoprotein-130 and induction of tyrosine kinase activity in trophoblasts to produce hCG.

▶ Multiple factors influence trophoblast function, specifically the production of hCG. Here we see cytokines being actively involved in this process. Cytokines, which are ubiquitous, are also produced by the trophoblast. This study examines the effect of IL-6 and its soluble receptor.

In these elegant studies, it has been determined, first, that the soluble receptor is increased in the sera of pregnant women. We next see that a complex forms between IL-6 and its receptor, thus activating the tyrosine kinase transduction system to stimulate the production of hCG. Figure 4 aptly shows that the highest levels of hCG production occur with the combination of IL-6 and the soluble IL-6 R. Then genistein, a potent inhibitor of the tyrosine kinase system, was shown to block the stimulation. Thus, it was determined that this production is mediated via tyrosine kinase.

You will notice also in the figure that gonadotropin-releasing hormone agonist does stimulate hCG production as well. This is not mediated through the tyrosine kinase system and was not affected by the addition of genistein. Gonadotropin-releasing hormone is known to be produced by the trophoblast. These systems operate in a paracrine and possibly an autocrine fashion in trophoblast tissue. Although the effects can be mediated externally, these results stress the importance of multiple collaborating systems within the trophoblast of early pregnancy.

R.A. Lobo, M.D.

Rapid Deoxyribonucleic Acid Analysis by Allele-Specific Polymerase Chain Reaction for Detection of Mutations in the Steroid 21-Hydroxylase Gene
Wilson RC, Wei J-Q, Cheng KC, Mercado AB, New MI (New York Hosp-Cornell Med Ctr)
J Clin Endocrinol Metab 80:1635–1640, 1995   13–3

Background.—Classic 21-hydroxylase deficiency is the most common form of congenital adrenal hyperplasia. Researchers have located the 21-hydroxylase gene on the short arm of chromosome 6 and identified a corresponding inactive pseudogene 98% homologous to the active gene. Gene conversion appears to occur during meiosis, in which deleterious point mutations are transferred from the pseudogene to the active gene, and results in complete or partial inactivation of 21-hydroxylase activity. Previously, allele-specific dot blot hybridization was performed to detect these single nucleotide point mutations by DNA analysis. This procedure is very time consuming. A rapid DNA analysis based on allele-specific polymerase chain reaction (PCR) using mutation site–specific primers was developed and performed on patients and, when possible, their parents.

Methods and Findings.—Seventy-eight patients were included in the study. The results of the new method were visualized immediately after the PCR run by ethidium bromide–stained agarose gel electrophoresis. Allele-specific PCR enabled mutations to be identified on 148 of 160 affected chromosomes. Although mutations were found on only 1 chromosome of 11 patients, their parents had a consistent pattern on DNA analysis. One exception was a family in which the parents each had a detectable mutation with a mutation identified on only 1 allele of the patient. In this case, there was probably a mutation in the patient's other allele that could have arisen de novo or was inherited from the parent but was not evident in the transmitting parent's phenotype.

Conclusion.—Allele-specific PCR is as accurate as the dot blot technique in detecting mutations. The advantages of the new method are that it is faster, it is less labor-intensive, and it does not involve radioactivity.

▶ This paper was abstracted merely to update the practitioner on the new techniques available for the diagnosis of defects in 21-hydroxylase. What is described here is allele-specific PCR, which is able to pick up at least 8 of the most common mutations in the gene for 21-hydroxylase deficiency. This can be detected rapidly by ethidium bromide–stained agarose gel electrophoresis. The advantage of this over the original blot methods is that it is far more rapid and less laborious for the technician. Speed and reproducibility are particularly important for the prenatal diagnosis of congenital hyperplasia in families so affected. Because there are no specific mutations but a series of possible mutations, it is important to have accurate, detailed methods that can be obtained rapidly to make this diagnosis.

R.A. Lobo, M.D.

The Biochemical and Phenotypic Characterization of Females Homozygous for 5α-Reductase-2 Deficiency

Katz MD, Cai L-Q, Zhu Y-S, Herrera C, DeFillo-Picart M, Shackleton CHL, Imperato-McGinley J (Cornell Univ, New York; Universidad Nacional Pedro Henriquez Urena, Santo Domingo, Dominican Republic; Children's Hosp Oakland Research Inst, Calif)
J Clin Endocrinol Metab 80:3160–3167, 1995   13–4

Background.—Inherited 5α-reductase-2 deficiency syndrome was first described in 1974 in 24 male pseudohermaphrodites from a large Dominican Republic kindred. The biochemical and phenotypic characteristics of 3 females from that kindred were reported.

Methods and Findings.—The women were found to be homozygous for a point mutation on exon 5 of the 5α-reductase-2 gene by single-strand DNA conformational polymorphism analysis and DNA sequence analysis. The women's body hair was reduced. None had a history of acne. All the women were fertile, despite delayed menarche. Two women had twins. Increased urinary $5\beta/5\alpha$ C_{19} and C_{21} steroid metabolite ratios were documented. The women had normal to increased plasma testosterone levels with low 5-αdihydrotestosterone (DHT), resulting in an increased testosterone/DHT ratio. The patients also had decreased 3α,5α-androstanediol glucuronide levels. Two women underwent menstrual cycle profiling, which revealed ovulatory gonadotropin peaks. The women's sebum production was normal, suggesting regulation by the 5α-reductase-1 isoenzyme (Figs 4 and 5).

Conclusion.—The study of these homozygous women with 5α-reducatse-2 deficiency shows that DHT has a role in the growth of normal body hair in females. The delayed menarche in these women suggests a regulatory role for 5α-reductase-2 in initiating puberty at the hypothalamic/pituitary and/or gonadal level. The women had ovulatory menstrual cycles and were fertile. Because 2 of the women had twins, it is possible that the number of mature ovarian follicles per cycle is regulated by the ratio of

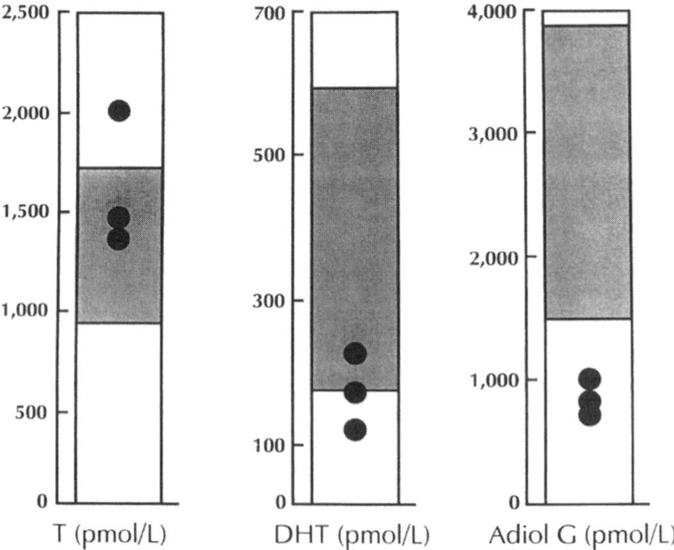

FIGURE 4.—Plasma androgen levels in women homozygous for 5α-reductase-2 deficiency. The mean of 3 plasma samples from 1 subject and 2 plasma samples from the other 2 subjects are shown. *Shaded area* represents the mean ± standard deviation for 26 samples from 15 control women. (Courtesy of Katz MD, Cai L-Q, Zhu Y-S, et al: The biochemical and phenotypic characterization of females homozygous for 5α-reductase-2 deficiency. *J Clin Endocrinol Metab* 80:3160–3167, Copyright 1995, The Endocrine Society.)

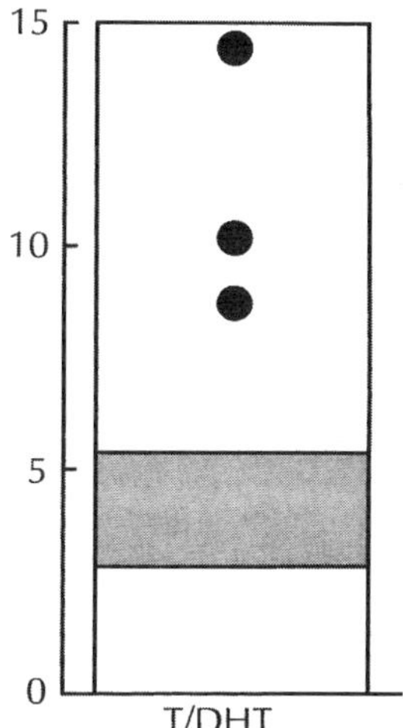

FIGURE 5.—The testosterone/5α-dihydrotestosterone ratio in women homozygous for 5α-reductase-2 deficiency. The mean of 3 plasma samples from 1 subject and 2 plasma samples from the other 2 subjects are shown. *Shaded area* represents the mean ± standard deviation for 26 samples from 15 control women. (Courtesy of Katz MD, Cai L-Q, Zhu Y-S, et al: The biochemical and phenotypic characterization of females homozygous for 5α-reductase-2 deficiency. *J Clin Endocrinol Metab* 80:3160–3167, Copyright 1995, The Endocrine Society.)

DHT to estradiol—a decreased ratio resulting in superovulation and an increased ratio leading to anovulation.

▶ We are just beginning to understand the role of 5α-reductase activity in men and women. There are 2 isoenzymes of 5α-reductase; type 2 is the predominant genital form that is responsible for prostatic enlargement and for which finasteride (Proscar) is an effective treatment.

Type 1 appears to affect the skin of the body, at least in part, and is also responsible for acne production. It is a natural experiment of nature, therefore, to see what happens with a homozygous deficiency in 5α-reductase type 2 in women. We see that body hair, at least in part, is affected by type 2, and this is consistent with data on the use of finesteride in women, in whom it is partially effective in the treatment of hirsutism. Moreover, there seem to be fertility consequences which are of great interest. Gonadotropin levels have not been measured specifically but, apparently, there is an increased level in these individuals.

If more mature follicles are produced, it would suggest that type 2 is somehow involved in the uncoupling of aromatase activity and 5α-reductase activity, which would normally lead to the atresia of many of the follicles during the normal cycling process. Also, the fact of delayed menarche suggests that 5α-reductase type 2 may also be involved in the gonadotropin-initiating event around the time of puberty. 5α-Reductase activity has been thought to be responsible for some of the progesterone actions during the cycle, and this, in part, may be the mechanism responsible for some of the gonadotropin changes observed at midcycle (specifically, the positive feedback of progesterone on luteinizing hormone).

This is an extremely interesting phenomenon observed in its natural state, but by understanding some of the roles of these enzymes, particularly the differences between type 1 and type 2 isoenzymes of 5α-reductase activity, we may be able to use this to our advantage to manipulate the natural cycle. 5α-reductase deficiency, however, does not appear to affect progesterone levels during the luteal phase. (See Abstract 13–5).

R.A. Lobo, M.D.

Women With Steroid 5α-Reductase 2 Deficiency Have Normal Concentrations of Plasma 5α-Dihydroprogesterone During the Luteal Phase

Milewich L, Mendonca BB, Arnhold I, Wallace AM, Donaldson MDC, Wilson JD, Russell DW (Univ of Texas, Dallas; Univ of Sao Paulo, Brazil; Royal Infirmary, Glasgow, Scotland)
J Clin Endocrinol Metab 80:3136–3139, 1995   13–5

Background.—Males with 5α-reductase deficiency (type 2), an autosomal recessive disorder, have defective virilization of their external genitalia during embryogenesis and are usually thought to be female at birth. 5α-Reduction converts a weak androgen (testosterone) to a more potent androgen (dihydrotestosterone). 5α-Reduction also converts progesterone to 5α-dihydroprogesterone, a major circulating hormone in women during the luteal phase of the menstrual cycle and during pregnancy. Steroid 5α-reduction is mediated by 2 isoenzymes, type 1 and type 2. Two families, each with 1 adult female with 5α-reductase-2 deficiency, were evaluated.

Subjects.—The male proband in this Brazilian family is homozygous for the G183S mutation in the steroid 5α-reductase-2 gene. His 41-year-old homozygous sister underwent normal sexual development. Her physical examination is unremarkable and she has had 3 uneventful pregnancies.

The male proband in this Scottish-Pakistani family is the offspring of a first-cousin marriage. He is homozygous for a splice junction abnormality at exon 4/intron 4 (designated the 5R2-Glasgow allele). However, his affected brother is a compound heterozygote with a splice abnormality on 1 allele and an R246Q mutation on the other allele. Their 31-year-old mother is a compound heterozygote who underwent 4 uneventful pregnancies. She has normal genitalia and regular menstrual cycles. One sister of the proband is a compound heterozygote and another sister is a homozygote.

Results.—The 2 adult women are endocrinologically normal but profoundly deficient in steroid 5α-reductase-2 activity. The patient from the Brazilian family is homozygous for the G183S mutation in steroid 5α-reductase. The patient from the Scottish-Pakistani family is a compound heterozygote for the R246W/755+1, G→T splice junction abnormality in the same gene. Both women have low rations of 5α- to 5 β-reduced steroids in their urine. However, they have normal levels of progesterone and 5α-dihydroprogesterone during the luteal phase of their menstrual cycles.

Conclusion.—These 2 women with different forms of 5α-reductase-2 deficiency underwent normal sexual development and pregnancies, and they have normal levels of 5α-dihydroprogesterone during the luteal phase of their menstrual cycles. Thus, 5α-reductase-2 deficiency is not clinically apparent in either woman. This appears to be associated with the fact that circulating 5α-dihydroprogesterone (secreted by the corpus luteum) is largely derived from the steroid 5α-reductase-1 isoenzyme.

▶ Here we see that fertility per se is normal in patients who are homozygous for the deficiency of 5α-reductase-2. The important point is made in this paper that there are several different mutations responsible for deficiency of the 5α-reductase enzyme. It has been described previously that there are separate genes for type 1 and type 2 5α-reductase, which are encoded on different chromosomes. Different tissues also have different levels of expression of 5α-reductase-1 and 5α-reductase-2. In that 5α-reductase progesterone levels were normal in women with documented 5α-reductase-2 deficiency suggests that in the corpus luteum of these patients, type 2 is not the predominant form for progesterone metabolism and that type 1 is the predominant form. However, the real proof of this would require that tissue from the corpus luteum be probed for both type 1 and type 2 isoenzymes. Because progesterone and its metabolites have CNS effects, data such as these will be important in determining whether blocking type 1 or 2 isoenzyme may be able to modulate the effects of progesterone on the CNS.

R.A. Lobo, M.D.

Postmenopausal Hormonal Replacement Decreases Plasma Levels of Endothelin-1

Ylikorkala O, Orpana A, Puolakka J, Pyörälä T, Viinikka L (Helsinki Univ)
J Clin Endocrinol Metab 80:3384–3387, 1995   13–6

Background.—Hormone replacement therapy (HRT) in postmenopausal women decreases their risk for myocardial infarction by 40% to 60%, but the mechanism is uncertain. Endothelin (ET)-1, the most potent known vasoconstrictor, is produced by endothelial cells, and increased levels have been reported in patients with acute myocardial infarction. To learn whether HRT affects plasma levels of ET-1, postmenopausal women were studied before and after receiving HRT.

Methods.—Twenty-six postmenopausal women (mean age, 52 years) complaining of climacteric symptoms were randomized to 2 groups. One group received continuous oral estradiol (2 mg/day) and norethisterone acetate (1 mg/day). The other group received continuous transdermal estradiol (50 µg/day) and periodic 12-day courses of medroxyprogesterone

(10 mg/day). Blood samples were drawn at baseline and periodically during the 12-month trial. Plasma ET-1 levels were measured by specific radioimmunoassay after concentrating the sample by solid phase extraction.

Results.—After 12 months of HRT, plasma levels of estradiol rose from a mean baseline level of 11.8 pg/mL to 65.3 pg/mL, climacteric symptoms were alleviated, and blood pressure and weight levels were essentially unchanged. The effects of the oral and transdermal treatments were similar. The mean plasma ET-1 levels fell significantly at both 6 months (1.05 pmol/L) and at 12 months (1.10 pmol/L), compared with the mean baseline levels (1.28 pmol/L). Plasma ET-1 levels were similar in both treatment groups.

Conclusion.—At least in part, the protective effect of HRT in postmenopausal women may be the result of suppression of ET-1 production. The fact that sublingual estradiol helps prevent exercise-induced myocardial ischemia suggests that it rapidly suppresses ET-1 production.

▶ There are multiple effects of estrogen on the cardiovascular system. This paper describes the effects of estrogen on ET-1. The endothelins, collectively, are among the most potent vasoconstrictors known to man and act at the level of the endothelium. These effects probably oppose those of endothelium-derived relaxing factor, or nitric oxide, which causes vasodilatation. Some of these effects are mediated via the estrogen receptor and some via progesterone receptor.

This study describes the effects of exogenous sex steroids on levels of ET-1 in postmenopausal women. The significance of these data, which were reported as Rapid Communications, is that both estrogen and estrogen plus progestin, and oral or as well as transdermal therapy, affect ET-1 in the same way by lowering levels. This should afford some degree of heart protection. The fact that progestins did not have any attenuating effect may suggest that the mechanisms of these sex steroids on ET-1 may not be receptor mediated. The authors' contention that the effect of sublingual estradiol may be mediated through ET-1 is unfounded at the present time.

R.A. Lobo, M.D.

The Role of Endothelin-1 in Regulating Human Granulosa Cell Proliferation and Steroidogenesis *In Vitro*
Kamada S, Blackmore PF, Kubota T, Oehninger S, Asada Y, Gordon K, Hodgen GD, Aso T (Eastern Virginia Med School, Norfolk; Tokyo Med and Dental Univ)
J Clin Endocrinol Metab 80:3708–3714, 1995   13–7

Background.—There is evidence that the potent vasoconstrictive peptides named endothelins (ETs) modulate ovarian function. Although ET-1 is present in high concentration in the rat corpus lutein, the effects of ETs on luteinized granulosa cells (GCs) and luteal cell function are not understood.

Objective and Methods.—In vitro studies were performed to assess the effects of ET-1 on intracellular calcium, cell proliferation, and basal and gonadotropin-stimulated steroid production in freshly isolated and cultured luteinized human GCs. Cells were from patients undergoing in vitro fertilization. Calcium concentrations were estimated using a fluorescent indicator and cell proliferation using bromodeoxyuridine. In addition, the expression of messenger RNA for ET receptor was studied.

Results.—Intracellular calcium concentrations were elevated by ET-1 in a dose-related manner, regardless of whether calcium was present extracellularly. This effect was much less marked with ET-3. Endothelin-1 significantly and dose-dependently stimulated the proliferation of luteinized GCs (Fig 8). Stimulation was blocked by BQ-123, a potent ET_A receptor antagonist. Both ETs reduced basal and gonadotropin-stimulated secretion of progesterone (Fig 10), but they did not alter basal or gonadotropin-stimulated secretion of estradiol by luteinized human GCs.

Conclusion.—Endothelin-1 may stimulate the proliferation of luteinized human GCs by increasing the intracellular calcium concentration via a receptor-mediated action.

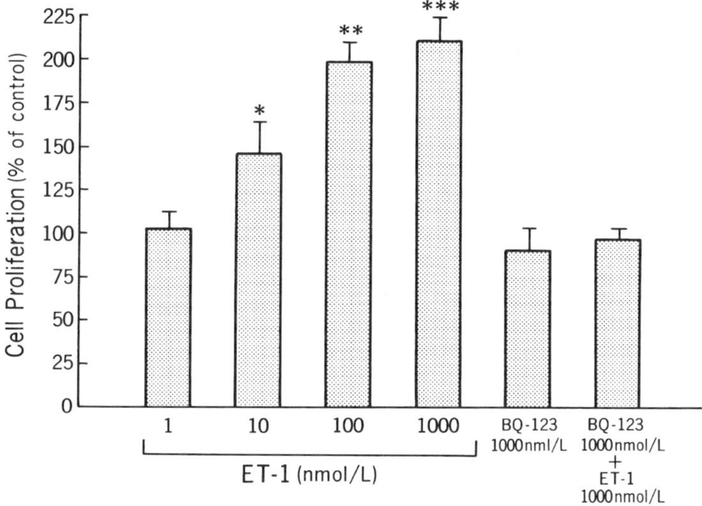

FIGURE 8.—Effects of endothelin (*ET*)-1 and BQ-123 on cell proliferation in luteinized human granulosa cells for a 48-hour incubation. After a 48-hour preincubation, cells were incubated in 100/µL of medium without fetal bovine serum in the presence of ET-1 with or without BQ-123 (1,000 nmol/L) for 48 hours. Cells were then labeled with 5-fluoro-2'-deoxyuridine for 30 hours. Data are expressed as the percentage of control (100%) that was cultured in the absence of ETs. Values are the mean ± standard error of between 4 and 6 separate experiments, each performed in quadruplicate. ***$P < 0.001$; **$P < 0.01$; *$P < 0.05$ vs. control. (Courtesy of Kamada S, Blackmore PF, Kubota T, et al: The role of endothelin-1 in regulating human granulosa cell proliferation and steroidogenesis *in vitro. J Clin Endocrinol Metab* 80:3708–3714, Copyright 1995, The Endocrine Society.)

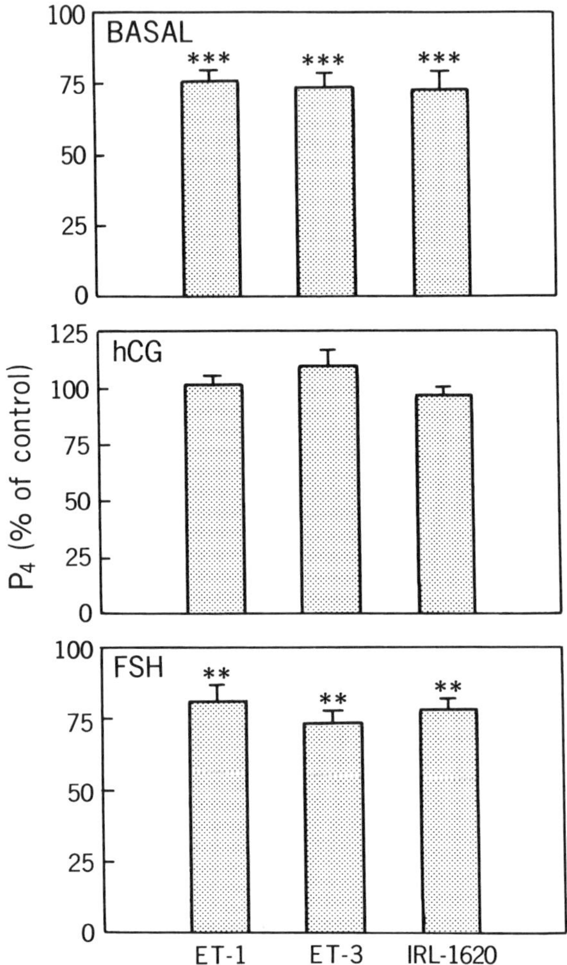

FIGURE 10.—Effects of endothelin (*ET*)-1, ET-3, and IRL-1620 (100 nmol/L) on basal (**top**), human chorionic qonadotropin (*hCG*)-stimulated (**center**), and follicle-stimulating hormone (*FSH*)-stimulated (**bottom**) P_4 secretion from luteinized human granulosa cells (*L-HGCs*). After 48 hours of incubation in medium, the cells were incubated with or without ETs in the absence or presence of hCGs (20 IU/mL) or FSH (1.5 IU/mL) for 24 hours. Data are expressed as the percentage of control (100%). Values are the mean ± standard error of between 4 and 6 separate experiments, each performed in quadruplicate. P_4 levels in control cultures of L-HGCs for 24-hour incubation were 749.2 ± 42.9 (basal), 1167.1 ± 106.2 (hCG-stimulated), and 1162.3 ± 73.8 (FSH-stimulated) nmol/mg of protein, respectively. ***$P < 0.01$ vs. control. (Courtesy of Kamada S, Blackmore PF, Kubota T, et al: The role of endothelin-1 in regulating human granulosa cell proliferation and steroidogenesis *in vitro*. *J Clin Endocrinol Metab* 80:3708–3714, Copyright 1995, The Endocrine Society.)

▶ In the previous report (Abstract 13–6) we described the effect of sex steroids on levels of ET-1 in the plasma of postmenopausal women. Endothelin is known to be extremely important to ovarian function as well, although the details of this relationship have not been well worked out. Granulosa cells were examined in this study where ET and its receptors are expressed. What role ET has in the ovary has not been clearly established, although high levels of ET are known to be present in follicular fluid. It has been suggested that ET may be an inhibitor of luteinization as well as having a possible role in progesterone production.

In this study, the effects of ET via its receptors, types A and B, were examined. The conclusion was that the type A receptor appears to have a predominant role. The figures first show the follicular effect of endothelin and, secondarily, the effect on progesterone production. In Figure 8, the proliferation is noted to be particularly inhibited by the type A–specific inhibitor BQ-123, and this is thought to be through a calcium-mediated mechanism. Contrast this with Figure 10 in which IRL-1620, which is a selective inhibitor of endothelin B, does not have a predominant effect. In the future, the multiple roles of endothelin in the ovary will be visited further.

R.A. Lobo, M.D.

Endothelin Synthesis and Receptors in Human Endometrium Throughout the Normal Menstrual Cycle

Kubota T, Taguchi M, Kamada S, Imai T, Hirata Y, Marumo F, Aso T (Tokyo Med and Dental Univ)
Hum Reprod 10:2204–2208, 1995

13–8

Introduction.—Endothelin (ET) has vasoconstrictive activity. It has been suggested that ET-1 may also play a role in the female reproductive system. This possibility was investigated by studying the expression of messenger RNA (mRNA) for the precursor of ET-1 (prepro-ET-1) and the bioactivity of ET-1 in endometrial cells during different stages of the menstrual cycle.

Methods.—Endometrial tissue was obtained from 20 ovulatory women undergoing hysterectomy in whom the day of the menstrual cycle was estimated. Total RNA was extracted from endometrial tissue samples, and the levels of prepro-ET-1 mRNA and the human receptor subtypes ET_A and ET_B were determined with Northern blot analysis. Endothelin-1 was measured by radioimmunoassay in cultured endometrial stromal cells. Stromal cells in the proliferative phase were incubated for 4 hours with ET-1, after which the concentration of cyclic adenosine monophosphate (cAMP) was assayed with estradiol and medroxyprogesterone.

Results.—The precursor of ET-1 mRNA had higher levels during the menstrual and proliferative phases than during the ovulatory and secretory phases. Oral treatment with estradiol and progesterone caused expression of prepro-ET-1 mRNA in the decidualized endometrium similar to the levels characteristic of the menstrual phase. Incubation with estradiol and medroxyprogesterone caused significantly attenuated ET-1 release (Fig 2). Expression of ET_A receptor mRNA was greater during the proliferative phase than during the secretory phase, and expression of ET_B receptor mRNA was greatest during the menstrual phase. Stromal cell incubation with ET-1 caused a dose-dependent increase in extracellular accumulation of cAMP and in DNA synthesis.

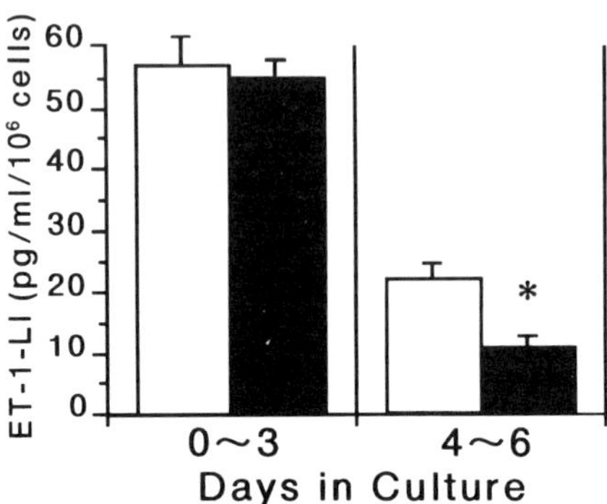

FIGURE 2.—Release of endothelin (*ET*)-1–like immunoreactivity (*ET-1-LI*) from human endometrial stromal cells in the proliferative phase in the absence (*open bar*: control) or presence (*solid bar*) of 10^{-6} mol of estradiol and 10^{-7} mol of medroxyprogesterone acetate during the first 3 days (*left panel*) and second 3 days (*right panel*). Cells were cultured at 37°C in RPMI-1640 serum-free medium for 6 days. Each bar represents the mean of 4 wells (+ standard deviation). *$P < 0.01$ compared with control. (Courtesy of Kubota T, Taguchi M, Kamada S, et al: Endothelin synthesis and receptors in human endometrium throughout the normal menstrual cycle. *Hum Reprod* 10:2204–2208, 1995, by permission of Oxford University Press.)

Conclusion.—Human endometrial cells synthesize and release ET-1 and have ET_A and ET_B receptors whose function is related to phosphoinositide breakdown and adenylate cyclase through increased cAMP. Therefore, ET-1 may have an autocrine and/or paracrine function, playing a role in endometrial re-epithelialization.

▶ This interesting paper is another report that follows data on ET in the endothelium and ovary. Endothelin, one of the most potent vasoconstrictors, is known to be a product of the endothelium and has important consequences in terms of coronary and other vascular blood flow. However, it is produced by glandular tissues as well and has been shown to function in the granulosa cell as abstracted previously.

In this study, the role of the stromal cell in ET production is investigated as is the message for its precursor protein prepro-ET-1. It being a vasoconstrictor, it is logical that these levels would be expressed together with its 2 receptors, ET 1A and 1B, during the menstrual and early follicular phases of the menstrual cycle. Expression of the receptor type A was more prevalent in the proliferative phase of the menstrual cycle and type B during the menstrual phase. Therefore, the action of ET would be surmised to be greatest at this phase, when vasoconstriction is important for cessation of menstrual bleeding.

As shown in Figure 2, this ET activity is inhibited by steroids. Thus, we see that the level of message for ET is reduced during the mid-menstrual phase and during the luteal phase of the menstrual cycle. These data provide important baseline information for understanding bleeding during the menstrual cycle and will be important in the groundwork for understanding ovulatory and anovulatory forms of dysfunctional uterine bleeding, as well as in other pathologic states.

R.A. Lobo, M.D.

Estrogen- But Not Androgen-Dominant Human Ovarian Follicular Fluid Contains an Insulin-Like Growth Factor Binding Protein-4 Protease
Chandrasekher YA, van Dessel HJHM, Fauser BCJM, Giudice LC (Stanford Univ, Calif; Erasmus Univ, Rotterdam, The Netherlands)
J Clin Endocrinol Metab 80:2734–2739, 1995   13–9

Introduction.—The insulin-like growth factor (IGF) system appears to play a role in regulating ovarian follicular development. Ligand-binding studies show that estrogen-dominant follicular fluid (FF_e) and granulosa-luteal cell conditioned media—unlike androgen-dominant FF (FF_a)—contain barely detectable levels of IGF-binding protein-4 (IGFBP-4). If there were an IGFBP-4 protease in FF_e, it might make the IGFBP-4 undetectable by ligand-binding techniques. This possibility was investigated in a series of experiments.

Methods.—The study used FF_e and FF_a from regularly menstruating women, as well as FF_e obtained during in vitro fertilization procedures. For mixing experiments, the substrate was human recombinant IGFBP-4 or IGFBP-4 in nonpregnancy serum (NPS), and the source of the hypothesized protease was FF.

Results.—Incubation of NPS in the presence of FF_e reduced IGFBP-4 to barely detectable levels, according to Western ligand blotting, with no change in the levels of other binding proteins. Levels of IGFBP-4 were unchanged by incubation of NPS in the presence of FF_a. Disappearance of IGFBP-4 in the presence of FF_e was optimal at a pH of 7 to 9. The hypothesized protease appeared to be a metalloserine protease because it was inhibited by aprotinin, ethylenediaminetetraacetic acid, and 1,10-phenanthroline. After incubation of recombinant IGFBP-4 in the presence of FF_e, Western immunoblotting detected a proteolytic fragment of approximately 17-18 kd. The protease in FF_e appeared to be specific for IGFBP-4.

Conclusion.—An IGFBP-4–specific metalloserine protease appears to be present in FF_e but not in FF_a. In estrogen-dominant follicles, the decreased levels of inhibitory IGFBP-4 and the resultant increased availability of IGF peptides may result from proteolytic cleavage. As a result, the dominant follicle may have more IGFs to stimulate estradiol production in synergy with gonadotropins and to inhibit this synergy in androgen-dominant and atretic follicles.

▶ There has been a growing interest in the effect of binding proteins on the expression of IGF action at the level of the ovary. This is 1 paper from a prominent group that epitomizes this explosion of information with which we must contend. Basically, IGF is bound by 6 binding proteins expressed in the ovary, and here we see that there are specific proteases as well that inhibit the action of binding proteins, thus allowing "free" IGF action at the level of the ovary. One such binding protein that has a putative role is BP4. Binding proteins 2 and 4 have been shown to be prominent in atretic and androgen-dominant follicules. This increase in binding proteins would mean that in these follicles, IGF action would be somewhat inhibited.

The data suggest that in FF_e there is an increase in protease activity, thereby limiting the action of BP4. The protease appears to be specific for the action of BP4 on IGF and, therefore, FF_e allows relatively uninhibited IGF action. However, there are other binding proteins as well, and it is the synergy between the different systems that results in the observed action.

R.A. Lobo, M.D.

Ovaries in Sexual Precocity

Bridges NA, Cooke A, Healy MJR, Hindmarsh PC, Brook CGD (Middlesex Hosp, London)
Clin Endocrinol 42:135–140, 1995   13–10

Background.—Pelvic ultrasound plays an important role in the management of sexually precocious girls. Ultrasound examination of the ovaries can help identify the specific type of precocious puberty, the treatment of which is increasingly affected by the appearance of the ovaries. Ultrasound scans of girls with sexual precocity were reviewed to determine the ovarian volume and the prevalence of polycystic ovaries.

Methods.—There were 25 girls with untreated central precocious puberty; 29 with central precocious puberty treated with gonadotropin-releasing hormone (GnRH) analogue, with or without recombinant human growth hormone (GH); 12 who had stopped treatment with GnRH analogue and GH; 15 with premature thelarche or thelarche variant; and 14 with premature adrenarche. Ovarian volume determinations and assessments of polycystic criteria were compared with those of a control group.

Results.—All of the precocious puberty groups had higher ovarian volume standard deviation (SD) scores than the control group. The mean ovarian volume SD score was +1.72 in the girls treated with GnRH analogue and GH, compared with +1.24 in the girls treated with GnRH analogue alone. Eighty-three percent of the girls who had stopped treatment with GnRH analogue and GH had ovaries with a polycystic appearance. Among the girls with precocious puberty, those with premature adrenarche had a lower ovarian volume SD score than those with untreated central precocious puberty.

Conclusion.—Ultrasound scans show that girls with central precocious puberty have greater ovarian volumes than expected for age, which do not return to normal after treatment. For girls treated with GnRH analogue and GH, the ovaries are very large after treatment is stopped, and most have a polycystic appearance. It is unknown whether the increased prevalence of polycystic ovarian appearance in these patients results from central precocious puberty or its treatment.

▶ Ultrasound has really revolutionized our thinking in reproductive endocrinology. This study is another clear example of this. In the past, we treated patients blindly, and now with ultrasound we are seeing things that we do not completely understand. It is clear that monitoring the size and appearance of the ovaries is important in terms of understanding function. In patients with precocious puberty despite gonadotropin suppression, the ovaries remain enlarged and it appears that whatever triggers sexual precocity also triggers ovarian growth which, once enlarged, does not regress.

The authors here have skirted around the issue as to why some ovaries become polycystic in appearance and, perhaps, even more so when treated with GnRH analogues and GH. Remember that once GnRH analogues are used to suppress sex steroids, skeletal growth is inhibited and one of the side effects of this treatment is a reduction in height. Therefore, GH therapy is often used in conjunction with GnRH analogue treatment. Large doses of GnRH analogues are sometimes needed to completely suppress the gonadotropin drive.

Here we see that these patients with larger ovaries had a higher prevalence of polycystic changes. However, it is suggested that the reason might be an exaggeration of the insulin-like growth factor (IGF) axis secondary to GH therapy. We know that GH enhances IGF-I secretion, and this certainly can stimulate androgen production as well and contribute to the appearance of these ovaries. More, I am sure, will come out of this work, as we are only beginning to understand how growth maturation, polycystic changes of the ovary, and pathophysiologic consequences are all starting to link together.

R.A. Lobo, M.D.

Immunization of Monkeys With Recombinant Complimentary Deoxyribonucleic Acid Expressed Zona Pellucida Proteins

VandeVoort CA, Schwoebel ED, Dunbar BS (Univ of California, Davis; Baylor College of Medicine, Houston)
Fertil Steril 64:838–847, 1995   13–11

Background.—The possibility that immunization could be used as a birth control method has prompted several studies for developing safe, effective contraceptive vaccines. Immunization with some zona pellucida (ZP) immunogens can change ovarian development and hormone function in animals. In human beings, antibodies are needed that inhibit sperm binding or penetration to the ZP without adversely affecting ovarian follicular development. Identifying distinct antigenic regions of ZP molecules to generate antibodies that interfere specifically with fertilization without changing ovarian endocrine function is crucial.

Methods.—Monkeys were immunized and boosted at regular intervals with ZP proteins produced with recombinant complementary DNA (cDNA) methods. The main outcome measures were urinary estrogen, P, serum antibody levels, sperm-ZP binding, and ovarian morphology.

Findings.—Antibodies that interfered with ovarian follicular development and ovarian cyclicity were produced by monkeys immunized with a recombinant rabbit 75-kd ZP protein expressed from a partial cDNA in the pEX bacteria expression system. By contrast, antibodies inhibiting homologous sperm binding that did not affect ovarian follicular development or subsequent ovarian hormonal cyclicity developed in monkeys immunized with a recombinant rabbit 55-kd ZP protein.

Conclusion.—Recombinant cDNA techniques may be used to express proteins that can be used to differentiate ZP protein immunogens that may be effective for human contraceptive vaccines from those that can be used for animal sterilization. These techniques are also useful tools for studying the immunologic basis of infertility and ovarian dysfunction.

▶ This interesting paper suggests a novel approach to contraception.

R.Z. Sokol, M.D., F.A.C.P.

Endocrine and Exocrine Effects of Testicular Torsion in the Prepubertal and Adult Rat

Becker EJ Jr, Turner TT (Univ of Virginia, Charlottesville)
J Androl 16:342–351, 1995   13–12

Background.—Clinical experience indicates that spermatic cord torsion lasting longer than 6–10 hours results in irreversible damage to the ipsilateral testis. Most experimental studies have used adult animals, despite the fact that, in human beings, torsion affects mainly adolescent and younger males. There is evidence that the potential for contralateral testicular damage may differ in adult and prepubertal males.

Objective and Methods.—The effects of unilateral testicular torsion on both testes were examined in adult Sprague-Dawley rats and in prepubertal animals 35 days of age. Either 360- or 720-degree torsion was imposed for 1, 2, or 4 hours, and the testes were examined histologically 1 and 2 months later. Daily sperm production was monitored and testosterone concentrations estimated in testicular venous blood.

Results.—In adult rats, the ipsilateral testis became significantly lighter within 30 days of 720-degree torsion, even when imposed for only 1 hour. A similar effect was seen in prepubertal animals 2 months after torsion. At 1 month, in contrast to that of adult animals, daily sperm production and the testicular venous testosterone level were not significantly reduced. Torsion for 2 or 4 hours did produce these effects in prepubertal animals. Neither adult nor prepubertal rats regained any lost function 2 months after torsion. Torsion of 360 degrees did not injure the ipsilateral testis in either age group. There was no evidence that the contralateral testis was affected in any group.

Implications.—The prepubertal testis may be more resistant to the effects of brief torsion than is the adult organ. Age apart, torsion does not damage the contralateral testis.

▶ Spermatic cord torsion is a urologic emergency. Clinically, duration of torsion and degree of torsion are correlated with disruption of testicular function. The germ cells are the most vulnerable to testicular ischemia, followed by the Sertoli cells and, finally, the Leydig cells. Periods of torsion exceeding 6–10 hours usually result in irreversible damage to the torsed testicle. Based on these and other animal studies, the conclusion emerges that ipsilateral torsion does not result in contralateral testicular damage in either adult or prepubertal animals. These findings are consistent with the clinical observation that fertility is preserved in the man with a history of unilateral torsion.

R.Z. Sokol, M.D., F.A.C.P.

Gene Expression in the Aging Brown Norway Rat Epididymis
Viger RS, Robaire B (McGill Univ, Montreal, Quebec, Canada)
J Androl 16:108–117, 1995   13–13

Background.—Mammalian spermatozoa mature in the epididymis and are stored there. The few studies done on the aging epididymis of rats and rabbits have shown reduced numbers of sperm and decreased motility, as well as accumulation of lipofuscin pigment and cytoplasmic vacuoles.

Methods.—Age-related changes were examined in the Brown Norway rat, which does not exhibit the many age-related pathologic changes common in other rat strains. Expression of a number of markers of epididymal function was quantified in the caput-corpus and cauda regions of the epididymis at 6-month intervals from ages 6–30 months. Relative concentrations of messenger RNA (mRNA) were determined by Northern blot analysis using specifc complementary DNAs for 5α-reductase isozymes 1 and 2, proenkephalin, androgen receptor, epididymal proteins, and sulfated glycoprotein-2 (SGP-2).

Findings.—The expression of types 1 and 2 5α-reductase in the caput-corpus region decreased significantly by one third or more at age 6–12 months and, subsequently, by as much as two thirds. No such changes occurred in the cauda epididymidis. Proenkephalin mRNA was identified only in the caput-corpus epididymis of rats aged 6 months. There were no significant age-related changes in levels of mRNA for androgen receptor or epididymal proteins B/C and D/E. Levels of SGP-2 mRNA doubled in the cauda epididymis at age 6–18 months and then declined sharply.

Conclusion.—Aging of Brown Norway rats is accompanied by region-specific changes in the expression of genes for specific markers of epididymal function.

▶ This article expands on previous studies that used the Brown Norway rat as a model for reproductive aging studies. Zirkin and co-workers reported age-related changes in testosterone levels and the seminiferous epithelium.[1] Viger and Robaire report here that 5α-reductase mRNAs change significantly in the aging rat, probably independently of the decrease in testosterone. However, androgen receptor mRNA expression does not change significantly in the aging epididymis. This finding is consistent with the ability of testosterone to restore epididymal sperm in old rats.

R.Z. Sokol, M.D., F.A.C.P.

Reference

1. Zirkin BR, Santulli R, Strandberg JD, et al: Testicular steroidogenesis in the aging Brown Norway rat. *J Androl* 14:118–123, 1993.

The Effect of Androgen on Nitric Oxide Synthase in the Male Reproductive Tract of the Rat

Chamness SL, Maguire MP, Ricker DD, Burnett AL, Crone JK, Chang TSK, Dembeck CL (Johns Hopkins Univ, Baltimore, Md)
Fertil Steril 63:1101–1107, 1995   13–14

Background.—Nitric oxide synthase has recently been localized to various structures of the male rat reproductive tract. Because nitric oxide synthase is present in androgen-dependent organs, nitric oxide synthase itself may be affected by androgens.

Methods.—Nitric oxide synthase activity was determined in the reproductive organs of mature, unoperated control rats, 1-week castrates, and 1-week castrates given testosterone capsules at the time of surgery. The nitric oxide synthase–specific inhibitor *N*-nitro-L-arginine methyl ester (L-NAME), was used to confirm the presence of nitric oxide synthase activity.

Findings.—After castration, nitric oxide synthase activity was significantly decreased by 88% in the caput, 73% in the corpus, and 54% in the cauda epididymidis. In addition, nitric oxide synthase activity declined by 45% and nitric oxide synthase protein by 57% in the penis. Nitric oxide synthase activity rose significantly after castration from undetectable levels in the control rats in the seminal vesicle and lateral prostate. Castration had no effect on nitric oxide synthase activity in the coagulating gland and ventral and dorsal prostate. T-cell replacement prevented the changes in nitric oxide synthase activity in all organs after castration. In all 3 groups of animals, the activity measured in every organ was more than 90% inhibited by L-NAME.

Conclusion.—Androgen affects nitric oxide synthase activity differentially in the male reproductive tract. This is the first study to show that androgen influences nitric oxide synthase in any tissue.

▶ Androgen withdrawal by castration differentially affects nitric oxide synthase activity within the male reproductive tract. These changes were prevented by testosterone replacement at the time of surgery. Of note is the decrease in penile nitric oxide synthase after castration. Nitrous oxide is thought to be a mediator of penile erection. As the authors suggest, change in the penile nitric oxide synthase activity after castration may be related to the reported loss of erectile ability after androgen withdrawal.

R.Z. Sokol, M.D., F.A.C.P.

The Effects of Recombinant Follicle-Stimulating Hormone on the Restoration of Spermatogenesis in the Gonadotropin-Releasing Hormone-Immunized Adult Rat

McLachlan RI, Wreford NG, de Kretser DM, Robertson DM (Monash Univ, Clayton, Australia)
Endocrinology 136:4035–4043, 1995   13–15

Introduction.—The role of follicle-stimulating hormone (FSH) in spermatogenesis in the adult mammal is not well understood. The gonadotropin-releasing hormone (GnRH)–immunized rat, which is gonadotropin-deficient, was used to test the role of FSH in the restoration of spermatogenesis.

Methods.—Adult male rats were immunized with GnRH to induce gonadotropin deficiency. Regression of testes was monitored by palpation and was complete by 12 weeks. Recombinant human FSH was administered for 7, 14, or 21 days. Testes were fixed and germ cells counted by the optical disector technique.

Results.—By the seventh day of FSH administration, testis weight had increased by 43%. There were no further increases in weight with continued FSH administration for up to 21 days. Germ cell numbers were significantly restored within the testis up to the elongated spermatid stage. Continued admistration of FSH beyond 7 days did not increase production of elongated spermatids. The incorporation of bromodeoxyuridine and the number of Sertoli cells were not affected by any treatment used in this study. Follicle-stimulating hormone treatment restored serum inhibin levels but did not increase serum or testicular levels of androgen.

Conclusion.—In the gonadotropin-deficient adult male rat model, addition of recombinant human FSH partially restores spermatogenesis, up through the round spermatid stage. Spermatid elongation was not restored by this addition of exogenous FSH. This indicates the need for additional factors, such as testosterone, to promote complete spermatogenesis.

▶ This study clarifies the role of FSH in the restoration of spermatogenesis. Recombinant human FSH, which eliminates the issue of luteinizing hormone contamination, was administered to animals rendered FSH-deficient by GnRH immunization. Although serum FSH levels in response to daily subcutaneous administration of FSH were 14 and 104 IU/L for the 10 and 50 IU/Kg doses respectively, spermatogenesis proceeded only to the round spermatid stage. Follicle-stimulating hormone exerted trophic effects on the tubular components: Tubule cross-sectional area and length increased significantly. However, only a modest increase in testicular weight was noted, and the testicular content of elongated spermatids was only 0.1% of the control value. These findings are consistent with a failure in spermiogenesis. Thus, disruption of spermatogenesis need not be accompanied by a decrease in testicular size. These data support the conclusion that testosterone is required to enable spermatogenesis to proceed to completion.

R.Z. Sokol, M.D., F.A.C.P.

Induction of Spermatogenesis by Androgens in Gonadotropin-Deficient (*hpg*) Mice

Singh J, O'Neill C, Handelsman DJ (Univ of Sydney, Australia; Royal Prince Alfred Hosp, Sydney, Australia)
Endocrinology 136:5311–5321, 1995

13–16

Background.—The *hpg* mouse, known to have complete congenital functional gonadotropin deficiency caused by major deletions in the gonadotropin-releasing hormone (GnRH) gene but an otherwise normal reproductive tract, represents a new experimental model for investigating the hormonal regulation of spermatogenesis. This model was used to determine the role of testosterone and dihydrotestosterone (DHT) in the initiation of spermatogenesis.

Methods.—Weanling homozygous *hpg* male mice were used. Mice received subdermal Silastic brand implants, ranging between 0 and 2 cm in length, which had been filled with either testosterone or DHT. Phenotypically normal (N/N or N/*hpg*) and untreated *hpg/hpg* mice served as positive and negative controls.

Results.—Both testosterone and DHT stimulated testis size by approximately 14-fold after 8 weeks. Qualitatively complete spermatogenesis was also induced by testosterone and DHT, even in the presence of reduced intratesticular androgen levels and undetectable circulating follicle-stimulating hormone (FSH). A dose-dependent increase in the absolute numbers of all germ cell types induced by both testosterone and DHT were noted on stereologic quantitation of Sertoli and germ cells. Germ cell numbers expressed per Sertoli cell and homogenization-resistant elongated spermatid expressed per milligram of testis rose to greater than 80% of non-*hpg* control values at maximal androgen doses. Both testosterone and DHT

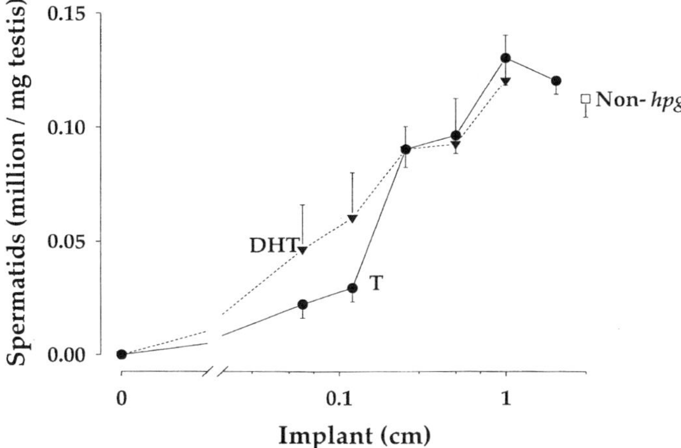

FIGURE 7.—Numbers of elongated spermatids (including spermatozoa) expressed as million per milligram of testis in *hpg* mice (*n* = 6–8) treated for 8 weeks with increasing implant lengths of testosterone (*solid circle*) or dihydrotestosterone (*solid triangle*) compared with those in untreated non-*hpg* control mice (*n* = 12–15) indicated by *open square*. *Error bars* indicate the standard error of the mean unless smaller than the corresponding symbol. *Abbreviation: DHT*, dihydrotestosterone. (Courtesy of Singh J, O'Neill C, Handelsman DJ: Induction of spermatogenesis by androgens in gonadotropin-deficient (*hpg*) mice. *Endocrinology* 136:5311–5321, Copyright 1995, The Endocrine Society.)

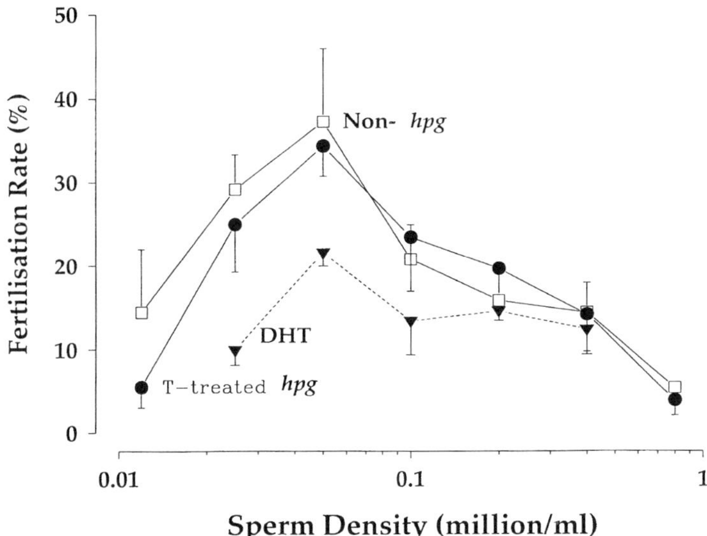

FIGURE 8.—Fertility of testosterone-treated *hpg* mice (*solid circle*), dihydrotestosterone-treated *hpg* mice (*open triangle*), and non-*hpg* control mice (*open square*) tested in an in vitro fertilization assay at different sperm concentrations. *Error bars* represent the standard error of the mean unless smaller than the corresponding symbol. *Abbreviation: DHT*, dihydrotestosterone. (Courtesy of Singh J, O'Neill C, Handelsman DJ: Induction of spermatogenesis by androgens in gonadotropin-deficient (*hpg*) mice. *Endocrinology* 136:5311–5321, Copyright 1995, The Endocrine Society.)

were found to induce quantitatively normal fertilizing capacity of the sperm in *hpg* males, as demonstrated by in vitro fertilization assay (Figs 7 and 8).

Conclusion.—Androgens alone, acting through the androgen receptor and without need for aromatization, lead to quantitatively and qualitatively complete spermatogenesis in the *hpg* mouse, including fertile sperm. This can occur even when intratesticular androgen levels are low and circulating blood FSH levels are absent.

▶ Data presented in this article support the conclusion reached in Abstract 13–15. Androgen-dependent induction of spermatogenesis can proceed despite low intratesticular androgen levels in the absence of detectable immunoreactive FSH in the blood. Follicle-stimulating hormone and testosterone may well act synergistically to maintain normal spermatogenesis in the human being.

R.Z. Sokol, M.D., F.A.C.P.

14 Polycystic Ovarian Syndrome

Transvaginal Ultrasonographic Morphology in Polycystic Ovarian Syndrome
Takahashi K, Okada M, Ozaki T, Uchida A, Yamasaki H, Kitao M (Shimane Med Univ, Izumo, Japan)
Gynecol Obstet Invest 39:201–206, 1995   14–1

Introduction.—A common cause of infertility is polycystic ovarian syndrome (PCOS), which can be evaluated with transvaginal ultrasound. Variable results have been seen in the criteria for the diagnosis of PCOS, such as ovarian size, number and size of cysts, and consistency of stroma. Morphologic findings based on transvaginal ultrasound were assessed in patients with clinically documented PCOS.

Methods.—The study included 47 women with clinical PCOS: 20 had secondary amenorrhea, 25 had oligomenorrhea, and 2 had anovulatory cycle. Thirty fertile women served as the controls. Each woman had a pelvic ultrasound examination, and each ovary was measured in 3 planes. Using conventional radioimmunoassays, luteinizing hormone, follicle-stimulating hormone, testosterone, Δ^4-androstenedione, and dehydroepiandrosterone sulfate was measured.

Results.—Women with PCOS had high mean ovarian volume (range of 3.1 to 41.1 mL with a mean of 10.3 ± 6.2 mL) and more follicles (range of 3 to 21 with a mean of 10.6) than the controls. In the ovaries of women with PCOS, the most prominent features were an ovarian volume greater than 6.2 mL and more than 10 follicles with a diameter of 2–8 mm; 94% of the women with PCOS had these findings. In about 50% of the women with PCOS, marked asymmetry of the 2 ovaries was seen, with a considerable overlap between the 2 groups in the ovarian volume and the number of follicles. In the women with PCOS, most of the endocrine parameters were significantly higher, except follicle-stimulating hormone.

Discussion.—Normal ovarian volume and normal number of follicles were observed in 3 (6%) of women. A woman with PCOS is difficult to distinguish from a woman without the syndrome based solely on transvaginal ultrasound criteria using the number of follicles or ovarian volume. Nevertheless, for the screening of PCOS, these criteria could be clinically useful.

▶ The diagnosis of PCOS has previously been established on the basis of clinical and endocrinologic abnormalities. With the use of sonographic visualization of the ovaries, it has been shown that the majority of women with the clinical and endocrinologic characteristics of this syndrome have enlarged polycystic ovaries. However, because these investigators found that about 30% of women with the endocrinologic changes of polycystic ovaries did not have an ovary with more than 10 small follicles, it is perhaps better to use the term chronic hyperandrogenic anovulation to describe the syndrome and to restrict the term PCOS to women who also have morphologic findings of polycystic ovaries as determined sonographically. If ovarian enlargement (with less than 10 small follicles) is also used as a morphologic criterion for diagnosis, one or the other of these abnormalities was found in more than 90% of the women in this study with the clinical and endocrinologic abnormalities consistent with the diagnosis. Thus, the presence of both of these morphologic changes—ovarian enlargement and multiple small follicles—should be documented when performing sonographic examination of women with suspected PCOS. The incidence of these changes in other endocrinologic abnormalities such as hyperprolactinemic anovulation also needs to be ascertained.

D.R. Mishell, Jr., M.D.

Polycystic Ovary Syndrome: The Spectrum of the Disorder in 1741 Patients
Balen AH, Conway GS, Kaltsas G, Techatraisak K, Manning PJ, West C, Jacobs HS (Univ College London)
Hum Reprod 10:2107–2111, 1995   14–2

Objective.—The criteria for diagnosing polycystic ovarian syndrome (PCOS) remain controversial, but in England it is generally agreed that the detection of polycystic ovaries by ultrasound scanning constitutes a unifying criterion. The clinical features were reviewed in a group of 1,714 women in whom ultrasonography demonstrated at least 10 follicles 2–8 mm in diameter, arranged around an echo-dense central stroma. The women also had signs and symptoms of PCOS.

Findings.—Thirty-eight percent of women were overweight. The serum luteinizing hormone (LH) was elevated in 40% of the group, and the serum testosterone was elevated in 29%. Only 30% of patients had normal menstrual cycles, and 19% were amenorrheic. Forty-six percent of women had moderate or severe hirsutism. Approximately one third of patients had acne, and 2.5% had acanthosis nigricans.

Correlations.—The body mass index (BMI) correlated significantly with ovarian volume and the cross-sectional area of the uterus, as well as with the serum testosterone and the presence of hirsutism. Obesity (BMI greater than 25 kg/m²) also was associated with infertility and a disordered menstrual cycle. Only 25% of 465 evaluable women had proven fertility; 49% had primary and 26% had secondary infertility. The risk of infertility increased with the serum LH concentration. Ovarian volume correlated with the serum LH and testosterone levels as well as with the BMI.

Implications.—The morphology of the ovaries is seemingly the most sensitive marker of PCOS. Women who are overweight and are able to lose weight may expect improvement in symptoms of menstrual disorder as well as infertility and hyperandrogenism.

▶ There is disagreement regarding the criteria used for the diagnosis of PCOS. In Britain, the diagnosis is usually made when more than 10 small follicles (less than 8 mm in diameter) are visualized in an ovary at the time of sonographic examination in a woman with at least one of the symptoms of PCOS: menstrual irregularity, infertility, or hyperandrogenism. In the United States, the diagnosis is usually made by the presence of the endocrinologic abnormalities present in the syndrome; elevated serum LH and/or testosterone together with anovulation. In this large study, the presence of obesity was directly correlated with a higher incidence of infertility, menstrual irregularity, and hirsutism. Therefore, women with PCOS and these symptoms who are obese should be told that weight reduction by means of caloric restriction and exercise will likely result in improvement of their abnormal symptoms.

D.R. Mishell, Jr., M.D.

Adjuvant Growth Hormone for Induction of Ovulation With Gonadotrophin-Releasing Hormone Agonist and Gonadotrophins in Polycystic Ovary Syndrome: A Randomized, Double-Blind, Placebo Controlled Trial
Homburg R, Levy T, Ben-Rafael Z (Tel Aviv Univ, Israel)
Hum Reprod 10:2550–2553, 1995   14–3

Background.—Growth hormone (GH) and a mediator of GH action, insulin-like growth factor-I, target the ovary. Women with polycystic ovarian syndrome (PCOS) have abnormal GH kinetics. The hypothesis that the disturbance in normal GH kinetics in women with PCOS may be corrected when GH therapy is given concurrently with human menopausal gonadotropin (hMG) for ovulation induction was examined.

Methods.—Thirty women with PCOS-associated anovulatory infertility who had failed to ovulate when given clomiphene were recruited. All the patients were given a gonadotropin-releasing hormone agonist, followed 2 weeks later with individually adjusted doses of hMG. Human chorionic gonadotropin, 10,000 IU, was given intramuscularly when at least 1 follicle larger than 16 mm was seen on ultrasound. On days 3, 7, and 11 after the injection of human chorionic gonadotropin, 50 mg of IM progesterone was given. For a single cycle, the 30 patients were randomized in a double-blind fashion to receive either a placebo or IM GH (12 IU) daily for 7 days from the first day the hMG was given.

Results.—No difference was found between the patients receiving GH or placebo in the number of ampules, duration of treatment, or daily effective doses of hMG required to cause ovulation. Only one of the 15 patients in each group failed to ovulate; 4 clinical pregnancies were achieved in the placebo group and 3 in the GH group. No patient had ovarian hyperstimulation syndrome develop. Mean fasting serum insulin concentrations increased more than fourfold and mean serum insulin-like growth factor-I concentrations more than twofold after 5 daily injections of GH. These values did not change significantly in the placebo group.

Conclusions.—In these women with clomiphene-resistant PCOS, adding GH therapy to a regimen of gonadotropin-releasing hormone agonist and hMG did not influence follicular development and did not appear to offer any clinical benefit.

Insulin Resistant and Non-Resistant Polycystic Ovary Syndrome Represent Two Clinical and Endocrinological Subgroups

Meirow D, Yossepowitch O, Rösler A, Brzezinski A, Schenker JG, Laufer N, Raz I (Hebrew Univ, Jerusalem)
Hum Reprod 10:1951–1956, 1995   14–4

Purpose.—Polycystic ovarian syndrome (PCOS) is diagnosed on the basis of typical clinical and endocrine features, although not all patients will have all the features at the same time. Among the various groups of patients with hyperandrogenism and hyperinsulinemia with insulin resistance, patients with PCOS are the most frequently seen and the least understood. Obesity is a major contributor to insulin resistance. Body composition and endocrine findings were compared in PCOS patients with and without insulin resistance.

Methods.—Thirty-five patients with PCOS were studied in an infertility unit. The patients' insulin and glucose responses to a standard 75-g oral glucose load were measured to assess the presence or absence of insulin resistance. Anthropometric measurements were performed, including body mass index, percentage of body fat, and waist-to-hip ratio. The degree of hirsutism was assessed by the Ferriman-Gallwey method, and the women's endocrine profiles were taken.

Results.—Insulin resistance was present in 18 patients—14 of unknown origin and 4 resulting from a type A insulin receptor mutation—and absent in 17. The women with insulin resistance were significantly more obese and more hirsute. They also had higher testosterone concentrations than the non–insulin-resistant women—2.65 vs. 1.37 nmol/L—but lower sex hormone–binding globulin concentrations–19.48 vs. 30.61 nmol/L. The luteinizing hormone–to–follicle-stimulating hormone ratio was elevated in the non–insulin-resistant patients but normal in the insulin-resistant patients (1.34 vs. 2.94).

Conclusions.—The findings suggest that there may be 2 approximately equal subpopulations of women with PCOS: one with insulin resistance of various causes and one without insulin resistance. The 2 groups of patients have differing anthropometric and endocrine characteristics. Oral glucose tolerance testing can easily determine whether a woman with PCOS has insulin resistance. Further research must be done to determine the best medical surveillance and treatment for both patient subgroups.

▶ This paper represents one of many in the field looking at variations in patients with PCOS who have or do not have insulin resistance. In fact, the data here are not novel but have been abstracted to give the reader a summary of what is going on in the field. Insulin resistance is thought to be central to the pathophysiology of the syndrome, yet a substantial proportion of the population may not be insulin resistant, at least according to some authors. Indeed, it is in the eyes of the beholder to determine who is and who is not insulin resistant, which depends largely on how testing is carried out. The authors of this study have used relatively crude methods, the oral glucose tolerance test, to assess in vivo insulin sensitivity. This can only be adequately accomplished in a subtle way with clamp techniques or with the IV insulin tolerance test with frequent sampling. The authors have therefore divided patients into 2 groups on the basis of insulin resistance, finding a large proportion of patients not to be insulin resistant. It has also been suggested that the more obese the patient, the more insulin resistant she is, which is certainly true.

Certain metabolic aberrations (hypertriglyceridemia, for example) are also more common in those who are insulin resistant. It is also thought to be more common in those patients who have a menstrual disturbance as opposed to those who have normal menses. Indeed, a spectrum exists here, and insulin resistance, if liberally diagnosed by sensitive techniques, probably occurs in the majority of patients but probably not in all patients with the syndrome. The worse the insulin resistance, the more likely additional clinical symptomatology will be encountered, such as the severity of the menstrual aberrations. In Table 3 in the original article, it is suggested that the associated parts of this spectrum that will be encountered as patients progress toward insulin resistance include: an elevated fasting insulin level, increased body mass index or body weight, altered waist–hip ratio, increased percentage of body fat, an increase in the incidence of hirsutism, and, paradoxically, a normal luteinizing hormone/follicle-stimulating hormone ratio, where it is often increased in the non–insulin-resistant group. Also encountered are a higher testosterone level and a lower sex hormone–binding globulin level. In general, androgens are higher, with the exception of dehydroepiandrosterone sulfate, which almost has a reciprocal relationship with insulin.

R.A. Lobo, M.D.

Diurnal Variation of Sex Hormone Binding Globulin and Insulin-Like Growth Factor Binding Protein-1 in Women With Polycystic Ovary Syndrome

Hamilton-Fairley D, White D, Griffiths M, Anyaoku V, Koistinen R, Seppälä M, Franks S (United Med and Dental School, London; St Mary's Hosp Med School, London; Helsinki Univ)
Clin Endocrinol 43:159–165, 1995   14–5

Background.—Research has shown that insulin inhibits the hepatic production of sex hormone–binding globulin (SHBG) and insulin-like growth factor binding protein-1 (IGFBP-1). If both SHBG and IGFBP-1 are regulated by insulin, then SHBG levels may show a diurnal variation, especially in hyperandrogenic women. The diurnal variation in SHBG and the interrelationships of insulin, insulin-like growth factor (IGF)-1, SHBG, and IGFBP-1 for 24 hours were investigated in women with anovulatory polycystic ovarian syndrome (PCOS).

Methods.—Ten anovulatory women with PCOS and 10 weight-matched control subjects were included. Serum samples were collected every 2 hours for 24 hours, and concentrations of SHBG, IGFBP-1, insulin, and IGF-1 were measured.

Findings.—The median body mass index (BMI) was 25.2 kg/m² in the women with PCOS and 24.3 kg/m² in the control group. Serum testosterone (T) and luteinizing hormone (LH) levels were increased significantly in the women with PCOS compared with those in the control group. No diurnal variation in SHBG was observed. The PCOS group had a lower median peak SHBG concentration, those values being 29.4 and 52.1 nmol/L. The fasting levels of insulin at 6 A.M. were 6.6 mU/L in patients and 6.2 mU/L in control subjects, this difference being nonsignificant. However, the peak median levels did differ significantly, being 66.1 mU/L in the PCOS group and 40 mU/L in the control group. A diurnal variation was found in insulin concentrations in the control group but not in the PCOS group. The diurnal variation in IGFBP-1 in the 2 groups was comparable, but the peak median levels were lower in the women with PCOS. The decrease in IGFBP-1 levels was correlated with the increase in insulin levels. The 2 groups had comparable IGF-1 concentrations. Insulin and SHBG were significantly negatively correlated, as were insulin and IGFBP-1 (Fig 1).

Conclusions.—Concentrations of SHBG show no diurnal variation. However, there is a marked diurnal variation in IGFBP-1 levels. Compared with control subjects, anovulatory women with PCOS have an abnormal pattern of insulin secretion with an absence of diurnal variation. These findings provide further evidence of the relative insulin resistance, independent of weight, found in women with anovulatory PCOS. Insulin may be a regulator of the circulating levels of these binding proteins, although the difference in the time course of their response makes it unlikely that they are co-regulated.

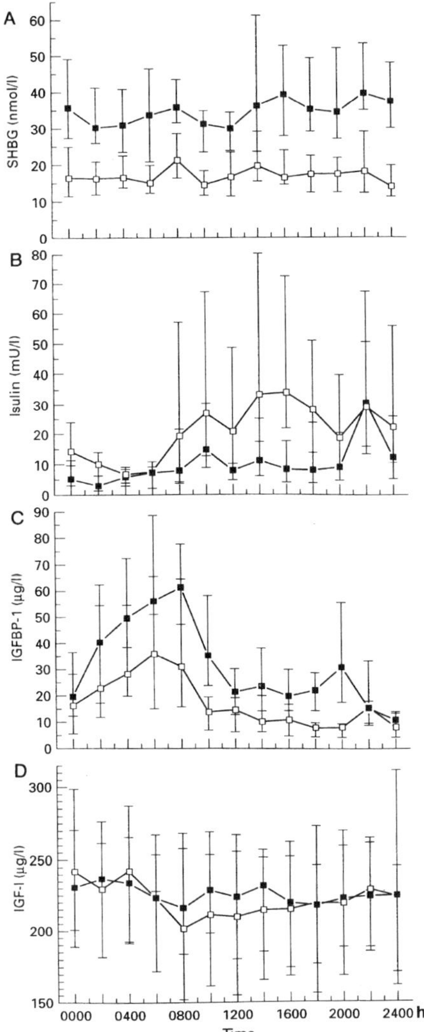

FIGURE 1.—Changes in the concentration of (**A**) sex hormone–binding globulin (*SHBG*); (**B**) insulin; (**C**) insulin-like growth factor binding protein-1 (*IGFBP-1*); and (**D**) insulin-like growth factor-I (*IGF-I*) (median [interquartile range]) over 24 hours (midnight to midnight). *Filled squares,* control; *open squares,* polycystic ovarian syndrome. (Courtesy of Hamilton-Fairley D, White D, Griffiths M, et al: Diurnal variation of sex hormone binding globulin and insulin-like growth factor binding protein-1 in women with polycystic ovary syndrome. *Clin Endocrinol* 43:159–165, 1995, Blackwell Science Ltd.)

▶ The importance of this paper is merely that it points out the fact that insulin is a major regulator of IGFBP-1 and SHBG. The importance of IGF-BP-1, which is both a circulating binding protein and has an action within the ovary, is that the lowering of IGFBP-1 results in high levels of "free IGFI." Conditions that are associated with lower IGFBP-1, such as obesity and

PCOS, are associated with elevated levels of "free" IGF-I. Together with the already elevated levels of insulin, increased levels of bioavailable IGF-I are thought to result in an increase in androgen action at the level of the ovary, among other phenomena. We would not have expected SHBG to be affected in this study, which looked at diurnal changes. Nevertheless, insulin and IGFBP-1 clearly did demonstrate changes, as shown in Figure 1. That SHBG levels, although lower in patients with PCOS, did not exhibit this diurnal variation is because of the rapidity of the changes in insulin. Sex hormone–binding globulin is a large molecule that turns over slowly and is synthesized by the liver. For example, estrogen therapy in postmenopausal women results in a significant change in only 10 days to 2 weeks. We would not expect changes to occur on a day-to-day basis. Even through the menstrual cycle, there are only minor changes in SHBG. The importance of the observations made in this paper, however, is that insulin is a major regulator of specific proteins; as seen in the next paper, insulin is also implicated in the appearance of the ovary, which in turn, may be caused by changes in the action of growth factors like IGF.

R.A. Lobo, M.D.

Follistatin Concentrations in Follicular Fluid of Normal and Polycystic Ovaries

Erickson GF, Chung D-G, Sit A, DePaolo LV, Shimasaki S, Ling N (Univ of California, San Diego; Stanford Univ, Calif; NIH, Bethesda, Md; et al)
Hum Reprod 10:2120–2124, 1995

14–6

Objective.—The activin/inhibin binding protein follistatin (FS) regulates growth and differentiation, presumably in an autocrine/paracrine manner. Aside from its presence, little is known about FS in human follicular fluid. Changes in follicular fluid FS concentrations during selection and atresia were studied, along with the follicular fluid FS concentrations of women with polycystic ovarian syndrome (PCOS).

Methods.—A radioimmunoassay was used to measure FS concentrations in follicular fluid samples. Samples were obtained from 4 groups of follicles: 5 dominant follicles from normal women; 11 nondominant, atretic follicles; 46 ovulatory follicles of in vitro fertilization (IVF) patients; and small graafian follicles from 3 patients with PCOS.

Results.—All follicular fluid samples had FS concentrations that were much higher than reported serum levels—on the order of 100 times higher. The normal dominant follicles had a mean FS concentration of 203 ng/mL, compared with 185 ng/mL for the atretic cohort follicles, 185 ng/mL for the IVF follicles, and 250 ng/mL for the PCOS follicles. These differences were nonsignificant. The follicular fluid FS concentration was not correlated with the estradiol, progesterone, or androstenedione concentration.

Conclusions.—High steady-state concentrations of FS are present in the microenvironment of human graafian follicles. This is true for healthy vs. atretic and for normal vs. PCOS follicles. The findings suggest that increases or decreases in follicular FS do not play a major role in selection, atresia, or PCOS. Follistatin binding could play a part in regulating intrinsic activin and inhibin activity.

▶ This paper is brought to the attention of the reader because measurements of FS are relatively novel. This is one of the family of peptides produced by the ovary that has significant implications in the ovarian microenvironment. Follistatin has been shown to be a binding protein for both activin and inhibin. Thus, just like the insulin-like growth factor family of peptides, in which there are specific binding proteins and changes in the binding proteins within the ovary have significant implications in terms of the insulin-like growth factor axis, in this case, the action of inhibin and activin may be influenced by FS. However, that it binds both activin and inhibin is somewhat at odds with its having a physiologic role, in that inhibin and activin generally have opposite modes of action physiologically. The importance of the observations here are that the concentrations are extremely high, one-hundredfold higher than levels in serum, and the values are in the 100–200 ng/mL range. Unfortunately, no differences were determined between the follicular fluid levels of different types of patients. Follistatin levels, which would be hypothesized to be low and would thereby result in higher inhibin content, locally, could not be shown in patients with PCOS in this study. Perhaps the concentrations of binding protein are important for follicular production and regulation of inhibin and activin in ways that cannot be determined at this point.

R.A. Lobo, M.D.

Metabolic Features of Polycystic Ovary Syndrome Are Found in Adolescent Girls With Hyperandrogenism

Apter D, Bützow T, Laughlin GA, Yen SSC (Univ of California, San Diego)
J Clin Endocrinol Metab 80:2966–2973, 1995
14–7

Background.—Augmented luteinizing hormone (LH) pulsatility and increased LH follicle-stimulating hormone (FSH) ratio with increased ovarian volume have been reported to accompany hyperandrogenism (HA) in adolescent girls. These neuroendocrine characteristics, along with greater levels of 17-hydroxyprogesterone, androstenedione, testosterone, and estrone, which are ovarian in origin, are the same as those observed in women with polycystic ovarian syndrome (PCOS). The metabolic features of hyperandrogenic teenaged girls were investigated.

Methods and Findings.—Thirteen girls aged 11–18 years with mild to moderate HA and 28 age-matched healthy control subjects were evaluated. Compared with the control group, the patients with HA had significantly increased fasting insulin levels but not plasma glucose concentrations. These values were 256 pmol/L in the patients and 103 pmol/L in the healthy girls. Insulin responses to IV glucose tolerance test and meals as well as 24-hour mean insulin concentrations were also increased in the patients with HA. The increased ratio of insulin and glucose suggests that hyperinsulinemia with normal fasting glucose levels in the patients may reflect insulin resistance. All insulin measures were associated with body mass index (BMI). However, insulin continued to be significantly higher in the patients after correcting for BMI, suggesting that factors in addition to BMI contributed to reduced insulin sensitivity. Twenty-four–hour insulin-like growth factor binding protein (IGFBP) levels demonstrated a diurnal pattern inversely associated with insulin. The 24-hour mean concentrations were 0.35 µg/L in the patients and 0.76 µg/L in the healthy girls. An inverse relationship was also found between decreased sex hormone–binding globulin and insulin levels. However, the groups had comparable growth hormone (GH) pulsatile characteristics, insulin-like growth factor (IGF)-I/IGFBP-3 levels, and GH responses to growth hormone–releasing hormone. The activity of the GH–IGF-I axis in patients with HA demonstrated age- and BMI-dependent decreases identical to those in the healthy girls. The HA group had larger ovarian volumes, which correlated independently with 24-hour mean LH and fasting insulin concentrations. Positive correlations were found between LH levels and basal serum concentrations of 17-hydroxyprogesterone, androstenedione, testosterone, and estrone. However, insulin had an independent influence on steroid levels during LH suppression by the gonadotropin-releasing hormone antagonist Nal-Glu.

Conclusions.—These adolescent girls with HA had no intrinsic abnormalities in the GH–IGF-I–IGFBP-3 axis. Their salient metabolic characteristic was hyperinsulinemia. Together with increased LH levels and reduced IGFBP-1 and sex hormone–binding globulin, this hyperinsulinemia may contribute to the development of manifestations of PCOS.

▶ A theory set out by Yen many years ago suggested that PCOS is initiated around the time of puberty or menarche. These data and subsequent studies during the past 20 years have corroborated this theory. In this nice study by Apter and associates we see an adolescent syndrome in which girls between the ages of 11 and 18 years have characteristic features of the adult. The cardinal feature here is the early emergence of insulin resistance. Figure 1 in the original article shows an exaggerated hyperinsulinemic response in the girls with HA after the IV administration of glucose. In Figure 2 in the original article, wide excursions of insulin throughout the day can be seen in hyperandrogenic girls with a reciprocal finding in IGFBP-1. Serum IGFBP-1 appears to be tightly regulated by insulin and is quite low in patients who have PCOS.

In this study, levels were not suppressed to the degree to which they often are in the adult population. Of interest, girls with HA had increased ovarian volume. We know that ovarian volume increases through childhood and peaks around the time of puberty, with full polycystic changes occurring as early as age 12–13 years. So we see a stage here during which this full-blown syndrome develops fairly early and apparently gets worse as the syndrome propagates over time. Another feature observed here is the lowering of sex hormone–binding globulin, which is tightly related to levels of insulin. This results in increased free steroids such as free testosterone and the emergence of the hyperandrogenic manifestations of the syndrome.

R.A. Lobo, M.D.

Normal Development and Metabolic Activity of Preimplantation Embryos *In Vitro* From Patients With Polycystic Ovaries

Hardy K, Robinson FM, Paraschos T, Wicks R, Franks S, Winston RML (Hammersmith Hosp, London; Kingsmill Hosp, Nottinghamshire, England; Imperial College of Science, Technology and Medicine, London)
Hum Reprod 10:2125–2135, 1995
14–8

Background.—Polycystic ovarian syndrome (PCOS) is associated with an increased miscarriage rate after spontaneous conception and with reduced fertilization, embryo cleavage, and pregnancy after in vitro fertilization (IVF). It has been hypothesized that PCOS is therefore associated with embryos with poor development potential. To investigate this hypothesis, the development of human embryos was prospectively compared in patients with ovulatory PCOS, anovulatory PCOS, and pure tubal disease by studying the blastocyst cell numbers and metabolic activity.

Methods.—Fifty-one patients, including 23 with pure tubal disease, 10 with anovulatory PCOS, or 18 with ovulatory PCOS who were awaiting IVF, were studied. Surplus embryos after IVF were incubated individually in medium between days 2 and 6. The depletion of pyruvate and glucose and the production of lactate were evaluated by measuring these nutrient concentrations in the embryo media and in medium alone. Cell numbers in the trophectoderm (TE) and in the inner cell mass (ICM) of blastocysts were determined using differential fluorescent labeling. The numbers of patients who became pregnant and of blastocyst cells, as well as metabolic activity, were compared in the 3 patient groups.

Results.—There were no significant differences among the 3 patient groups in the proportion of patients becoming pregnant or of embryo implantation. The percentage of embryos reaching the blastocyst stage by day 6 was also similar. However, embryos from patients with anovulatory PCOS were significantly more likely to have cavitated blastocysts by day 5 than were those from patients with tubal disease. Blastocysts from patients with anovulatory PCOS had significantly more cells than blastocysts from patients with tubal disease, and cell numbers in patients with ovulatory PCOS were between those 2 groups. There were no differences in mitotic activity or cell death rate in the 3 groups. Increases in pyruvate uptake by embryos were similar in the patient groups but were increased with a titrated ovulation induction protocol. Patients with tubal disease and PCOS also demonstrated similar patterns of embryonic glucose uptake, but embryonic lactate production was higher in patients with ovulatory PCOS than in the other 2 groups, particularly during the morula stage.

Conclusions.—Contrary to the hypothesized poor-quality embryos in patients with PCOS, these findings show that patients with PCOS produce preimplantation embryos of comparable or better quality than do patients with tubal disease. However, there were differences in embryo quality, rate of development, blastocyst cell number, and metabolism in embryos from different diagnostic groups and undergoing different ovulation induction regimens, suggesting that differences in the in vivo gonadotropin concentrations before oocyte maturation may affect preimplantation development. Therefore, successful IVF is dependent on using an individualized ovulation induction regimen.

▶ Some controversy exists regarding whether the embryos generated from patients who have PCOS are normal or abnormal. The weight of evidence suggests that even though more oocytes are produced, the overall success of pregnancy generated from these embryos may be decreased. This is in part because of a high miscarriage rate that has been ascribed to a reduction in embryo quality. Of interest in this study was that the patients with PCOS were divided into 2 groups, those who were anovulatory and those who were considered to have ovulatory function. The distinction here is characteristic of authors in England, and in general many of us in the United States do not diagnose PCOS in patients who have normal ovulatory menses. Clearly there are many women who have polycystic-appearing ovaries who do not have the full-blown syndrome.

Nevertheless, these data are provocative and suggest that there may be some early dysfunction in the environment leading to follicle growth that may subsequently affect embryo quality and thereby increase the implantation failure of patients with PCOS. The principal candidate for this dysfunction has been suggested to be an elevated serum luteinizing hormone (LH) level, as discussed in this report. Of interest, however, is the fact that these events were not easily ascertained. Embryos were allowed to grow, and cell number and metabolic production were observed after 6 days of culture. Figure 6 in the original article clearly demonstrates higher pyruvate uptake in patients with high basal LH with PCOS compared with those with normal LH. However, in general the data show few differences in the embryos of these patients, who all had LH downregulation before stimulation. The differences in LH levels are an interesting observation. Authors in England have suggested that LH values as high as 10 IU/L or 10 mIU/mL can be abnormal. The mean value of the anovulatory PCOS group was 9.3 and of the controls was 6.6 mIU/mL. If this theory is correct, only a very small amount of LH increase may be responsible for this abnormality.

R.A. Lobo, M.D.

The Prognostic Value of Basal Luteinizing Hormone: Follicle-Stimulating Hormone Ratio in the Treatment of Patients With Polycystic Ovarian Syndrome by Assisted Reproduction Techniques

Tarlatzis BC, Grimbizis G, Pournaropoulos F, Bontis J, Lagos S, Spanos E, Mantalenakis S (Aristotle Univ Thessaloniki, Greece; Infertility and IVF Ctr 'Geniki Kliniki', Thessaloniki, Greece)

Hum Reprod 10:2545–2549, 1995   14–9

Background.—Increased luteinizing hormone (LH) is one of the main endocrinologic disorders in patients with polycystic ovarian syndrome (PCOS), which results in a high LH–to–follicle-stimulating hormone (FSH) ratio. The relationship between the baseline LH:FSH ratio with the stimulation response and the miscarriage risk in women with PCOS stimulated for assisted reproduction techniques (ART) with and without gonadotropin-releasing hormone analogues (GnRHa) was investigated retrospectively.

Methods.—One hundred forty-eight patients were included in the analysis. Group 1 consisted of 20 patients and 20 cycles stimulated with human menopausal gonadotropin (hMG). Group 2 included 128 patients and 162 cycles stimulated with buserelin-long/hMG. In a preceding spontaneous or progestin-induced cycle, LH and FSH levels were assessed during the early follicular phase.

Findings.—The baseline LH:FSH ratio in group 1 was inversely related to the number of follicles developed, the number of oocytes obtained, and the percentage of mature oocytes. There was no correlation between the LH:FSH ratio and number of follicles and oocytes in group 2, because these numbers were relatively constant, regardless of baseline LH:FSH. However, the LH:FSH ratio was significantly inversely correlated with the percentage of mature oocytes. When the slopes of the curve were compared, there was a better correlation between the LH:FSH ratio and the percentage of mature oocytes in group 1 than group 2. Analysis of patients subgrouped on the basis of LH:FSH ratio of less than 3 or 3 or more confirmed these findings. The mean LH:FSH ratio was significantly greater in women who miscarried than in women giving birth to a live infant.

Conclusions.—A high basal LH:FSH ratio appears to have an adverse effect on the number of follicles and oocytes and on oocyte maturity in patients with PCOS stimulated with hMG. However, GnRHa administration in a long protocol seems to reverse this detrimental effect on follicle and oocyte development. Greater LH:FSH ratios appear to predict a greater possibility for miscarriage, despite GnRHa administration.

▶ Others have also shown that elevated LH levels in women with PCOS are associated with an increased risk of early pregnancy loss. It has been suggested that women with elevated LH levels wishing to conceive be treated with a GnRH agonist to reduce the rate of spontaneous abortion. The results of this study indicate that such therapy may not be beneficial for reducing the abortion rate when such women are treated by in vitro fertilization. Gonadotropin-releasing hormone agonist therapy appears to increase oocyte development rate. Therefore, such therapy may be useful when treating anovulatory women with PCOS and elevated LH levels with hMG to induce ovulation.

D.R. Mishell, Jr., M.D.

Initial Estradiol Response Predicts Outcome of Exogenous Gonadotropins Using a Step-Down Dose Regimen for Induction of Ovulation in Polycystic Ovary Syndrome

Schoot DC, van Dessel TJHM, Hop WC, Fauser BCJM, de Jong FH (Erasmus Univ, Rotterdam, The Netherlands)
Fertil Steril 64:1081–1087, 1995   14–10

Background.—Infertile, anovulatory, clomiphene-resistant patients with polycystic ovarian syndrome (PCOS) are commonly given exogenous gonadotropins in stepwise incremental doses (step-up regimen). However, step-up regimens may result in multiple follicles and multiple ovulation. Ovarian responses during gonadotropin-induced cycles using a modified step-down regimen were prospectively evaluated in such patients with PCOS.

Methods.—On the first day of menstrual bleeding (progesterone withdrawal or spontaneous), 28 patients with PCOS were started on GnRH-agonist treatment (buserelin acetate, 400 µg intranasally 3 times per day). Three weeks later, randomized patients either received human menopausal gonadotropin (hMG, Humegon) or purified urinary follicle-stimulating hormone (FSH, Metrodin) at an initial dose of 150 IU IM. When transvaginal sonography showed $\geq$ 1 follicle exceeding a diameter of 9 mm, the dose of gonadotropins was first reduced to 112 IU/day for 2 days and then to 75 IU/day. When 1–3 follicles reached a diameter of $\geq$ 18 mm, the buserelin acetate and gonadotropins were stopped and the patient was given a single injection of 10,000 IU of IM human chorionic gonadotropin.

Results.—Because the endocrine and sonographic findings were similar, the data from the hMG and the purified urinary FSH groups were pooled. After 3 weeks of buserelin acetate treatment, serum E_2 and lutenizing hormone levels were lowered significantly. Follicle-stimulating hormone levels showed no significant changes. After the gonadotropins were started, the FSH levels increased 2.1-fold and peaked at day 4. Subsequently, the FSH levels decreased about 10% per day for 4 days. In 22 patients, ovarian follicle growth was sustained and ovulation occurred. Differences in ovarian sensitivity to FSH stimulation were suggested by a large variability of the increased levels of E_2 on day 3. A marked increase of E_2 on day 3 was strongly correlated with ovulation. E_2 levels on the day of gonadotropin dose reduction predicted the chances of late follicular phase E_2 levels exceeding 871 pg/mL.

Conclusions.—Data obtained from this study using a step-down regimen for induction of ovulation in patients with PCOS suggest the following: (1) after dose reductions of gonadotropins, serum FSH levels decreased significantly; (2) although the FSH levels decrease, dominant follicle growth continues and ovulation occurs; (3) variable initial estrogen production may reflect differences in intraovarian abnormalities; and (4) initial increases of E_2 may predict low response or hyperresponse and may be used to guide gonadotropin dose adjustments.

▶ The step-down regimen for gonadotropin stimulation is of interest. This group had previously reported that the step-down regimen in women with polycystic ovaries resulted in less hyperstimulation. However, rigorous trials suggesting the efficacy of this approach over conventional low-dose therapy have still to be carried out. This also was not a randomized study. In addition, the gonadotropin regimens used both FSH and hMG. However, this would not be expected to vary the results because these 2 agents have not been shown to be different. These data suggested that this kind of step-down regimen is clearly a different way to stimulate the ovaries and may be efficacious. What caught my interest was the use of FSH levels in serum to determine the overall ability of the ovaries to be stimulated.

These data are similar to data also generated from The Netherlands by the Schoemaker group,[1] where levels of FSH above a certain threshold level determined the follicular response. It was also interesting that, whereas high levels were initially predictive of a stimulatory response, with stimulation there was a lowering of FSH as a result of negative feedback. In spite of this, follicular activity continued because of the increased sensitivity of the follicles. Also of interest is the fact that the rapid rise of E_2 within the first 3 days was somewhat predictive of a good follicular response. Clearly more data are needed on these interesting points. In an era when we want to measure less for cost containment, some measurements may still be useful.

R.A. Lobo, M.D.

Reference

1. 1994 Year Book of Infertility and Reproductive Endocrinology, pp 139–141.

The Prevalence of Polycystic Ovaries in the Hepatic Glycogen Storage Diseases: Its Association With Hyperinsulinism
Lee PJ, Patel A, Hindmarsh PC, Mowat AP, Leonard JV (Middlesex Hosp, London; King's College Hosp, London)
Clin Endocrinol 42:601–606, 1995   14–11

Background.—There is controversy regarding the contribution of abnormalities of luteinizing hormone secretion and insulin resistance to the development of polycystic ovaries. Hyperinsulinism could be a very important factor, although it may be linked primarily with obesity. Women and girls with abnormalities of insulin secretion were studied to determine their ovarian morphologic findings and insulin/androgen status.

Methods.—The cross-sectional study included 27 patients. Thirteen patients, ranging in age from 3 to 27 years, had hepatic glycogen storage disease type Ia (GSD-Ia); 14 patients, ranging in age from 4 to 31 years had GSD-III. None of the patients had clinical hyperandrogenism, and only 2 of the 13 adults in the study had irregular menstruation. Each patient underwent ovarian ultrasound examination, oral glucose tolerance testing, and measurement of gonadotropins and androgens. The findings were compared with those of 9 normal women.

Results.—The ovaries were polycystic in appearance in all patients with GSD older than 5 years. Among prepubertal patients, basal and 2-hour blood glucose and plasma insulin concentrations were lower in those with GSD-Ia than in those with GSD-III. These values were no different between adults with GSD-Ia and those with GSD-III. However, they were significantly higher in the adult patients with GSD than in the normal controls. Few abnormalities in serum gonadotropins, androgens, insulin-like growth factor I, or sex hormone–binding globulin were noted.

Conclusions.—Even before they reach puberty, girls with glycogen storage disease may have a polycystic ovarian appearance. Polycystic ovaries are linked with hyperinsulinism in patients with GSD-III and in adult patients with GSD-Ia, suggesting a possible causative association. Valuable insight into the mechanisms of ovarian physiology and development could be gained using inborn errors of carbohydrate metabolism as a model.

▶ This paper was abstracted, even though it appears to be relatively esoteric, to emphasize the importance of insulin in understanding ovarian morphology. Insulin is a major regulator of sex hormone–binding globulin as well as binding protein-1. We know that lower levels of binding protein-1, which are in turn related to elevated insulin levels, are a major feature of polycystic ovarian syndrome. Here we see women and prepubertal individuals who have hepatic storage disease, and thus abnormalities in carbohydrate metabolism and hyperinsulinemia, who have polycystic ovaries by classic criteria. These women did not have luteinizing hormone or androgen measurements that would make these women similar to those with traditional polycystic ovarian syndrome. However, of note was the finding of the ovarian morphology, which was classified as polycystic. Thus insulin, which has been shown previously to correlate with total ovarian volume, is seen to result in structural abnormalities of the polycystic type as well. This could be related to insulin directly or to reductions in binding protein-1. However, it appears that carbohydrate metabolism, and specifically hyperinsulinemia and its consequences, are intrinsically involved in ovarian morphologic abnormalities, which occur even prepubertally and progress through puberty. The problem with some of these data is that there is a background prevalence of polycystic ovaries in women. This has been suggested to occur in up to 20% to 25% of all women. It is unclear whether any of these "normal" women in the population also have a form of insulin resistance. Do all women who happen to have polycystic ovaries, regardless of their underlying abnormality, have insulin resistance?

R.A. Lobo, M.D.

Effectiveness of a Somatostatin Analogue in Lowering Luteinizing Hormone and Insulin-Stimulated Secretion in Hyperinsulinemic Women With Polycystic Ovary Disease

Fulghesu AM, Pierro E, Lanzone A, Caruso A, Andreani CL, Mancuso S (Universita' Cattolica del Sacro Cuore, Rome; Oasi Inst for Research, Troina, Enna, Italy)

Fertil Steril 64:703–708, 1995   14–12

Rationale.—Hyperinsulinism is a frequent feature of polycystic ovarian disease (PCOD), and it may contribute to ovarian hyperandrogenism in these patients. In addition, normal regulation of gonadotropin secretion is disrupted in PCOD. In principle, somatostatin could restore normal secretion of both insulin and gonadotropins.

Study Design.—The somatostatin analogue octreotide was given to 20 consecutive women 19–30 years of age in whom PCOD was diagnosed and who had plasma androgen levels at or above the upper limit of normal. The patients received 100 mg of octreotide subcutaneously twice a day for 6 weeks.

Results.—Five patients had diarrhea for a few days when treatment began. None had spontaneous menstrual bleeding. Twelve of the 20 women were considered to be hyperinsulinemic. Eight of these women and 2 who had normal insulin responses on glucose tolerance testing were obese. Octreotide therapy significantly reduced the responses of both insulin and luteinizing hormone (LH) to gonadotropin-releasing hormone in hyperinsulinemic women. In addition, circulating levels of androstenedione and testosterone were reduced in these women. Endocrine responses to octreotide did not relate to body weight.

Conclusion.—Octreotide may prove helpful for normalizing the secretion of both insulin and LH in hyperandrogenic women with PCOD.

▶ It is becoming more and more clear that insulin plays a major role in the pathogenesis of polycystic ovarian syndrome (PCOS), which is incorrectly called a disease in this paper. The effects of somatostatin therapy were evaluated using the analogue octreotide. Octreotide is known to inhibit insulin levels as well as IGF-I levels, and octreotide therapy with the possibility of lowering insulin and IGF-I levels would be attractive in patients who have PCOS. The effect of octreotide, which in the past has been shown to lower LH and androgen levels, was confirmed in this study using alternate approaches. Of interest in this study, the effects of LH and androgen were only noted in the patients who were hyperinsulinemic. This is demonstrated for LH in Figure 2. The study therefore is not simple, and several variables influence the elevated androgen and LH levels of patients with PCOS, regardless of whether they are hyperinsulinemic. Thus, the dominant player in this arena, insulin, does not appear to be the sole contributor to the endocrine abnormality.

R.A. Lobo, M.D.

Effect of Laparoscopic Ovarian Electrocautery on Ovarian Response and Outcome of Treatment With Gonadotropins in Clomiphene Citrate-Resistant Patients With Polycystic Ovary Syndrome

Farhi J, Soule S, Jacobs HS (Univ College London)
Fertil Steril 64:930–935, 1995   14–13

Study Group.—Forty-three women with polycystic ovarian syndrome (PCOS) underwent ovarian electrocautery treatment by the laparoscopic approach. Twenty-two of them subsequently presented for further treatment. The patients (average age, 31 years) had been infertile for 4 years on average. Infertility was primary in 15 cases and secondary in 7. The women were followed for an average of 26 months after electrocautery. At the time of the procedure, all of them were oligomenorrheic or amenorrheic. All patients had failed to ovulate when given clomiphene and, in some cases, human menopausal gonadotropin (hMG) or follicle-stimulating hormone (FSH).

TABLE 2.—Characteristics of Ovulation Induction Treatment Cycles Before and After Laparoscopic Ovarian Electrocautery

	Before laparoscopic ovarian electrocautery	After laparoscopic ovarian electrocautery	P
No. of gonadotropin cycles*	74	59	
No. of ovulatory cycles†	27 (36)	46 (78)	< 0.01
No. of pregnancies per total no. of cycles†	3 (4.0)	14 (23.7)	< 0.01
hMG			
No. of cycles	48	38	
No. of ampules‡	23.7 ± 8.2	14.8 ± 6.9	< 0.01
Daily effective dose‡	2.0 ± 0.8	1.2 ± 0.3	< 0.05
Days of treatment per cycle‡	16.0 ± 4.2	10.1 ± 3.4	< 0.01
Ovulation per cycle (%)	48 (23/48)	71 (27/38)	< 0.05
Pregnancy rate per cycle (%)	2 (1/48)	23 (9/38)	< 0.01
FSH			
No. of cycles	26	21	
No. of ampules‡	12.5 ± 8.3	11.8 ± 6.0	NS
Daily effective dose‡	2.4 ± 0.5	1.1 ± 0.3	< 0.01
Days of treatment per cycle‡	13.2 ± 6.2	12.0 ± 4.8	NS
Ovulation per cycle (%)	50 (13/26)	71 (15/21)	NS
Pregnancy rate per cycle (%)	7 (2/26)	23 (5/21)	NS

* Gonadotropin, hMG, or FSH.
† Values in parentheses are percentages.
‡ Values are means ± standard deviation.
Abbreviations: hMG, human menopausal gonadotropin; *FSH,* follicle-stimulating hormone; *NS,* not significant.
(Courtesy of Farhi J, Soule S, Jacobs HS: Effect of laparoscopic ovarian electrocautery on ovarian response and outcome of treatment with gonadotropins in clomiphene citrate-resistant patients with polycystic ovary syndrome. *Fertil Steril* 64:930–935, 1995. Reproduced with permission of the publisher, the American Society for Reproductive Medicine [The American Fertility Society].)

Management.—Hydrotubation was done with methylene blue before applying unipolar cautery at 4 points on each ovary. Regardless of the status of menstrual function, women who failed to conceive within 6 months of electrocautery received hMG or FSH.

Results.—Normal menstrual cycles returned in 41% of patients after electrocautery treatment. The overall results were significantly improved compared with previous gonadotropin therapy (Table 2). Doses of both hMG and FSH were reduced after electrocautery. No hormonal differences were apparent between the women who responded and those who did not, either at baseline or after electrocautery. One of 3 women having a "second-look" laparoscopy because of continued infertility was found to have adhesions and occlusion of both tubes.

Conclusions.—Infertile women with PCOS become more sensitive to gonadotropin therapy after laparoscopic ovarian electrocautery. This procedure may prove more effective than medical treatment alone in some clomiphene-resistant patients.

▶ The initial treatment of infertile anovulatory women with PCOS is clomiphene citrate. Unfortunately, a high percentage of women with PCOS and elevated serum luteinizing hormone levels do not ovulate after treatment with clomiphene citrate. For such women, subsequent treatment can either be a combination of gonadotropin-releasing hormone agonists and hMG or partial ovarian destruction with cautery or laser. Laparoscopic ovarian cautery produces spontaneous ovulatory cycles in the majority of women so treated. A high percentage of the remaining anovulatory women ovulate after treatment with clomiphene citrate. If hMG is necessary to achieve ovulation in those women who do not respond to clomiphene citrate after ovarian electrocautery, the amount of drug necessary to achieve ovulation is less than is needed before cautery and the chance of ovarian hyperstimulation and multiple gestation is also markedly reduced. Thus, anovulatory women with PCOS who fail to respond to clomiphene citrate should be given the option of having ovarian cautery instead of one or more courses of hMG.

D.R. Mishell, Jr., M.D.

Laser Vaporization of the Ovarian Surface in Polycystic Ovary Disease Results in Reduced Ovarian Hyperstimulation and Improved Pregnancy Rates

Fukaya T, Murakami T, Tamura M, Watanabe T, Terada Y, Yajima A (Univ of Tohoku, Sendai, Japan)
Am J Obstet Gynecol 173:119–125, 1995   14–14

Background.—The incidence of polycystic ovarian disease is high among infertile women with anovulation. Treatment of this disease generally consists of clomiphene citrate, human menopausal gonadotropin (hMG), or human chorionic gonadotropin (hCG). Successful treatment outcomes can, however, be difficult to achieve because of ovarian hyperstimulation syndrome, particularly with hMG stimulation. The effect of laser vaporization on patients with polycystic ovarian disease who were not ovulating spontaneously and who could not undergo successful ovarian stimulation because of severe ovarian hyperstimulation syndrome was determined.

Patients and Methods.—Twenty-six infertile women with polycystic ovarian disease who had ovarian hyperstimulation caused by stimulation with hMG and who had failed to conceive were included. Twenty to 30 vaporizations were performed with potassium titanyl phosphate and neodymium-yttrium-aluminum-garnet laser. Treatment with either clomiphene citrate or hMG was administered to patients not ovulating spontaneously after vaporization.

Results.—Spontaneous ovulation occurred in 6 patients after laser vaporization. Of the remaining 20 patients, 3 were given clomiphene citrate and 17 received hMG for ovulation induction. In all patients, the stimulation regimen was completed without the occurrence of severe ovarian hyperstimulation syndrome. Clinical pregnancy occurred in 19 of the 26 patients. Of these, 5 conceived after a spontaneous ovulation, 2 after ovulation induction with clomiphene citrate, and 12 after stimulation with hMG.

Conclusions.—Laser vaporization appears to aid in the prevention of ovarian hyperstimulation syndrome and helps improve pregnancy outcome in patients with polycystic ovarian disease who have had ovarian hyperstimulation syndrome. Ovulation stimulation was, however, required in approximately 77% of the patients after vaporization. This may be because the benefits of laser treatment become less effective with time.

▶ Ovarian hyperstimulation syndrome (OHSS) is an iatrogenic condition produced by exogenous ovarian stimulation that results in perfusion of fluid from the vascular to the extracellular compartment with resultant hemoconcentration. Serious complications, including venous thrombosis, renal failure, and adult respiratory distress syndrome, can occur. Use of hMG to induce ovulation in women with polycystic ovarian syndrome (PCOS) is associated with an appreciable risk of OHSS. In this study, women with PCOS who had previously developed OHSS with hMG treatment before multiple laser vaporization of the ovarian surface either ovulated spontaneously after such treatment or did not develop moderate or severe OHSS with use of hMG after laser vaporization. If women with anovulation resulting from PCOS fail to ovulate after use of clomiphene citrate, it may be better to use multiple laser or coagulation treatment of the ovarian surface instead of treating them with hMG to reduce the risk of OHSS.

D.R. Mishell, Jr., M.D.

Subject Index*

A

A23187
  spermatozoa responses to, and
    acrosome reaction, *94:* 71
Abortion
  induced, effect on subsequent fertility,
    94: 51
  spontaneous
    active immunization with third party
      leukocytes in, *95:* 101
    after in vitro fertilization, rate
      increase in polycystic ovary and
      reduction in pituitary
      desensitization with buserelin,
      94: 208
    first trimester prediction, ratio of
      mean sac diameter to crown rump
      length vs. embryonic heart rate,
      95: 221
    rate reduction with GnRH agonist, in
      polycystic ovary syndrome,
      94: 153
    recurremt, anticardiolipin antibody
      prevalence in, *94:* 246
    recurrent, antibodies to lipoprotein,
      oxidized low density, and
      cardiolipin in, *96:* 189
    recurrent, antiphospholipid antibodies
      and beta$_2$-glycoprotein I in,
      96: 190
    recurrent, contributing factors and
      outcome of subsequent pregnancies,
      94: 244
    recurrent, couples with,
      immunogenetics of, *96:* 7
    recurrent, early, luteinizing hormone
      and ovarian steroids hypersecretion
      in, *94:* 243
    recurrent, early, of unknown etiology,
      fibrinolytic activators and inhibitors
      in, *94:* 256
    recurrent, histocompatibility antigens
      in, and leukocyte immunotherapy,
      94: 250
    recurrent, HLA-DR types in,
      maternal, *94:* 253
    recurrent, immunotherapy and,
      95: 227
    recurrent, in first trimester,
      antithyroid antibodies in, *94:* 254
    recurrent, in first trimester, ultrasound
      of live fetus in, *94:* 258

    recurrent, informative protocol for
      investigation of, *95:* 226
    recurrent, sperm morphology and,
      95: 229
    recurrent, with paternal leukocyte
      immunotherapy, flow cytometric
      crossmatch and early pregnancy
      loss in, *94:* 252
    (*See also* Pregnancy loss)
Acrosome reaction
  inducibility predicting in vitro
    fertilization success, *96:* 88
  insufficiency, and pentoxifylline for
    sperm improving fertilizing ability,
    94: 114
  to ionophore challenge test, in assisted
    reproduction program, *95:* 65
  sperm, characterization and frequency
    distribution, *96:* 89
  of spermatozoa, and platelet activating
    factor, *95:* 67
  and spermatozoa responses to A23187,
    94: 71
ACTH
  adrenal responses to, in hirsutism in
    3β-hydroxy-delta^5-steroid
    dehydrogenase deficiency, *94:* 24
Activin
  A
    in DNA synthesis during seminiferous
      epithelial cycle (in rat), *95:* 257
    human recombinant, altering pituitary
      LH and FSH secretion, follicular
      development and steroidogenesis
      during menstrual cycle (in
      monkey), *94:* 5
    inhibin system mRNA and protein and
      in ovarian follicles in polycystic
      ovarian syndrome, *95:* 275
Adenosine
  monophosphate, cyclic, responsive
    element modulator functional
    switch during spermatogenesis,
    FSH directing, *94:* 276
Adhesiolysis
  microsurgical, Interceed to prevent
    adhesion reformation after, *95:* 168
Adhesions
  absorbable adhesion barrier, Interceed,
    to prevent adhesion reformation
    after microsurgical adhesiolysis,
    95: 168

** All entries refer to the year and page number(s) for data appearing in this and previous
editions of the* YEAR BOOK.

D

Death
  of embryo, in early pregnancy, first
    trimester study, *95:* 220
Decidua
  insulin like growth factors and receptors
    in, mRNA encoding, *94:* 269
Dehydroepiandrosterone
  sulfate, weight reduction by diet
    disparate effects on, in obesity,
    96: 30
Deletion
  Xp22.3, in Kallmann's syndrome,
    isolated familial, *94:* 266
  of Y chromosome in azoospermia,
    94: 79
Delivery
  successful, after in vitro fertilization,
    cost of, *95:* 198
2-Deoxyadenosine
  for sperm in mouse in vitro fertilization,
    95: 260
Diabetes mellitus
  with neuropathy in men
    erectile response induction to film and
      fantasy in, *94:* 99
    pituitary gonadal hormones in,
      94: 97
    semen analysis in, *94:* 95
Diathermy
  ovarian, laparoscopic, *94:* 157
Diet
  weight reduction by, disparate effects on
    dehydroepiandrosterone sulfate
    levels in obesity, *96:* 30
Diethylstilbestrol
  prenatal exposure in men, fertility after,
    96: 46
5 alpha-Dihydroprogesterone
  normal concentrations during luteal
    phase, in women with steroid five
    alpha reductase 2 deficiency,
    96: 200
Dihydrotestosterone
  concentration, in male pattern baldness,
    effect of finasteride on, *95:* 20
  regulation of semen in male
    pseudohermaphroditism, with
    5alpha-reductase-2 deficiency,
    95: 33
DNA
  expressed zona pellucida protein,
    recombinant complimentary,
    immunization with (in monkey),
    96: 209

  rapid analysis by allele specific
    polymerase chain reaction, for
    mutations detection in steroid
    21-hydroxylase gene, *96:* 196
  synthesis during seminiferous epithelial
    cycle, activin A, inhibin A and
    transforming growth factor beta 1
    in (in rat), *95:* 257
Doppler
  color, hysterosalpingography, for
    fallopian tube patency evaluation,
    95: 56
  ultrasound (*see* Ultrasound, Doppler)
Drugs
  fertility, and ovarian cancer risk,
    epithelial, *95:* 143
Dysphoria
  premenstrual, fluoxetine for, *96:* 18
Dystrophic
  peritoneal calcification, and *Chlamydia
    trachomatis* immunoglobulin
    gamma titers, *95:* 157

E

Ectopic
  endometrium, hormonal responsiveness
    of, *94:* 171
  pregnancy
    after in vitro fertilization and embryo
      transfer, prediction, *96:* 188
    cervical, conservative treatment
      results, *95:* 225
    fertility after, *94:* 49
    reproductive prognosis after,
      determinants of, *95:* 224
Edetic acid
  infusion response, and estrogen, in
    postmenopausal osteoporosis,
    95: 27
Egg yolk
  in binding capacity of spermatozoa to
    zona pellucida, *95:* 72
Eggs
  number available, correlating with
    pregnancy outcome after
    intracytoplasmic sperm injection,
    96: 126
Ejaculate
  fertile, epididymis in development of,
    96: 87
  leukocytic infiltration into, and semen
    quality, oxidative stress and sperm
    function, *95:* 90
  non-sperm cell excess in, and motile
    spermatozoa morphometric
    characteristics in subfertile men,
    95: 82